Veterinary Biochemistry and Biotechnology

NIPA® GENX ELECTRONIC RESOURCES & SOLUTIONS P. LTD.
New Delhi-110 034

About the Editor

Dr. Tanmoy Rana obtained his Bachelor of Veterinary Sciences and Animal Husbandry degree (B.V.Sc. & A.H.) and Masters (M.V.Sc) in Veterinary Medicine, Ethics & Jurisprudence from West Bengal University of Animal and Fishery Sciences, Kolkata, India. He secured his Doctor of Philosophy (Ph.D.) in Veterinary Science from the University of Calcutta, Kolkata, India. He works currently as an Assistant Professor of the Veterinary Clinical Complex at West Bengal University of Animal and Fishery Sciences, Kolkata, India. Previously he has also worked as a Veterinary Officer, Animal Resources Development Department, Government of West Bengal, India. He is actively engaged in teaching and clinical practices in veterinary medicine and research related to animal health, production, and disease monitoring regimes. His research interests involve arsenic toxicity, molecular diagnosis, molecular toxicology and medicine, oxidative stress, immunopathology, nanoparticles, Echinococcosis, and microbes. He has published several research articles in reputed international and national journals along with review articles in international journals. He is an editorial board member (especially BMC Veterinary Research, Associate Editor of Frontier in Veterinary Science), and a reviewer of international and national journals. He is a member of many international scientific societies and organizations importantly the West Bengal Veterinary Council (WBVC), The Indian Society for Veterinary Medicine (ISVM), the Association of Public Health Veterinarians, and The Indian Science Congress Association (ISCA). He is also an associate of the West Bengal Academy of Science & Technology, West Bengal, India. He is an editor and author of so many national and international books.

Veterinary Biochemistry and Biotechnology

Tanmoy Rana, Ph.D.
AFWAST, FVASc., Assistant Professor
Veterinary Clinical Complex
Veterinary Medicine, Ethics & Jurisprudence
Department of Veterinary Clinical Complex
West Bengal University of Animal & Fishery Sciences
Kolkata-700037, West Bengal, India

NIPA® GENX ELECTRONIC RESOURCES & SOLUTIONS P. LTD.
New Delhi-110 034

NIPA® GENX ELECTRONIC RESOURCES & SOLUTIONS P. LTD.

101,103, Vikas Surya Plaza, CU Block
L.S.C. Market, Pitam Pura, New Delhi-110 034
Ph : +91-11-43860225, Mob.: +91 9717133558, 9540816132
E-mail: newindiapublishingagency@gmail.com
Website: www.nipaersources.com

Print ISBN: 978-93-58875-20-1

ebook ISBN: 978-93-58873-61-0

NIPA® also publishes books in a variety of electronic formats. Some content that appears in print may not be available in electronic books, and vice versa.

Composed and Designed by NIPA®.

Preface

This book entitled "**Veterinary Biochemistry and Biotechnology**" is Multiple Choice Questions in Biochemistry and Biotechnology and it has been written to introduce a comprehensive question bank to students and academicians covering nearly the entire syllabus in Biochemistry as well as Biotechnology. MCQ book is a backbone for all entrance/competitive examinations throughout the globe with a best approach for the constitution of an important method for objective assessment of an examinee's knowledge. Every chapter has been written and reviewed by experienced fallible teacher of relevant subject matter with a good attempt to provide best answer at the bottom of the questions. The book is formed in concise, up-to-date, accurate and reliable fashion for the readership. The book covers thirty one chapters covering almost all of the biochemistry and biotechnology syllabus with a validation from the reference biochemistry and biotechnology books. The book is especially mainly structured for the undergraduate, postgraduate, MBBS medical biochemistry students, academicians and researcher and other allied courses. The book is very useful for the students preparing University exam, PG entrance exam, NET examinations, State PSC, to make it as simplest ones to real brain teasers. The book is planned on the basis of the current pattern of exam, and will be benefitted for the students preparing any competitive examination confidently and successfully. The book is organized in a simple lucid language so that the students can easily understand the same and also choose the correct option from those. Henceforth, when errors or serious omissions are detected and examined, or if any clarity of presentation of the chapter should be improved, constructive feedback would also be genuinely appreciated.

Editor

Acknowledgement

I convey my sincere gratitude to Hon'ble Vice Chancellor, West Bengal University of Animal & Fishery Sciences for providing me opportunity to edit the book. I also convey sincere thanks to all contributors who wholeheartedly helped me by sending their chapters in proper time. I am really grateful to all colleagues for their useful ideas, and suggestion in this regard. I am also helpful to all the personnel at publisher for helping me with the opportunity to act as editor for this MCQ book. I am also grateful to family members for providing a great support and the time to finalize the book.

Editor

Contents

1

General Aspects of Biochemistry Scope and Importance

M.K. Vidya[1], C.N. Darshan[2], N.R. Srikanth[3] and Tanmoy Rana[4]

[1]*Department of Physiology and Biochemistry, Veterinary College, Hassan KVAFSU - Karnataka Veterinary, Animal and Fisheries Sciences University*

[2]*Department of Animal Husbandry and Veterinary Services, Karnataka*

[3]*Division of Veterinary Biochemistry, Livestock Research Station, Lam, Guntur Sri Venkateswara Veterinary University*

[4]*Department of Veterinary Clinical Complex, West Bengal University of Animal & Fishery sciences, Kolkata, India*

Introduction

"Bio" means pertaining to life and "Chemistry" is the Study of chemicals and chemical reactions. So Biochemistry may be defined as the study of chemical processes within and relating to, living organisms. It is a field of science that explores the chemical processes and substances within living beings. Biochemistry bridges the gap between biology and chemistry, aiming to understand how biological molecules give rise to the complex processes of life. In other words "Biochemistry is the science dealing with various molecules that are present in living cells and organisms and their chemical reactions."

Scope of Biochemistry

As a life itself, the scope of biochemistry is vast and ever changing. It has its influence on vide range of fields playing a major role in understanding and influencing living organisms. Here some of the fields were put forth that have applications of biochemistry.

Human and Medical Healthcare

Nutrition and metabolism: As they say, we are what we eat; nutrition is a prime aspect of the being and knowing how the body process what it eats is a necessary knowledge that comes from biochemical aspect of nutrition. The dietary component of the beings converting into energy, protein and other essential bodily macro and micro molecules is a great knowledge imparted by biochemistry aspect of nutrition. Metabolism which broadly includes anabolism and catabolism deals with various activities of the physiological systems with in the body. Knowledge of biochemistry is very essential these days as the metabolic diseases are very much prevailing. Biochemistry imparts basic to complex know-hows about various metabolic processes and their derailments.

Diagnostics: However the latest is the diagnostics in the field of medical sciences may be, still the prime part of it is by analysing the biochemical molecules. In a way it is not wrong to say that biochemistry and diagnostics are inseparable. To name a few, blood glucose level, enzyme profiles, hormone profiles, estimation of vitamins and minerals occupy a major portion among diagnostics besides the imaging sciences. All these analysis and estimations involve biochemistry and its applications to a vast range.

Drug discovery and development: Biochemistry unfurls the knowledge behind the molecular basis of a disease. Based on the molecular reason of the disease a Biochemist can effectively design a drug using the necessary molecules and its structural isotopes. Targeted drugs can be designed to treat the ailments and can be developed with the knowledge of biochemistry, which gives the acquaintance of the molecules, their structures and their interaction with in the body to treat the diseases.

Agriculture and food science

Though every step of agriculture and food science involve intricately the biochemical aspects, herewith we discuss two of the main and latest points of them.

Genetic engineering: Keeping in view of the exploding human population in the world, day by day vanishing of agricultural lands, it is a herculean task to make hands reach mouth of this humongous population. With latest technologies like genetic engineering, the crop yield can be increased instantaneously unlike in plant breeding experiments which take plant generations to wait. Plant pests and diseases are concerning areas with the changing environments. Genetic engineering is a sustainable solution to counteract these hurdles and to provide food for the world Genetic engineering is the science that involves the biochemistry of macro molecules like DNA, RNA and proteins and their structural engineering to provide better yields.

Food processing and preservation: Almost from the advent of human civilization, it is evident that humans did preserve their food to increase their shelf-life. Though they might have followed these preserving techniques without knowing the intrinsic biochemistry, we all know today that they did their best to preserve the otherwise easily perishable food and the same knowledge was passed onto generations that reached us till date. They followed the basic yet very strong biochemical rules of preservation. Through latest science technology their knowledge was studied in aspects of biochemistry of food, food chemistry and preservation technological interventions and many approaches are being followed to preserve the food and to increase the shelf-life and quality.

Biotechnological industries: In a way it is not wrong to say that the biotechnology and the latest sciences like molecular biology have their roots from biochemistry. Fermentation is another one of the science that is passed from the almost first of human ancestors to us. The fermentation sciences involve the biochemistry of microorganisms and industrial production of products and by-products that help in betterment of human and animal life, in a large scale. Not only food produces but the best of the vaccines can be produced by harnessing the power of microbe biochemistry. Biofuels can be produced from the bio wastes and at the same time environment pollutants can be handled in a smart and non-toxic way by use of latest biotechnological interventions. Also, biomaterials are being developed that have their applications everywhere from heart valves to space rockets. The bimolecular biochemical knowledge and its applications in the material science does these wonders.

Academics, Research and other areas: As one can observe there is no scientific field that is devoid of biochemistry. Biochemistry gradually metamorphosed as biotechnology and molecular biology. Now a days the latest research in medical and related sciences is so much interrelated and interdisciplinary courses play major role in academics and research. The best of the interdisciplinary courses is molecular biology which effectively bridges the gaps between various departments and the biochemical knowledge of the subject involved in the study so deep till the molecular level. Many other wings of sciences like forensics and environmental sciences have no say without the involvement of biochemistry.

Importance of Biochemistry: Biochemistry is a basic biological and medical science that provided working knowledge of cell biology, microbiology, nutrition, physiology, pathology and pharmacology at a molecular level. Biochemistry holds the instructional manual of life. It's a blueprint of life which deciphers the structure and function of minutest of molecules like DNA, RNA, proteins, carbohydrates and rest of the molecules, with which one could gain insights into how living organisms function at the most fundamental and molecular level. It is the key to unlock the mysteries of life. Of course many mysteries where unfurled by this key of knowledge and many more to come.

1. Discipline that uses the principles and language of chemistry to explain biology
   a. Biomechanics b. Biology
   c. Biochemistry d. Anatomy
2. Chemicals produced in living organisms had been identified by the end of
   a. 17th century b. 18th century
   c. 19th century d. 20th century
3. Friedrich wohler synthesized the organic compound urea by heating the inorganic compound
   a. Ammonium carbonate b. Ammonium silicate
   c. Aluminium silicate d. Ammonium cyanate
4. Discovery of stereoisomers
   a. Friedrich Wohler b. Louis Pasteur
   c. Joseph Lister d. Edward Buchner
5. Lock and key model is proposed by
   a. Emil Fisher b. Friedrich Wohler
   c. Louis Pasteur d. Edward Buchner
6. Biological reaction occur in faster rate
   a. Without catalyst b. With catalyst
   c. With enzyme d. Both b and c
7. Avery, MacLeod and McCarty extracted DNA from pathogenic strains of
   a. Streptococcus pneumoniae b. Streptococcus pyogenus
   c. E coli d. Staphylococcus aureus
8. Molecular biology is a discipline of
   a. Chemistry b. Biochemistry
   c. Physiology d. Physical chemistry

9. Unidirectional flow of information from nucleic acid to proteins
   a. Biomolecular flow b. Diffusion
   c. Central dogma d. Active transport
10. Major component of cell
   a. Water b. Carbohydrates
   c. Proteins d. Lipids
11. Common linkages found in fatty acids and lipids
   a. Ether linkage b. Ester linkage
   c. Both a and b d. None of the Above
12. Amide linkages found in
   a. Protein b. Carbohydrates
   c. Fats d. None of Above
13. Phosphoanhydride linkage found in
   a. Nucleiosides b. Nucleiotides
   c. Proteins d. All of the above
14. Starch is a polymer of
   a. Lactose b. Sucrose
   c. Galactose d. Glucose
15. Relative molecular mass is defined as
   a. Mass of a molecule relative to $1/12^{th}$ the mass of an atom of the carbon isotope
   b. Mass of a molecule relative to $1/24^{th}$ the mass of an atom of the carbon isotope
   c. Mass of a molecule relative to $1/12^{th}$ the mass of an atom of the hydrogen isotope
   d. Mass of a molecule relative to $1/24^{th}$ the mass of an atom of the hydrogen isotope
16. Which of the following is correct regarding relative molecular mass (Mr)
   a. Dimensionless quantity
   b. It is also called as molecular weight
   c. Both of the Above
   d. None of the Above
17. 1 mole is equal to
   a. 6.022*10^23 molecules b. 1.027*10^23 molecules
   c. 6.022* 10^24 molecules d. 1.027*10^24 molecules
18. The bond between the carbon atom of one amino acid residue and nitrogen atom of next residue is called as
   a. Glycosidic bond b. Peptide bond
   c. Phosphodiester bond d. None of the Above
19. The function of the proteins depends on
   a. One dimensional conformation b. Two dimensional conformation
   c. Three dimensional conformation d. Quaternary conformation

20. Polymers of monosaccharides is called as
    a. Disaccharides
    b. Polypeptide
    c. Polynucieotides
    d. Polysaccharides
21. Linear representation of monosaccharides is
    a. Fischer projection
    b. Haworth projection
    c. Ring structure
    d. None of the above
22. Storage polysaccharides are
    a. Starch and Glucose
    b. Glycogen and Galactose
    c. Glucose and Galactose
    d. Starch and Glycogen
23. Structural polysaccharide
    a. Glycogen
    b. Cellulose
    c. Cellulobiose
    d. Starch
24. Nucleosides consists of
    a. Nitrogenous base and phosphate group
    b. Nitrogenous base and 6 carbon sugar
    c. Phosphate group and 5 carbon sugar
    d. Nitrogenous base and 5 carbon sugar
25. The linkage between the carbons of adjacent nucleotides is called as
    a. Phosphoester linkage
    b. Phosphodiester linkage
    c. Both of the Above
    d. None of the Above
26. Myriad reaction in which organic compound are synthesized and degraded and useful energy is extracted, stored and used, is termed as
    a. Anabolism
    b. Catabolism
    c. Metabolism
    d. None
27. Biochemical reactions are
    a. Mostly reversible
    b. Always reversible
    c. Mostly irreversible
    d. Always irreversible
28. For a biochemical to be spontaneous DG has to be
    a. More than zero
    b. Less than zero
    c. Equal to zero
    d. Both a and b
29. In case of reversible reaction the activation energy is the difference of
    a. Energy peak and the energy of the reactant
    b. Energy peak and the energy of the product
    c. Energy of reactant and energy of product
    d. Both a and b
30. In case of reversible reaction, DG >0 then the activation energy for forward reaction is _________ that of reverse reaction
    a. Higher than
    b. Lower than
    c. Same as
    d. Half of

31. A typical eukaryotic cell has a diameter of about
    a. 2.5μm b. 25μm
    c. 250μm d. 0.25μm
32. Plant cell walls are mostly composed of
    a. Hemicellulose b. Lignin
    c. Cellulose d. Chitin
33. ________is the major site of RNA synthesis
    a. Endoplasmic reticulum b. Nucleolus
    c. Golgi bodies d. Mitochondrion
34. _______and ________organelle play major role in energy transduction
    a. Endoplasmic reticulum and Golgi body b. ER and ribosome
    c. Nucleus and ribosome d. Mitochondria and ribosome
35. ________is responsible for modification and sorting of proteins.
    a. ER b. Golgi
    c. Ribosome d. lysosome
36. ________is the main site for energy transduction in aerobic eukaryotic cells.
    a. Mitochondria b. Cytoplasm
    c. Nucleus d. Cell wall
37. Mitochondrion oxidise organic acids, fatty acids and amino acids to _______ and ________
    a. Glucose and fructose b. Acetic acid and lactic acid
    c. Pyruvate and acetyl CoA d. CO_2 and H_2O
38. The energy released in mitochondrion as a result of oxidation is conserved as
    a. ATP in mitochondrial matrix
    b. Heat
    c. Proton concentration gradient across mitochondrial membrane
    d. Starch
39. ATP is require for ________
    a. Biosynthesis b. Transport of molecules
    c. Muscle contraction d. All of the above
40. Which of the following not true for chloroplast
    a. Membrane is double walled
    b. Contains circular DNA
    c. Granum suspends in stroma
    d. Thylakoid membrane surround the entire stroma and granum
41. Molecular evolution studies shows mitochondria derived from a particular group of bacteria called
    a. Proteobacteria b. Probacteria
    c. Cyanobacteria d. Mycobacteria

42. Chloroplast are descended from bacteria called
    a. Proteobacteria
    b. Probacteria
    c. Cyanobacteria
    d. Chlorobacteria
43. Eukaryotic cells contain specialised digestive vesicle called
    a. Ribosome
    b. Golgi vesicles
    c. Lysosome
    d. Vacuoles
44. Acidity in lysosome is maintained
    a. Ions like Cl^-, HCO^{3-}
    b. Proton pump on membrane
    c. Acidic proteins
    d. Membrane wall proteins
45. lysozymes enzymes mostly active in
    a. Basic condition
    b. Acidic condition
    c. Neutral condition
    d. Around neutral condition
46. ________keeps lysosomal enzyme away from accidentally catalyzing degradation of macromolecules in cytosol
    a. Ions like Ca^{++}, Mg^{2+}
    b. Proton pump inhibitors in lysosome
    c. Protein around lysozyme
    d. Compartmentalisation of enzymes
47. ________enzyme degrade H_2O_2 into H_2O and O_2 present in peroxisomes
    a. Peroxidase
    b. Oxidase
    c. Catalase
    d. Hydroxylase
48. The vesicle acting on storage site for water, ions nutrients, are
    a. Peroxisomes
    b. Vacuoles
    c. Lysozomes
    d. Phagosomes
49. ________is a protein scaffold required for support, internal organisation and even movement of cell
    a. Cell wall
    b. Cytoskeleton
    c. Cell membrane
    d. Nucleolus
50. The cytoskeleton consists of
    a. Actin filament
    b. Microtubule
    c. Intermediate filament
    d. All of the above
51. Which is the most abundant component of cytoskeleton
    a. Actin filament
    b. Microfilament
    c. Microtubule
    d. Both a and b
52. Microtubule are composed of which protein
    a. Actin
    b. Myosin
    c. Tubulin
    d. Both a and b

53. ________forms mitotic spindle during mitosis of cell

a. Microtubule b. Microfilament

c. Actin d. Intermediate filament

54. Structures like cilia and flagella are composed of

a. Microfilament b. Microtubule

c. Intermediate filament d. Actin filament

55. ________lines the in side of nuclear envelope and extend outward from the nucleus to the periphery of the cell and helps the cell resists external mechanical stress

a. Microfilament b. Microtubule

c. Intermediate filament d. Actin filament

56. What is the right order of diameter of the protein filament of cytoskeleton

a. Actin>intermediate>microtubule

b. Microtubule>intermediate>actin

c. Intermediate>actin>microtubule

d. Intermediate>microtubule>actin

57. Prokaryote are divide into ------- and ------ domain

a. Probacteria and protobacteria b. Eubacteria and protobacteria

c. Archaea and eubacteria d. Probacteria and eubacteria

59. ________acts as attachment site for cell-cell interaction

a. Cell wall b. Cell membrane

c. Pili d. Cilia

60. Charles and Darwin published ------------on this theory of evolution by natural selection

a. The voyage of the beagle b. The origin of species

c. Species plantarum d. System naturae

61. Most of biochemical reaction are

a. Zero order b. First order

c. Second order d. Third order

62. Dr. Edward buchner got nobel prize for discovery of

a. Aerobic respiration b. Cell free fermentation

c. Urea cycle pathway d. Protein synthesis pathway

63. First protein structures were solved by

a. Watson and crick b. M. Delbruch and Salvatore

c. C. Kendrew and M. Perutz d. Schwan and Schleiden

64. Deoxyribose sugar lacks the one hydroxyl group at________compared to ribose sugar

a. c-2 b. c-3

c. c-5 d. c-1

65. Under most biological condition -COOH AND -NH2groups exist as________ and________

a. -COOH AND -NH2 b. -COO- AND -NH3 +

c. -COOH AND -NH3+ d. -COO- AND -NH2

66. Who got noble prize for his work in sugar and purine synthesis

a. Avery b. Watson

c. E. Fisher d. H.C crick

67. Molecular mass of a typical protein

a. 3000 Dalton b. 10,000 Dalton

c. 38000 Dalton d. 400000 Dalton

68. Sugars on nucleic acid are connected with other

a. Hydrogen bond b. Phosphodiester linkage

c. Peptide bond d. Glycosidic bond

69. ________is not a lipid

a. Steroid b. Wax

c. Acetic acid d. Aspartic acid

70. Correct order of central dogma theory is

a. dNA –RNA--PROTEIN b. DNA—PROTEIN—RNA

c. RNA—DNA—PROTEIN d. PROTEIN—RNA--DNA

71. ________is the region on an enzyme where chemical reaction takes place

a. Reaction centre b. Active site

c. Reaction site d. Allosteric site

72. THE NITROGEN BASES of nucleonic acids are linked with sugars at

a. c-1 b. c-2

c. c-3 d. c-5

73. For a reaction to be at equilibrium, delta G =

a. >0 b. <0

c. =0 d. Both a and c

74. Standard Ph for biochemistry reactions are

a. 2-5 b. 5-7

c. 7 d. 7-10

75. Primitive chordate from which modern human evolved

a. Opabinia b. Pibia

c. Anomalocaris d. Trilobite

76. The structure that separates the contents of the cell from surrounding is called

a. Cell wall b. Plasma membrane

c. Plasma lemma d. None of these

77. As cell size increases; what happens to the surface to volume ratio
    a. Increase b. Decrease
    c. Remains constant d. None of these
78. The archaebacteria are found in
    a. Salt lakes b. Hot springs
    c. High acidic bogs d. All of these
79. The diameter of plant and animal cell are
    a. 5 - 100 micrometer b. 10 - 25 micrometer
    c. 1 - 2 micrometer d. 0.5 - 10 micrometer
80. The organisms that die when exposed to oxygen
    a. Facultative anaerobes b. Obligate anaerobes
    c. Both of these d. None of these
81. The organisms that utilise carbon from carbondioxide are
    a. Heterotrophs b. Autotrophs
    c. Lithotrophs d. Organotrophs
82. The organisms which utilise energy from inorganic compounds is called as
    a. Lithotrophs b. Organotrophs
    c. Both a & b d. None of these
83. The organisms which utilise energy from organic compounds is called as
    a. Autotrophs b. Organotrophs
    c. Lithotrophs d. None of these
84. The polymer that gives the cell it's shape and rigidity is called as
    a. Polypeptide b. Phospholipase
    c. Peptidoglycan d. All of these
85. Thick peptidoglycan layer is present in
    a. Gram negative bacteria b. Gram positive bacteria
    c. Cyanobacteria d. Archaebacteria
86. The cytoplasm contains small, circular segment of DNA called
    a. Nucleolus b. Plasmid
    c. Vacuoles d. Nucleus
87. The component present in animal cell is
    a. Starch granules b. Lysosome
    c. Vacuoles d. Glyoxysome
88. The types of cytoplasmic filaments are
    a. Actin filaments b. Microtubules
    c. Intermediate filaments d. All of these
89. The protein filaments crisscrossing the eukaryotic cell forming an interlocking 3D meshwork is called
    a. Cytoskeleton b. Microtubules
    c. All of these d. None of these

90. Actin filaments bundle together to form
   a. Cytoskeletal filaments
   b. Intermediate filaments
   c. Stress fibres
   d. None of these
91. Haemoglobin consists of
   a. 600 amino acid subunits in 2 long chains
   b. 300 amino acid subunits in 3 long chains
   c. 300 amino acid subunits in 6 long chains
   d. 600 amino acid subunits in 4 long chains
92. The monomeric subunits of proteins, nucleic acids and polysaccharides are joined by
   a. Hydrogen bond
   b. Ionic bond
   c. Non covalent bond
   d. Covalent bond
93. Non covalent bonds are
   a. Hydrogen bond
   b. Ionic bond
   c. Van der waals interaction
   d. All of these
94. The study of arrangement of molecule's constituent atom in 3D is known as
   a. Molecular chemistry
   b. Stereochemistry
   c. Biochemistry
   d. None of these
95. Maleic acid is an example for
   a. Cis isomer
   b. Trans isomer
   c. Enantiomer
   d. Diasteriomer
96. Fumaric acid is an example for
   a. Enantiomer
   b. Cis isomer
   c. Diasteriomer
   d. Trans isomer
97. Carbon atom with 4 different substituent group is said to be asymmetric; and symmetric carbon are called
   a. Enantiomeric carbon
   b. Isomeric carbon
   c. Chiral carbon
   d. None of these
98. Sterioisomers which are mirror images of each other is called
   a. Diasteriomers
   b. Racemic mixtures
   c. Enantiomers
   d. None of these
99. Sterioisomers which are not mirror images of each other is called as
   a. Diasteriomers
   b. Enantiomers
   c. Trans isomers
   d. Cis isomers
100. Equimolar solution of 2 enantiomers which shows no optic rotation is know as
   a. Chiral mixture
   b. Racemic mixture
   c. Geometric mixture
   d. None of these

101. Living organisms exist in which state?
   a. Steady state b. Equilibrium
   c. Dynamic state d. Dynamic steady state
102. Free energy content of a thermodynamic reaction was given by which scientist
   a. Williard Gibbs b. Schrodinger
   c. Kliensmith d. Kornberg
103. Which of the following equations represents Gibbs free energy?
   a. G = H - TS b. G = H + TS
   c. G = H - TS + P d. G = H + TS - P
104. Change in randomness of any system is indicated by
   a. Entalpy change b. Entropy change
   c. Both d. None
105. Which law states as following "In any physical or chemical change, the total amount of energy in the universe remains constant, although the form of energy may change"
   a. First law of thermodynamics b. Second law of thermodynamics
   c. Third law of thermodynamics d. Zeroth law of thermodynamics
106. In which of the following equations does the equilibrium constant (K eq) for a reaction relate to the Gibbs free energy change (AG°)?
   a. AG° = -RT In(K eq) b. AG° = RT In(K eq)
   c. AG° = -K_eq RT d. AG° = K_eq RT
107. The reactions which require energy are known as
   a. Endergonic reactions b. Exergonic reactions
   c. Both a and b d. None of the above
108. The study of energy transformations in living systems is known as
   a. Biogenesis b. Biogenetics
   c. Bioenergitics d. None of the above
109. According to the principles of thermodynamics, what is the relationship between the change in enthalpy (ΔH) and the change in entropy (AS) for a reaction to be spontaneous?
   a. $\Delta H < 0$ and $\Delta S < 0$ b. $\Delta H > 0$ and $\Delta S > 0$
   c. $\Delta H < 0$ and $\Delta S > 0$ d. $\Delta H > 0$ and $\Delta S < 0$
110. The mojor carrier of chemical energy in living cell is
   a. ADP b. ATP
   c. AMP d. None of the above
111. Remarkable property of living organisms is
   a. Growth b. Reproduction
   c. Cell division d. All of the above

112. _________ promotes the sequence of chemical reactions
   a. Hormones b. Enzymes
   c. Both a and b d. None
113. "Omnis cellula e cellula is given by
   a. Rudolph virchow b. Charles Darwin
   c. Carolus Linnaeus d. George Mendel
114. Which molecule was considered as 1st gene or 1st catalyst
   a. DNA b. RNA
   c. Aminoacids d. None of the above
115. Changes in the nucleotide sequence of the DNA leads to
   a. Replication b. Transcription
   c. Translation d. Mutation
116. The capacity of an enzyme to selectively lower the activation barrier is obtained by
   a. Multiplicity b. Specificity
   c. Susceptibility to regulation d. All of the above
117. In exergonic reactions ΔG will be
   a. Negative b. Positive
   c. Zero d. None of the above
118. Theory of survival of the fittest under selective pressure was given by
   a. Charles Darwin b. Carlos Linnaeus
   c. Schwartz d. None of the above
119. The first cell found was probably
   a. Autotroph b. Heterotroph
   c. Chemo heterotroph d. Autoheterotroph
120. Which is present in prokaryotic cell
   a. Cell division b. Cytoskeleton
   c. Membrane bound organelles d. None
121. What is the process by which DNA is copied to RNA called?
   a. Replication b. Transcription
   c. Translation d. Mutation
122. The classic experiment on abiotic origin of organic biomolecules was carried out by
   a. Stanley Miller b. Carl Neuberg
   c. James D. Watson d. None of the above
123. If homologous genes appear in the same species they are said to be
   a. Paralogous b. Orthologous
   c. Metalogous d. None

124. Which of the following mutations involves the substitution of one nucleotide for another?
   a. Insertion b. Deletion
   c. Point mutation d. Frameshift mutation

125. The human genome is 99.9% identical to
   a. Monkeys b Chimpanzees
   c. Gorilla d All of the above

126. ________is the structure unit of living organisms
   a. Cell b. Tissue
   c. Organ d. Molecules

126. Science concerned with the chemical constituents of the living cells and with reaction and process they undergo
   a. Physiology b. Biochemistry
   c. Anatomy d. Pharmacology

127. The biochemistry of the nuclei acids lies at the heart of
   a. Immunology b. Genetics
   c. Pharmacy d. Toxicology

128. The study of body function overlaps with biochemistry almost completely
   a. Immunology b. Physiology
   c. Pharmacy d. Toxicology

129. Poisons act on biochemical reactions or processes
   a. Immunology b. Pharmacy
   c. Physiology d. Toxicology

131 State of complete physical mental and social well being and not merely the absence of disease or infirmity
   a. Health b. Disease
   c. Illness d. Fever

132. Methods of separating and purifying bio molecules
   a. Salt fractionation b. Chromatography
   c. Electrophoresis d. All of the above

133. Double helical nature of dna by
   a. Watson and crick b. Robert k Murray
   c. Harpers d. Daryl k granger

134. Mmajor causes of disease among the following
   a. Physical agents b. Therapeutic drugs
   c. Both a and b d. None of the above

135. Causes of diseases having defect in bio molecules
   a. Nuclic acids b. Lipids
   c. Cho d. Proteins

136. Among the which are physical agents that causes disease
  a. Electric shock b. Drugs
  c. Bacteria d. Molecular
137. Among the fallowing which are genetical disorders casuging agents
  a. Molecular b. Virus
  c. Drugs d. Bacteria
138. Among the fallowing major immunological reactions
  a. Autoimmune disease b. Fungi
  c. Drugs d. Toxins
139. Methods for determining bio molecular structure
  a. UV b. Visible light
  c. Infrared d. All the above
140. Among the fallowing which is the use of biochemical investigation and laboratory tests in relation to disease
  a. Reveal the fundamental causes and mechanisms of disease
  b. To suggest rational treatments of diseases based on above
  c. To act as screening tests for the early diagnosis of certain diseases
  d. All the above
141. Which two groups announced that over 90% of genome has been sequenced
  a. Waston and crick b. Consortium and celera genomics
  c. Robbins sl d. None of the above
142. Among the fallowing which causes disease by chemical agents
  a. Drugs b. Fungi
  c. Bacteria d. None of the above
143. According to Watson and crick DNA is
  a. Double helical b. Single helical
  c. Thriple helical d. None of the above
144. Any harmful devivation from the normal structure or functional state of an organism generally associated with certain signs and symptoms differing in nature from physical injury known as
  a. Disease b. Health
  c. Symptoms d. Injury
145. Biochemistry study association with disease known as
  a. Pathology b. Biochemistry
  c. Pharmacology d. Physiology
146. Use of plasma enzyme ALT monitoring the progress of ________
  a. Infectious hepatitis b. Nephritis
  c. Cystitis d. None of these

147. Measurement of blood carcinoembryonic antigen in certain patients who have been treated for cancer of the________

a. Colon
b. Liver
c. Heart
d. Kidney

148. Use of measurement of blood thyroxine or TSH in neonatal diagnosis of———

a. Congenital hypothyroidism
b. Myocardial infarction
c. Phenylketonuria
d. Cystic fibrosis

149. A diet low in phenylaline for treatment of ________

a. Phenylketonuria
b. Cystic fibrosis
c. Myocardial infarction
d. Hypothyroidism

150. ALT stands for

a. Alanine amino transferase
b. Alanine transferase
c. Amino alanine transferase
d. None of the above

151. Characteristic feature of eukaryotic cell

a. Lack of nucleus
b. Presence of ribosomes
c. Presence of membrane bound organelles
d. Single circular DNA molecule

152. Organalle responsible for energy production in eukaryotic cells

a. Nucleus
b. Ribosomes
c. Mitochondria
d. Lysosomes

153. Function of nucleus in eukaryotic cell

a. Energy production
b. Protein synthesis
c. Genetic material storage
d. Cellular respiration

154. Role of mitochondria

a. Photosynthesis
b. Protein modification
c. Cellular respiration
d. DNA replication

155. Organelle involved in synthesis of protein

a. Golgi apparatus
b. Ribosomes
c. Mitochondria
d. Lysosome

156. Organelle containing variety of hydrolytic enzymes responsible for digestion and to recycle cellular compounds

a. Mitochondria
b. Golgi apparatus
c. Nucleus
d. Lysosome

157. Membrane enclosed organelles that contain oxidative enzymes

a. Mitochondria
b. Peroxisomes
c. Lysosomes
d. Golgi apparatus

158. Organelle whose function is to protect sensitive cell components from oxidative attack by hydrogen peroxide
   a. Mitochondria b. Endoplasmic reticulum
   c. Golgi apparatus d. Peroxisomes
159. Following found in only plant cells and not in animal cells
   a. Mitochondria b. Ribosomes
   c. Chloroplasts d. Endoplasmic reticulum
160. Primary function of chloroplasts
   a. Protein synthesis b. Photosynthesis
   c. Energy production d. Lipid synthesis
161. Characteristic of plant cell
   a. Presence of rigid cell wall b. Absence of rigid cell wall
   c. Presence of chloroplasts d. Both a and c
162. Structure controls passage of materials in and out of the cell
   a. Cell wall b. Cytoplasm
   c. Plasma membrane d. Nucleus
163. Cell structure responsible for synthesis and modification of lipid and protein
   a. Mitochondria b. Endoplasmic reticulum
   c. Golgi apparatus d. Ribosomes
164. Structure provides support and shape to plant cells
   a. Plasma membrane b. Cytoskeleton
   c. Nucleus d. Cell wall
165. Component of cytoskeleton
   a. Lysosome b. Golgi apparatus
   c. Microtubules d. Ribosomes
166. Following is a characteristic of animal cell but not plant cell
   a. Vacuoles b. Cell wall
   c. Lysosomes d. Chloroplasts
167. Structure involved in synthesis of lipids
   a. Rough endoplasmic reticulum b. Smooth endoplasmic reticulum
   c. Ribosomes d. Golgi apparatus
168. Organelle responsible for degradation of worn-out organelles
   a. Peroxisomes b. Lysosome
   c. Golgi apparatus d. Mitochondria
169. Thylakoids are present in
   a. Mitochondria b. Chloroplasts
   c. Golgi apparatus d. Nucleus

170. Following domains of life includes all Eukaryotes
   a. bacteria b. Archaea
   c. Eukarya d. Protista
171. Group of eukaryotes that are most closely related to the ancestors of animals
   a. Plants b. Fungi
   c. Protista d. Algae
172. In which part of eukaryotic cell does glycolysis occur
   a. Nucleus b. Cytoplasm
   c. Endoplasmic reticulum d. Mitochondria
173. Primary function of photosynthesis in plants
   a. To breakdown glucose and produce ATP
   b. To convert light energy into chemical energy
   c. To degrade fatty acids
   d. To produce amino acids
174. Transcription process in eukaryotes occurs in
   a. Mitochondria b. Nucleus
   c. Cytoplasm d. Endoplasmic reticulum
175. Enzyme responsible for synthesizing RNA from DNA template
   a. DNA polymerase b. RNA polymerase
   c. Ligase d. Helicase
176. Theory of germplasm was given by
   a. Lamarck b. August Weismann
   c. Charles Darwin d. Mendel
177. During Cell division each chromosome attaches by its _____ to the mitotic spindle
   a. Centromere b. Chromatid
   c. Genes d. Allele
178. Exchange of corresponding section of homologous chromosome is called as____
   a. Zygote b. Fertilization
   c. Crossing over d. Cell division
179. ABO Blood group system is example for
   a. Incomplete dominance b. Codominance
   c. Over dominance d. None of above
180. Chromosomal theory of inheritance formulated by
   a. Walter suton b. Mendel
   c. Lamarck d. Weismann
181. Loosely packed chromtin fibres and lightly stained are called as
   a. Heterochromatin b. Euchromatin
   c. Centromere d. Polytene chromatids

182. Single chromatid chromosome move to opposite poles in _______
   a. Prophase
   b. Metaphase
   c. Anaphase
   d. Telephase
183. Genetic makeup of an individual with respect to particular trait is called ______
   a. Phenotype
   b. Genetics
   c. Genotype
   d. Hybrid
184. Phenotypic ratio of dihydrid cross of Mendel experiment
   a. 9:3:3:1
   b. 9:3:1:3
   c. 9:3:4:1
   d. 9:3:1:4
185. One pair of gene controlling one trait assort independently of members of other pair of gene during gamete formation is called
   a. Law of Segregation
   b. Law of Independent assortment
   c. Law of Mutual exclusive
   d. Law of Chromosomes
186. If an organism has two identical alleles for a particular trait, it is said to be
   a. Heterozygous
   b. Homozygous
   c. Dominant
   d. Recessive
187. In Mendel's experiment what type of plant did he use to study inheritance
   a. Tomato plants
   b. Pea plants
   c. Corn plants
   d. Sunflower plants
188. What does the law of independent assortment state?
   a. Genes for different traits are inherited together
   b. Genes for different traits can segregate independently during the formation of gametes
   c. Genes are passed from parent to offspring
   d. Genes are located on the same chromosome
189. Which of the following is true regarding plasmids in bacteria?
   a. They are always essential for bacterial survival
   b. They are composed of RNA molecules
   c. They are linear DNA molecules
   d. They often carry antibiotic resistance genes
190. 'V' shaped chromosomes are:
   a. Metacentric
   b. Sub metacentric
   c. Acrocentric
   d. Telocentric
191. One of the following principles was not proposed by Mendel. It was the law of __________.
   a. Segregation
   b. Blending inheritance
   c. Dominance
   d. None of above

192. If the blood group of both the parents is AB, then the possible blood group of their children will be:

   a. A, B, AB and O
   b. A, B and AB
   c. A and B
   d. A, B and O

193. The percentage of people that cross over is higher when

   a. The genes are in a distinct cell
   b. There is no relationship between genes
   c. Connected genes are near to one another
   d. Related genes are separated by a large distance

194. __________ test indicates whether two recessive traits are allelic

   a. Dihydrid
   b. Cross
   c. Complementation
   d. Molecular

195. Which scientist proposed the chromosomal theory of inheritance?

   a. Gregor Mendel
   b. Thomas Hunt Morgan
   c. Alfred Wallace
   d. Charles Darwin

196. Which experiment by Thomas Hunt Morgan provided strong evidence for the chromosomal theory of inheritance?

   a. Pea plant experiments
   b. Drosophila (fruit fly) experiments
   c. Mouse breeding experiments
   d. Bacterial transformation experiments

197. During which process does crossing over occur, contributing to genetic diversity?

   a. Mitosis
   b. Fertilization
   c. Meiosis
   d. DNA replication

198. What is the main idea of the chromosomal theory of inheritance?

   a. Traits are passed on through blending inheritance.
   b. Genes are located on chromosomes and their behavior during meiosis and fertilization accounts for inheritance patterns.
   c. Only maternal traits are inherited
   d. Traits are determined solely by environmental factors.

199. Which phenomenon violates Mendel's law of independent assortment and supports the concept of gene linkage?

   a. Incomplete dominance
   b. Codominance
   c. X-linked inheritance
   d. Polygenic inheritance

200. What happens during nondisjunction?

   a. Chromosomes fail to separate properly during meiosis, leading to gametes with abnormal chromosome numbers.
   b. Crossing over occurs between non-homologous chromosomes.
   c. Linked genes undergo independent assortment.
   d. Chromosomes replicate before cell division.

201. ________is the generation time of E.coli.

a. 20 min
b. 30 min
c. 50 min
d. 10 min

202. Viruses are infectious particles consisting of a molecule.

a. Amino acid
b. Nucleic acid
c. Protein
d. Carbohydrates

203. Are usually detected by their ability or inability to grow under Certain conditions.

a. Mutants
b. Recombination
c. Transformation
d. All of the above

204. Mutants that are unable to synthesize amino aci d.

a. Leucine
b. Lysine
c. Threonine
d. Methionine

205. Mutants in which they become temperature sensitive grow at 30°C but not at________°C

a. 50°C
b. 67°C
c. 42°C
d. 37°C

206. Replication of viral chromosome take place in,

a. Host cell
b. Viral call
c. Both a & b
d. None

207. Presence of viable bacteriophages is conveniently indicated by ________.

a. Plaques
b. Bacteria
c. Screening
d. All of the above

208. T4 chromosome, consists of two adjacent complementation groups designated________& ________.

a. rIIA & rIIB
b. rIIIA & rIF
c. rIIC & rIE
d. None

209. The structures that appear as beads-on-string in the chromosomes are

a. Nucleosome
b. Chromosome
c. Chromatid
d. None

210. Theory of evolution was originated by ________.

a. Charles Darwin
b. Benzer
c. Aristotle
d. James Chadwick

211. Radioactive dating studies indicate that Earth formed________years ago.

a. ~4.6 billion
b. ~4.6 million
c. ~2.6million
d. ~2.6 billion

212. The is the most accepted theory regarding the origin of the planet earth and the existence of different life forms on it.

a. Big Bang Theory
b. Darwin Theory
c. Both a & b
d. General theory

213. Is the element to make three or more bonds and thus to form chains.
   a. Carbon b. Hydrogen
   c. Helium d. Sodium
214. The valence electrons of Boron is
   a. 4 b. 6
   c. 3 d. 1
215. Is large atomic radius
   a. Silicon b. Boron
   c. Carbon d. Zinc
216. The general electronic configuration of p block elements is________.
   a. $ns^2 np^{1}$–6 b. $ns^3 np^{1-10}$
   c. $ns^0 np^{0-1}$ d. All of the above
217. In periodic table group VIII A is classified as________.
   a. Noble gases b. Halogen
   c. Alkali metals d. Alkali Earth metals
218. ________&________are mostly composed, condensed to form sun.
   a. Hydrogen & helium b. Hydrogen & sodium
   c. Sodium & chloride d. Sodium & helium
219. Electrodes are used in the synthesis of organic compounds on the prebiotic Earth.
   a. Tungsten b. Copper
   c. Zinc d. Silver
220. Hypothesis suggest that life did not originate on earth but was brought here by meteorites from elsewhere in the universe.
   a. Panspermia b. Clay hypothesis
   c. RNA world d. All of the above
221. How many map unites for mutant vestigial wings________.
   a. 67 map unites b. 61 map unites
   c. 55 map unites d. 60 map unites
222. Produce urine that darkens alarmingly on exposure to air, a consequence of the oxidation of the Homogentisic acid they excrete.
   a. Alkaptonuria b. Oligonuria
   c. Both a & b d. None of the above
223. Who gave the semi-conservative type of hypothesis of DN a.
   a. James Watson & Francis Crick b. Alfred Hershey & Martha chase
   c. Mendel d. All of the above
224. What is the formula of the Chargaff rule
   a. A + G = T + C / A + U = G + C b. A + C = G + T
   c. A + U = U + G d. All of the above

225. Who gave the germ plasm theory________.
   a. August Weismann
   b. Lamarck
   c. Charles Darwin
   d. None of the above
226. Which type of cell has membrane enclosed nucleus
   a. Prokaryotes
   b. Eukaryotes
   c. Both
   d. None
227. Why viruses are not classified as living
   a. They have relatively simple structures
   b. They are mainly unicellular
   c. They lack ability to reproduce outside the host
   d. They are large molecular aggregates
228. bacterial cells allows them to survive in adverse conditions
   a. Spores
   b. Flagella
   c. Cilia
   d. Mesosome
229. Whip like appendages on bacterial cells
   a. Pilli
   b. Cell wall
   c. Mesosome
   d. Flagella
230. Prokaryotes usually reproduce by
   a. Conjugation
   b. Budding
   c. Mating
   d. Binary fission
231. What is false about pilli
   a. Helps attachment of bacterium to host tissue
   b. Helps in sexual conjugation
   c. Aids in DNA transport from cell to cell
   d. None
232. Filamentous projection on bacterial cells helps in conjugation
   a. Flagella
   b. Pilli
   c. Cell wall
   d. Mesosome
233. Organisms which can synthesize all their cellular constituents from simple molecules
   a. Heterotrophs
   b. Lithotrophs
   c. Autotrophs
   d. Chemo lithotrophs
234. Organisms obtain energy through oxidation of inorganic compounds
   a. Heterotrophs
   b. Chemo lithotrophs
   c. Autotrophs
   d. Photo autotrophs
235. Organisms obtain energy through photosynthesis
   a. Photo autotrophs
   b. Heterotrophs
   c. Chemotrophs
   d. Lithotrophs

236. Organisms obtain energy through the oxidation of organic compounds
    a. chemotrophs b. Chemo autotrophs
    c. Photo autotrophs d. Heterotrophs
237. Organisms can grow in either presence or absence of oxygen
    a. Obligate anaerobes b. Facultative anaerobes
    c. Anaerobes d. Aerobes
238. Organisms that inhabit acidic hot springs
    a. Thermophiles b. Acidophiles
    c. Chemophiles d. Thermoacidophiles
239. Common eukaryotic secretory mechanism that is reverse of endocytosis
    a. Deglutition b. Agglutination
    c. Exocytosis d. Phagocytosis
240. Organisms which can live only in concentrated Brine solution
    a. Halobacteria b. Heyerobacteria
    c. Chemobacteria d. Chenobacteria
241. Size of eukaryotic cell ranges
    a. 10 – 100 micro meter b. 10-100 nano meter
    c. 10-100 Pico meter d. 10-100 milli meter
242. Partial metabolisation in intramolecular oxidation – reduction process is known as
    a. Fragmentation b. Fermentation
    c. Obligation d. Reduction
243. Organisms which are poisoned by presence of Oxygen
    a. Obligate aerobes b. Facultative Aerobes
    c. Facultative anaerobes d. Obligate anaerobes
244. What is the process by which organisms maintain a stable internal environment?
    a. Homeostasis b. Metabolism
    c. Evolution d. Adaptation
245. What type of organisms are typically composed of eukaryotic cells?
    a. Bacteria and Archaea b. Bacteria and Viruses
    c. Plants, Animals, Fungi, and Protists d. Only Fungi
246. Which of the following structures is found in both prokaryotic and eukaryotic cells?
    a. Mitochondria b. Endoplasmic reticulum
    c. Ribosomes d. Golgi apparatus
247. Which structure is present in plant cells but not in animal cells?
    a. Nucleus b. Chloroplast
    c. Mitochondrion d. Ribosome

248. What distinguishes eukaryotic chromosomes from prokaryotic chromosomes?
   a. Eukaryotic chromosomes are circular, while prokaryotic chromosomes are linear.
   b. Eukaryotic chromosomes are linear, while prokaryotic chromosomes are circular.
   c. Both types of chromosomes are circular.
   d. Both types of chromosomes are linear.

249. Where is the genetic material of a prokaryotic cell located?
   a. In the nucleus
   b. In the nucleoid region
   c. In the mitochondria
   d. In the chloroplasts

250. What type of cell division do prokaryotic cells undergo?
   a. Mitosis
   b. Meiosis
   c. Binary fission
   d. Budding

251. What is the primary type of bond that associates water molecules together?
   a. Covalent bond
   b. Ionic bond
   c. Hydrogen bond
   d. Metallic bond

252. In a hydrogen bond between two water molecules, what typically acts as the hydrogen bond donor?
   a. Oxygen atom
   b. Hydrogen atom in O-H
   c. Lone-pair electron cloud
   d. Nitrogen atom

253. What is the main reason hydrogen is central to hydrogen bonding?
   a. Its large size
   b. Its small size
   c. Its high electronegativity
   d. Its ability to form double bonds

254. What percentage of hydrogen bonds are considered to be covalent in character?
   a. 5%
   b. 10%
   c. 20%
   d. 50%

255. What is the typical distance of an O-H hydrogen bond in water?
   a. 0.5 Å
   b. 1.8 Å
   c. 2.6 Å
   d. 3.0 Å

256. What is the energy of a hydrogen bond compared to a typical covalent bond?
   a. Much higher
   b. Comparable
   c. Much lower
   d. Nearly the same

257. Why does water expand upon freezing?
   a. Decreased hydrogen bonding
   b. Open structure formed by hydrogen bonds
   c. Increased van der Waals forces
   d. Decrease in density due to temperature

258. What is the density of ice compared to liquid water?
   a. 1.10 g/ml
   b. 1.00 g/ml
   c. 0.92 g/ml
   d. 0.80 g/ml

259. What would happen if ice were denser than liquid water?
   a. Ice would float on water
   b. Ice would sink to the bottom of lakes and oceans
   c. Water bodies would remain liquid in winter
   d. Earth would experience warmer climates

260. What is the heat of sublimation of ice at 0°C?
   a. 20 kJ/mol b. 46.9 kJ/mol
   c. 100 kJ/mol d. 460 kJ/mol

261. What quantity of the heat of sublimation of ice can be attributed to the kinetic energy of gaseous water molecules?
   a. 46.9 kJ/mol b. 15 kJ/mol
   c. 41 kJ/mol d. 613 J/molp

262. What is the remaining 41 kJ/mol of the heat of sublimation of ice used for?
   a. Increasing kinetic energy
   b. disrupting hydrogen bonds in the ice crystal
   c. Forming covalent bonds
   d. Melting the ice

263. What percentage of hydrogen bonds are broken when ice melts?
   a. 10% b. 15%
   c. 20% d. 25%

264. Why is the boiling point of water much higher than that of methane (CH_4)?
   a. Water has a higher molecular mass b. Water forms hydrogen bonds
   c. Methane forms stronger bonds d. Methane is nonpolar

265. What is the average nearest-neighbor O-O distance in liquid water near 1°C?
   a. 2.76 Å b. 2.82 Å
   c. 3.5 Å d. 7.0 Å

266. What does the presence of a 3.5 Å intermolecular distance in liquid water indicate?
   a. An icelike structure
   b. A breakdown of the tetrahedral structure
   c. A decrease in density
   d. An increase in temperature

267. What is the average number of nearest neighbors surrounding each water molecule in liquid water?
   a. 2.4 b. 3.4
   c. 4.4 d. 5.4

268. How often does each water molecule reorient in liquid water?
   a. Once every 10 seconds b. Once every 10 milliseconds
   c. Once every 10 picoseconds d. Once every 10 nanoseconds

269. How are the hydrogen bonds in liquid water compared to those in ice?
   a. Stronger and more regular
   b. Weaker and more distorted
   c. The same strength but more numerous
   d. Fewer but stronger
270. What range of hydrogen bonds can each water molecule form in liquid water?
   a. 2 to 4
   b. 3 to 6
   c. 4 to 8
   d. 5 to 7
271. What types of rings are commonly formed in liquid water's hydrogen-bonded structure?
   a. 3 to 7-membered rings
   b. 4 to 6-membered rings
   c. 5 to 8-membered rings
   d. 6-membered rings only
272. What makes determining the instantaneous structure of liquid water difficult?
   a. The static nature of water molecules
   b. The rapid reorientation of water molecules
   c. The simple structure of liquid water
   d. The inability to form hydrogen bonds
273. What is a consequence of liquid water having a rapidly fluctuating structure?
   a. Liquid water has a constant, predictable structure
   b. Liquid water behaves exactly like ice
   c. Liquid water exhibits both icelike and non-icelike characteristics
   d. Liquid water cannot form hydrogen bonds
274. Why is water considered a "universal solvent"?
   a. It dissolves nonpolar substances easily
   b. It can dissolve more types of substances in greater amounts than any other solvent
   c. It can dissolve only ionic compounds
   d. It dissolves all types of substances
275. What is the main factor that contributes to the solubility of salts in water?
   a. The low molecular mass of water
   b. The high dielectric constant of water
   c. The lack of hydrogen bonding in water
   d. The ionic nature of water molecules
276. The living matter is composed of:
   a. Carbon, Hydrogen, Oxygen, Nitrogen, Phosphorus, Sulphur
   b. Calcium, Iron, Carbon, Hydrogen, Nitrogen, Sulphur
   c. Chlorine, Carbon, Hydrogen, Nitrogen, Phosphorus, Sulphur
   d. Carbon, Hydrogen, Oxygen, Nitrogen, Copper, Cobalt

277. Building block /Monomeric units of fat is/are:
  a. Fattyacids b. Ketone
  c. Glycerol d. Both a & b

278. What is serves as a storage form of energy to meet long term demands & structural components of membranes?
  a. Glycogen b. Protein
  c. Nucleotide d. Lipid

279. Which of the following is true for eukaryotes:
  a. Cells is enveloped by a rigid cell wall
  b. Cell division by fission & no mitosis
  c. Cell organelles and cytoskeleton is absent
  d. Enzymes of energy metabolism are located in mitochondria

280. What is the largest cellular organelle?
  a. Mitochondria b. Nucleus
  c. Nucleolus d. Endoplasmic reticulum

281. Diameter of nucleopore which is present in between two nuclear membrane:
  a. 40nm b. 90nm
  c. 80nm d. 60nm

282. Which of the following biomolecule is responsible for transmitting genetic information from one generation to next generation?
  a. RNA b DNA
  c. Proteins d Carbohydrates

283. Role of nucleus in a cell is:
  a. To synthesize proteins b. To store genetic information
  c. Regulate the cell growth & division d. To control cell singnaling

284. Eukaryotic DNA is associated with basic protein to form nucleosomes:
  a. 1:2 b. 2:1
  c. 3:2 d. 1:1

285. Which syndrome occur as a result of distortion of nuclear envelope due to accumulation protein lamina A.
  a. Hutchinson-Gilford Progeria Syndrome (HGP's)
  b. Zellweger syndrome
  c. Klinefelter syndrome
  d. Marfan syndrome

286. Nucleolus is rich in:
  a. DNA b. RNA
  c. RNA polymerase d. Protein

287. Choose the correct sentence among the following:
   a. Single bound organelle-Lysosome, Mitochondria, Golgi apparatus
   b. Single bound organelle-Lysosome, Golgi apparatus, Peroxisomes, Endoplasmic reticulum
   c. Double bound organelle-Mitochondria, Nucleus, Chloroplast, Endoplasmic reticulum
   d. Both b & c

288. ______is the principle producer of ATP.
   a. Mitochondria
   b. Golgi apparatus
   c. Nucleus
   d. ER

289. ______are the centers for the cellular respiration and energy metaobolism.
   a. Mitochondria
   b. Golgi apparatus
   c. Nucleus
   d. ER

290. Which of the statement is false about mitochondria?
   a. Mitochondrial matrix contains a circular dsDNA,RNA,Ribosomes.
   b. Mitochondria equipped with an independent protein synthesizing machinery.
   c. The component of ETC and Oxidative phosphorylation are buried in the outer mitochondrial membrane.
   d. Matrix enzymes involved in synthesis of heme & Ure a.

291. ________are the factories of protein synthesis.
   a. ER
   b. Golgi apparatus
   c. Lysosome
   d. Ribosome

292. Which of the following statement is true about smooth endoplasmic reticulum?
   a. Ribosomes studded on the SER.
   b. Involved in synthesis of lipids and metabolism of drug.
   c. Supplying Calcium for the cellular function
   d. both b&c

293. Eukaryotic cell contain a unique cluster of membrane vesicles known as_______ which in turn constitute golgi apparatus.
   a. Lysosomes
   b. Microsomes
   c. Peroxisomes
   d. Dictyosomes

294. Lysosomes are regarded as the ________.
   a. Digestive tract of the cell
   b. Urinary tract of the cell
   c. Respiratory tract of the cell
   d. Excretory tract of the cell

295. Lysosomal enzymes are categorized as:
   a. Catalases
   b. Hydrolases
   c. Ligases
   d. Reductases

296. ________ is the age pigment /wear and tear pigment.
   a. Melanin b. Haemosiderin
   c. Lipofuscin d. Ceroid
297. Inclusion cells(I-cells)disease occurs due to:
   a. Absence of catalase in lysosome
   b. Absence of reductase in lysosome
   c. Absence of hydrolase in lysosome
   d. Absence of ligase in lysosome
298. Peroxisomal enzyme is categorized as:
   a. Catalase b. Hydrolase
   c. Ligase d. Oxidase
299. Zellweger syndrome is categorized by the absence of ________
   a. Functional ribosomes b. Functional lysosomes
   c. Fuctional microsomes d. Fuctional peroxisomes
300. ________is the programmed cell death/cell sucide.
   a. Necrosis b Apoptosis
   c. Gangrene d Autophagy

Answer Key

1	c	2	c	3	d	4	b	5	a	6	d	7	a
8	b	9	c	10	a	11	c	12	a	13	b	14	d
15	a	16	c	17	a	18	b	19	c	20	d	21	a
22	d	23	b	24	d	25	b	26	d	27	d	28	b
29	d	30	a	31	b	32	c	33	b	34	d	35	b
36	a	37	d	38	c	39	d	40	d	41	a	42	c
43	c	44	b	45	b	46	d	47	c	48	b	49	b
50	d	51	d	52	d	53	c	54	a	55	b	56	c
57	b	58	c	59	c	60	b	61	b	62	c	63	c
64	a	65	b	66	c	67	c	68	b	69	d	70	a
71	b	72	a	73	c	74	c	75	b	76	b	77	b
78	d	79	a	80	b	81	b	82	a	83	b	84	c
85	b	86	b	87	b	88	d	89	a	90	c	91	d
92	d	93	d	94	b	95	a	96	d	97	c	98	c
99	a	100	b	101	d	102	a	103	a	104	b	105	a
106	a	107	a	108	c	109	c	110	b	111	b	112	b
113	a	114	b	115	d	116	d	117	a	118	a	119	c
120	a	121	b	122	a	123	a	124	c	125	b	126	a
127	b	128	b	129	b	130	d	131	a	132	d	133	a
134	d	135	a	136	c	137	a	138	a	139	a	140	a

141	d	142	d	143	a	144	a	145	a	146	a	147	a
148	a	149	a	150	a	151	c	152	c	153	c	154	c
155	b	156	d	157	b	158	d	159	c	160	b	161	d
162	c	163	c	164	d	165	c	166	c	167	b	168	b
169	b	170	c	171	b	172	b	173	b	174	b	175	b
176	b	177	b	178	c	179	a	180	b	181	c	182	c
183	c	184	a	185	b	186	b	187	b	188	d	189	d
190	a	191	b	192	b	193	d	194	c	195	b	196	b
197	c	198	b	199	c	200	a	201	a	202	b	203	a
204	a	205	c	206	a	207	a	208	a	209	a	210	a
211	a	212	a	213	a	214	c	215	a	216	a	217	a
218	a	219	a	220	a	221	a	222	a	223	a	224	a
225	a	226	b	227	c	228	a	229	a	230	d	231	d
232	b	233	c	234	b	235	a	236	d	237	b	238	d
239	c	240	a	241	a	242	b	243	d	244	a	245	c
246	c	247	b	248	b	249	b	250	c	251	c	252	b
253	b	254	d	255	b	256	c	257	b	258	c	259	b
260	b	261	a	262	b	263	d	264	b	265	b	266	b
267	b	268	d	269	b	270	a	271	a	272	b	273	c
274	b	275	b	276	a	277	d	278	d	279	d	280	b
281	b	282	b	283	b	284	d	285	a	286	b	287	b
288	a	289	a	290	c	291	d	292	d	293	c	294	a
295	b	296	c	297	c	298	a	299	d	300	b		

2

pH, Acid, Bases and Buffers

M.K. Vidya[1], N.R. Srikanth[2], C.N. Darshan[3] and Monoshree Sarma[4]

[1]Department of Physiology and Biochemistry, Veterinary College, Hassan KVAFSU - Karnataka Veterinary, Animal and Fisheries Sciences University

[2]Division of Veterinary Biochemistry, Livestock Research Station, Lam, Guntur Sri Venkateswara Veterinary University

[3]Department of Animal Husbandry and Veterinary Services, Karnataka

[4]Department of Veterinary Pharmacology and Toxicology, Institute of Veterinary Science and Animal Husbandry, Siksha 'O' Anusandhan, Bhubaneswar, Odisha

Introduction

pH is a quantitative measure of the concentration of hydrogen ions in a solution. The pH scale ranges from 0 to 14, with 7 being neutral. Lower pH indicates acidity, while higher pH indicated alkalinity. Pure water at 25°C has a pH of 7.0 as the concentrations of H_3O^+ and OH^-. pH is defined as potential of hydrogen and is a measure of how acidic or basic a substance or solution is. The concentration of Hydrogen (H^+) in a solution determines its pH. Higher concentrations of H^+ ions correspond to lower pH values (more acidic), and lower concentrations of H^+ ions correspond to higher pH values (More alkaline/basic). pH is an important measurement concept in many fields, including chemistry, biology, and environmental science. pH of blood and other fluids of the body, secretions *etc.*, determine the health status of an individual. Likewise, pH determines the quality of soil for plant growth. In medical sciences, pH plays a crucial role in maintaining a healthy internal environment for various bodily functions. Internal environment of an animal or human is tightly regulated more so the pH of different body fluids like blood, saliva and stomach acid.

pH balance is a very prime aspect to maintain homeostasis inside a biological system. Speaking of which the first thing that comes to mind is the enzyme function. Many enzymes have a specific pH range for optimal activity. Any deviation from this specific pH range not only significantly disrupt their function but also hinder biochemical processes involved. Most vital operations of a cell are nutrition transport and waste disposal *i.e.*, excretion. pH of the fluids surrounding cells impacts these activities; hence, maintaining a proper pH is vital for healthy cell function. Different organs of the body need to maintain different pH ranges for functioning accordingly. Stomach operates at acidic pH to digest the food material ingested whereas, blood need alkaline pH for optimal oxygen transport by RBC.

Acid is defined by Svante Arrhenius as early as 19th century as any substance that, when dissolved in water increases the concentration of hydrogen ions (H^+) in the solution. It is the most basic definition of acid. Johannes Bronsted and Thomas Lowry elaborated Arrhenius acid definition and theory. According to them an Acid is any substance that can donate a proton (H^+) to another substance (which is referred to as base). However, G. N. Lewis, in a completely different approach defined acid as any molecule or ion that can accept an electron pair from another molecule or ion (Lewis base). These three types of views on acid define three aspects of acid behaviour. The first of the above definitions of acid deal with proton transfer and the later one focuses on electron interactions.

Acids doesn't display same strengths. Some readily dissociate in water, exhibiting a high concentration of hydrogen ions (H^+). These are classified as strong acids. Hydrochloric acid, Sulphuric acid comes under this category. These acids ionize completely in water. However, weak acids partially dissociate in water, displaying a lower concentration her this category. The strengths of the acids play significant role in biochemical aspects of living beings. Strong acids due to their strength proved to be harsh and can denature proteins by altering their structure. Their typical dissociation makes them useful in controlled laboratory applications and experiments. Weak acids due to their lower ionization act as buffers to maintain pH of the body and bodily fluids.

If we go to the roots of the biochemistry there is a separate classification of the acids, not based on their strengths but on their origin. Organic and inorganic acids come under this classification. Organic acids are derived from living organisms and or their breakdown products. Citric acid, lactic acid and acetic acid to name a few. While inorganic acids mostly come from minerals, which include hydrochloric, sulphuric and phosphoric acids.

Bases are substances that dissociate in water to produce hydroxide ions (OH^-), according to Arrhenius theory. Sodium hydroxide and potassium hydroxide come under this category and are generally referred to as alkalis. However, according to Bronsted-Lowry theory, a base is a proton acceptor and under this theory along with Arrhenius bases other molecules or compunds can be referred a bases. One such example is Ammonia.

Just like acids, based on the strength, bases are classified as strong and weak bases Strong bases readily dissociate in water accepting protons and forming large concentrations of hydroxide ions. Sodium hydroxide and potassium hydroxide come under this category. When coming to weak bases, they partially dissociate in water forming rather lesser concentrations of hydroxide ions compared to stronger bases. They attain equilibrium with their undissociated form and conjugate acids. Ammonia and bicarbonate are the prime in this category. Base on the sources, even bases also can be classified as organic and inorganic bases. Amino group from proteins and certain vitamins occupy the organic category whereas, unlike organic bases, they are not part of any organic life but derive from minerals naturally. Sodium hydroxide and calcium carbonate come under the inorganic category.

Buffers are solutions that resist change in pH when small amounts of acids or bases are added to them. Buffers play a crucial role in organic systems to maintain homeostasis. Maintaining pH is utmost important in biological processes without buffer this feat cannot be achieved. We may say buffers are peacemakers between ever antagonising acids and bases. Buffers in general are weak acid and its conjugate with strong base or weak base and its salt with strong acid. The former one is called acidic buffer and the later one is a basic buffer. When a strong acid, such as HCl is added to the bicarbonate buffer solution, the increased hydrogen ions (from HCl) are buffered by HCO_3^- which form a weak base H_2CO_3. The opposite reaction will happen when strong base like Sodium Hydroxide is added. Sodium hydroxide reacts with H_2CO_3 to form weak base HCO_3^-. Thus even when strong acid and weak base are added to the buffer system, they will be converted to weak acid and weak base, respectively and hence the pH of the buffer system is maintained without any change. Bicarbonate and phosphate buffer systems are the main buffer systems in the biological systems. Also, proteins and haemoglobin function as buffer systems within the body.

1. Which of the following is not a macromolecular components of a cell
   a. Lipids b. Nucleic acids
   c. Enzyme d. Proteins
2. The physical properties of water allow it to act as
   a. Solution b. Solute
   c. Solvent d. All of the above
3. A water molecule is
   a. V shaped b. U shaped
   c. W shaped d. J shaped
4. The angle between [O-H] covalent bond of water
   a. 104.5 degree b. 105.5 degree
   c. 106 degree d. 107.5 degree
5. An 0xygen atom as
   a. 6 electrons b. 8 electrons
   c. 2 electrons d. 10 electrons
6. The uneven distribution of charge within a bond is known as
   a. Dipole b. Tripole
   c. Tetrapole d. None of the above
7. How much heat is required to disrupt hydrogen bond between water molecules
   a. 40 KJ/mol b. 10 KJ/mol
   c. 50KJ/mol d. 20KJ/mol
8. Hydrogen bonds are -------- interactions compared covalent bond
   a. Strong b. Weak
   c. Moderate d. None of the above
9. In water molecule each hydrogen atom can participate in only --------hydrogen bond
   a. One b. Two
   c. Three d. Four
10. The energy required to break a covalent O-H bond in water is
    a. 400KJ/MOL b. 300 KJ/MOL
    c. 460 KJ/MOL d. 500 KJ/MOL

11. The average energy required to break each hydrogen bondin ice has been estimated as
    a. 10 KJ/MOL
    b. 15 KJ/MOL
    c. 23 KJ/MOL
    d. 33 KJ/MOL
12. The water_______as the temperature drops below 4 degree
    a. Contracts
    b. Expands
    c. Remains same
    d. None of above
13. The amount of heat needed to raise the temperature of 1 gram of the substance by 1^celcius
    a. Latent heat
    b. Heat of vaporization
    c. Threshold heat
    d. Specific heat
14. Specific heat is also called as
    a. Heat capacity
    b. Latent heat
    c. Threshold heat
    d. Heat of vaporization
15. Molecules that dissociate to form ions are called
    a. Dipole
    b. Electrolytes
    c. Dissociative compounds
    d. All of the above
16. Substances that are easily dissolve in water are said to be
    a. Solvent
    b. Hydrophobic
    c. Hydrophilic
    d. None of the above
17. Water fearing substance are called
    a. Hydrophobic
    b. Hydrophilic
    c. Amphoteric
    d. None of the above
18. Extreme thermophiles live in
    a. 100°
    b. 0°
    c. 200°
    d. 121°
19. The shell of water molecules that surrounds each ion is called as
    a. Solution sphere
    b. Solvation sphere
    c. Sphere
    d. None of above
20. An increase in the number of polar groups in an organic molecule______its solubility
    a. Increases
    b. Decreases
    c. Remain same
    d. None of above
21. Collisions of solute with other molecules inhibit the diffusion due to the effect
    a. Molecular inhibition
    b. Molecular effect
    c. Molecular collision
    d. None of above
22. The pressure required to prevent the flow of solvent is called as
    a. Water pressure
    b. Diffusion pressure
    c. Threshold pressure
    d. Osmotic pressure

23. Movement of water molecules from a solution of higher concentration of water molecules to a solution of lower water molecules is called as
    a. Diffusion
    b. Passive transport
    c. Active transport
    d. Osmosis
24. The substance which acts as both acid and base is called as
    a. Dipole
    b. Amphoteric
    c. Hydrophilic
    d. All of the above
25. The energy required to break a covalent C-H bond is about
    a. 410 KJ/MOL
    b. 200KJ/MOL
    c. 500KJ/MOL
    d. 1000KJ/MOL
26. Which of the following forces is a variation of electrostatic interaction.
    a. Van der wales
    b. Hydrogen bonds
    c. Ionic bonds
    d. All of the above
27. Charge- Charge interaction of in proteins, where opposite groups attract one another is called
    a. Ion pairing
    b. Intermolecular H bonding
    c. Salt bridge
    d. Crystallization
28. Which of the following is the strongest non-covalent bond
    a. Hydrogen bond
    b. Van der Waals bond
    c. Peptide bond
    d. None
29. ______ bond is present between enzyme and substrate during formation of enzyme-substrate complex.
    a. Van der Waals bond
    b. Hydrogen bond
    c. Ionic bond
    d. Covalent bond
30. The strength of hydrogen bond between two nitrogen bases of DNA may be estimated as
    a. 60-70 kJ.mol-1
    b. 70-80 kJ. mol-1
    c. 25-30 kJ. mol-1
    d. 40-60 kJ. mol-1
31. The atoms forming hydrogen bond in close proximity maintain a distance of
    a. 0.2 um
    b. 0.2 nm
    c. 0.2 Å
    d. 20 nm
32. Van der Waals force is a force that is
    a. Always Attractive
    b. Always Repulsive
    c. Fluctuating between attraction and repulsion
    d. Acts as both attractive and repulsion depending on distance between molecules
33. ______ is also known as London dispersion force.
    a. Van der Waals force
    b. Hydrophobic force
    c. Nucleus electron force of atom
    d. Intranuclear force of atom

34. ______stabilize the double stranded DNA helix between the heterocyclic bases of nucleic acid.
 a. Hydrogen bond b. Van der Waals force
 c. Covalent bond d. Peptide bond

35. Micelles are stabilized by
 a. Van der Waals force b. Hydrogen bond
 c. Hydrophobic interaction d. Covalent bond

36. Water molecule act as
 a. Electrophile b. Nucleophile
 c. Proton donor d. Both a and c

37. Electrophiles are
 a. Electron rich b. Electronic deficient
 c. Neutron deficient d. None

38. Nucleophiles are
 a. Electron rich b. Electron deficient
 c. Nucleus loving d. Both a and c

39. Nitrogen atom in biological environment acts as
 a. Nucleophile b. Electrophile
 c. Proton donor d. None

40. The density of water at 0°C is
 a. 1 g/ml b. Less than 1g/ml
 c. 0.5 g/ml d. More than 1g/ml

41. Ionization of water
 a. A spontaneous process b. A reversible process
 c. Release heat d. All of the above

42. The equilibrium constant for ionization of water (25°C,1 atm) is
 a. 2.2 b. 1.8×10-16
 c. 1.8×1016 d. 6.023×1023

43. Which of the following is the strongest conjugate base
 a Cl— b COOH—
 c CH3COO- d C3H5COO-

44. The patient suffering from diabetes have a blood pH of
 a. 7.4 b. >7.4
 c. <7.4 d. Vary around 7.4

45. Purine and pyrimidines act as
 a. Weak acid and weak base b. Weak base and weak acid
 c. Weak acid only d. Weak base only

46. pH of a solution having H+ concentration of 10-8
 a. 8 b. 6.98
 c. 7.02 d. 6.8

47. Which of the following in basic in nature

a. Cow's milk
b. Coffee
c. Wine
d. None

48. pH equals pOH at H+ concentration of

a. 10-14
b. 107
c. 10-7
d. 1014

49. If the acid dissociation constant for an acid HA is 1.9×10-8, then the A- is a

a. Strong acid
b. Strong base
c. Weak acid
d. Weak base

50. Van der Waals force is highly repulsive at

a. Van der Waals radii
b. Interatomic distance
c. Intranuclear distance
d. More than van der Waals radii

51. Henderson - hasselbalch equation is ______

a. PH=PKa+log(proton acceptor)/(proton donor)
b. PH=PKa+log(proton donor)/(proton acceptor)
c. PKa=PH+log(proton acceptor)/(proton donor)
d. PKa=PH+log(proton donor)/(proton acceptor)

52. Phosphoric acid is a ______acid

a. Monoprotic acid
b. Diprotic acid
c. Polyprotic acid
d. Not a protic acid

53. If the PH of a solution remains nearly constant when small amount of strong acid or strong base are added the solution is called _______

a. Buffered
b. Equivalent
c. Acidity
d. Basicity

54. A excellent example of _____is found in the blood plasma of mammals which has remarkably ____ph

a. Acidity, constant
b. Acidity, increased
c. buffer, increase
d. Dbuffer, constant

55. PKa value of formic acid ____

a. 3.5
b. 3.6
c. 3.7
d. 3.8

56. A buffer solution contain 0.36M sodium acetate and 0.45M acetic acid,pka=4.8,what is the pH of the buffer solution?

a. 4.7
b. 6.3
c. 5.5
d. 4.2

57. If the pka=pH,the log of the ratio of dissociating acid and associated acid will be________

a. Equal
b. Zero
c. Greter than 1
d. Lesser than 1

58. Which of the following mixture is an example of buffer solution?
   a. KCl and HCl b. NH4Cl and HNO3
   c. NaNO2 and HNO3 d. NaCl and NaOH
59. A buffer solution is a mixture of _____
   a. Strong acid & weak base b. Weak acid & strong base
   c. Strong acid & conjugate base d. Weak acid & conjugate base
60. What is the PH of buffer solution?
   a. Same as if pka value b. Same as it's ka value
   c. Can't be calculated d. None of the above
61. The strength of weak acid is indicated by ____
   a. pH value b. Pka value
   c. Acidity d Bacisity
62. The major non-covolent interaction that determine the structure and function of biomolecules are _____ and _____
   a. Electrostatic interaction & hydrophilic interaction
   b. Hydrophilic interaction & electrostatic interaction
   c. Electrostatic interaction & hydrophobic interaction
   d. Hydrophobic interaction & electrostatic interaction
63. What is the pka value of lactic acid _____
   a. 3.8 b. 4.8
   c. 5.8 d. 6.8
64. A buffer job is to prevent large pH changes upon the addition of small amount of either ____or____
   a. Strong acid or weak base b. Weak acid or strong base
   c. Strong acid or strong base d. Weak acid or weak base
65. What is used to resist any change in pH?
   a. Acid b. Base
   c. Buffers d. Water
66. Dilution with water has _____effect on the pH of any buffer
   a. Increases b. Decreases
   c. Highly increased d. No effect
67. Henderson equation might not be applicable when associating with ____
   a. Weak bases b. Weak acid
   c. Both weak acid or weak base d. None
68. Assumption of the Henderson hasselbalch equation
   a. The acid, HA is monobasic
   b. The self-dissociation of water can be ignored
   c. The salt is completely dissociated in the solution
   d. All of above

69. Who created Henderson hasselbalch equation

a. Karl Albert hasselbalch
b. Lawrence Joseph Henderson
c. Robert hasselbalch
d. Robert Henderson

70. What are the factors affecting buffer solution?

a. Temperature
b. Ionic strength
c. Hydroniumion
d. All of the above

71. In humans blood,a constant pH 7.4 is mentaned by _____

a. CO_2, carbonic acid, bicarbonate buffer
b. O_2, carbonic acid , bicarbonate buffer
c. CO_2, O_2, bicarbonate buffer
d. both a and b

72. The acidity or basicity of an aqueous solution depends on the concentration of_____

a. H+
b. OH-
c. IINO3-
d. NH3

73. Within cell both _____&_____ contribute to intracellular buffering

a. Proteins & organic phosphate
b. Proteins & acid
c. Proteins & inorganic phosphate
d. Proteins & base

74. The pH of blood is controlled by the ratio of ____

a. HCO3- to pCO2
b. HCO3- to pO2
c. O2 to CO2
d. O2 to NH3

75. Hydrogen bonding contributes to the _____ & ____Of water

a. High specific heat & heat of vaporization
b. High specific heat & heat of atomisation
c. Heat of vaporization & solubility
d. None

76. Which is the most abundant substance in living systems

a. Water
b. Air
c. Soil
d. Light

77. The first living organisms arose in an ____________ environment

a. Acidic
b. Basic
c. Aqueous
d. Non aqueous

78. Among the following characteristics of water which are crucial for structure and function of biomolecules

a Attractive forces between water molecules
b. Ionizing capacity
c. Buffering capacity
d. All of the above

79. The product of ionization of water molecule are

a. H+ and OH-
b. H- and OH+
c. H+ and OH+
d. H- and OH-

80. What is the heat of vaporization of water
 a. 2260 J/g b. 1100 J/g
 c. 854 J/g d. 590 J/g
81. Force that make water a liquid at room temperature?
 a. Cohesive force b. Kinetic force
 c. Intermolecular forces d. Intramolecular forces
82. Which of the following for water is high?
 a. Melting point b. Boiling point
 c. Heat of vapourisation d. All of the above
83. Hydrogen bonds are relatively
 a. Strong b. Weak
 c. None of the above d. Both a and b
84. Water is __________ type of solvent
 a. Polar b. Non polar
 c. Both a and b d. None of the above
85. Compounds that dissolve in water are
 a. Hydrophobhic b. Hydrophilic
 c. Polar d. None of the above
86. Compounds that donot dissolve in water are
 a. Hydrophobic b. Hydrophilic
 c. Non polar d. All of the above
87. Non polar gases are _______ soluble in water
 a. Highly b. Poorly
 c. Very high d. None of the above
88. Stable structures of amphipathic compounds in water called
 a. Micelles b. Clusters
 c. Clathrates d. None of the above
89. Attraction between oxygen atom of one water molecule and hydrogen of other is
 a. Magnetic b. Electrostatic
 c. Electromagnetic d. None of the above
90. Type of arrangement in outer shell electron of oxygen atom of water is
 a. Pyramidal b. Planar
 c. Tetrahedral d. Octahedral
91. Each water molecule form how many hydrogen bonds in ice
 a. 1 b. 2
 c. 3 d. 4
92. Density of ice is ______ than water
 a. More b. Less
 c. Very high d. None of the above

93. Water makes _____ percentage of living organisms

a. 90 b. 70

c. 50 d. 60

94. The H----O----H bond angle is _____ degrees

a. 120 b. 104.5

c. 106 d. 180

95. When Nacl dissolves in water. The entropy becomes_____

a. Low b. High

c. Very low d. None of the above

96. Water soluble carrier protein is

a. Haemoglobin b. Myoglobin

c. both a and b d. None of the above

97. Carbon dioxide with water forms

a. Carboxylic acid b. Carbonic acid

c. Formic acid d. None of the above

98. Hydrophobic molecules among these are

a. Chloroform b. Benzene

c. Both a and b d. None of the above

99. Boiling point of water is______ degree Celsius

a. 100 b. 70

c. 75 d. 80

100. The density of liquid water is highest at ________ degree Celsius

a. 0 b. 4

c. -4 d. 10

101. The non covalent interactions are weaker than

a. Ionic bond b. Covalent bond

c. Hydrogen bond d. All of these

102. The amount of energy required to break a mole of C-C bond is

a. 350 kJ b. 450 kJ

c. 10 kJ d. 25 kJ

103. The amount of energy required to break a mole of C-H bond is

a. 460 kJ b. 310 kJ

c. 210 kJ d. 410 kJ

104. The energy required to disrupt a mole of typical Van der Waals interaction is

a. 2 kJ b. 3 kJ

c. 4 kJ d. 5 kJ

105. The non covalent binding of an enzyme to its substrate may involve

a. Hydrogen bond b. Ionic interaction

c. Van der Waals interaction d. All of these

106. The binding of hormone or a neurotransmitter to its cellular receptor protein is a result of

a. Strong interaction
b. Weak interaction
c. Depends on the hormone
d. None of these

107. How many chains of bound water molecules are present in proteins and cytochromef

a. 5
b. 4
c. 3
d. 2

108. The protons move through the membrane by a process called as

a. Proton transport
b. Proton exchange
c. Proton hopping
d. All of these

109. How many water molecules are hydrogen bonded to each other and to the functional group

a. 5
b. 7
c. 9
d. 11

110. Solutes of all kinds alter the physical properties of the solutes like vapour pressure, boiling point and melting point. This property is known as

a. Colligative properties
b. Tied together properties
c. Both a & b
d. None of these

111. The effect of solute concentration on the colligative properties of water is

a. Depends on the chemical properties of the solute
b. Independent on the chemical properties of the solute
c. Remains constant
d. None of these

112. The component that alters the colligative properties of aqueous solution by lowering the effective concentration of water is

a. Solvent
b. Diluent
c. Solute
d. All of these

113. 1.00 molal aqueous solution means

a. 1 mol of solute per 10g of water
b. 1 mol of solute per 100g of water
c. 1 mol of solute per 1000g of water
d. All of these

114. Water molecules move from a region of higher water concentration to lower water concentration is called

a. Osmosis
b. Diffusion
c. Facilitated diffusion
d. Active transport

115. Van't Hoffs equation says

a. $\pi = RT$
b. $\pi = iRT$
c. $\pi = cRT$
d. $\pi = icRT$

116. The term " ic " in Van't Hoffs equation is

a. Osmolality
b. Osmolarity
c. Formality
d. Normality

117. For non ionised solutes the value of Van't Hoffs factor ' i ' is
    a. 3 b. 2
    c. 1 d. 0
118. Solutions of equal osmolarity is said to be
    a. Isotonic b. Hypotonic
    c. Hypertonic d. None of these
119. What happens to the cell in case of hypertonic solution
    a. No changes in the cell b. Cell swells
    c. Cell shrinks d. Cell burst
120. In hypotonic solution, the osmolarity of the cytosol is _______ than that of the cell
    a. No change b. Higher
    c. Lower d. None of these
121. The organelle which pumps water out of the cell in certain freshwater protists is
    a. Contractile vacuole b. Food vacuole
    c. Both a & b d. None of these
122. There is no net water movement in
    a. Hypotonic solution b. Isotonic solution
    c. Hypertonic solution d. Both a & b
123. The effect of solute on osmolarity depends on
    a. Number of dissolved particles b. Number of water particles
    c. both a & b d. All of these
124. The pressure used by plants to achieve mechanical turgidity is
    a. Turgor pressure b. Osmotic pressure
    c. Both a & b d. None of these
125. Hydrogen ions formed in the water are immediately hydrated to
    a. Hydroniumion b. Hydrate ion
    c. Hydrogen d. None of these
126. Which of the property of water is due to hydrogen bonding
    a. High density b. High boiling point
    c. High solubility of nonpolar substances d. Low specific heat capacity
127. Density of water is highest at
    a. 0°C b. 100°C
    c. 4°C d. 40°C
128. What type of bond primarily responsible for structure of water molecule
    a. Ionic bond b. Covalent bond
    c. Hydrogen bond d. Metallic bond
129. Angle between H-O-H bonds in the water molecule is
    a. 90° b. 104.5°
    c. 120° d. 180°

130. Which of the following is not a property of water due to Hydrogen bonding
 a. High specific heat b. High boiling point
 c. Low solubility of salts d. Low density of ice
131. The structure of ice is due to cumulative strength of
 a. Covalent bonds b. Ionic bond
 c. Metallic bond d. Intermolecular Hydrogen bond
132. Property of water to resist changes in temperature is called
 a. Thermal conductivity b. Latent heat
 c. Specific heat d. Surface tension
133. Water ability to dissolve many substances is primarily due to its
 a. Non polar nature b. Polar nature
 c. High viscosity d. Low density
134. Which property of water is responsible for capillary action
 a. Cohesion b. Adhesion
 c. Surface tension d. Specific heat
135. In a water molecule, oxygen has a partial
 a. Positive charge b. Negative charge
 c. Double bond d. No charge
136. Proton mobility of water is due to
 a. Covalent bonding b. Hydrophobic interaction
 c. Vanderwall's forces d. Hydrogen bonding
137. Proton mobility in water contribute to
 a. Conductivity b. Viscosity
 c. Solubility of nonpolar substances d. Surface tension
138. In water protons are often found associated with
 a. Sodium ions b. Chloride ions
 c. Water molecule as Hydronium ions d. Carbondioxide
139. Which phenomenon enhances the rate of proton mobility in water
 a. Low temperature b. High ionic strength
 c. Low pH d. High viscosity
140. Presence of which ions enhances proton mobility
 a. K+ and Cl- b. Na+ and OH-
 c. H+ and OH- d. NO3- and $SO4^{2}$-
141. Proton mobility in water is affected by
 a. Water temperature b. pH level
 c. Ionic strength d. All of the above
142. Which of the following substances will water most likely dissolve
 a. Sugar b. Oil
 c. Wax d. Plastic

143. What is the pH scale used to measure
 a. Concentration of acids
 b. Concentration of bases
 c. H+ ion concentration
 d. Oxygen concentration

144. Formula for calculating pH
 a. pH = -log(OH-)
 b. pH= - log(H+)
 c. pH= H+/OH-
 d. pH = log(H+)

145. pH range of acidic solution
 a. 0 to 7
 b. 7 to 14
 c. 4 to 7
 d. 5 to 10

146. Which of the following substances can act as buffer
 a. Sodium chloride
 b. Sodium hydroxide
 c. Acetic acid and sodium acetate
 d. Hydrochloric acid

147. Which of the following is not a property of acids
 a. They taste sour
 b. They turn blue litmus paper to red
 c. They react with bases to form salts
 d. They feel slippery

148. Which type of reaction is used to prepare a buffer solution
 a. Precipitation reaction
 b. Redox reaction
 c. Neutralization reaction
 d. Decomposition reaction

149. In a neutral solution the pH is
 a. Less than 7
 b. Greatet than 7
 c. Zero
 d. Equal to 7

150. The acid dissociation (Ka) is used to quantify the strength of
 a. Strong acids
 b. Weak acids
 c. Strong bases
 d. Weak bases

151. Which of the following statement is correct regarding the pH Scale?
 a. It is the negative logarithm of the H+ ion concentration of a given solution.
 b. It is the positive logarithm of the H+ ion concentration of a given solution.
 c. It is a 10 point scale.
 d. pH is an example of an extrinsic property.

152. What is the neutral value of the pH scale?
 a. Less than 5
 b. Equal to 7
 c. Less than 8
 d. Less than 10

153. When a given solution turns red litmus blue, it indicates?
 a. The solution is alkaline
 b. The solution is acidic
 c. The solution is neither acidic nor basic
 d. None of the above

154. The pH of a solution is determined by
   a. Concentration of salt
   b. Relative concentration of acids and bases
   c. Dielectric constant of the medium
   d. Environmental effect

155. Molecules in which the atoms are held together by __________ bonds have the strongest chemical linkages.
   a. Noncovalent
   b. Covalent
   c. Ionic
   d. Hydrogen

156. Buffer solutions
   a. Will always have a pH of 7
   b. They are rarely found in living systems
   c Cause a decrease in pH when acids are added to them
   d. Tend to maintain a relatively constant pH

157. Strong acids will have
   a. High pka value
   b. Low pka value
   c. Zero pka value
   d. None of these

158. Physiological Buffers include
   a. Bicarbonate
   b. Orthophosphate
   c. Protein
   d. All of these

159. ___________Participate in Maintaining Molecular structure
   a. Salt bonds
   b. Hydrophobic interaction
   c. Van der Waals forces
   d. All of these

160. In the equation: HF + H2O H3O+ + F-
   a. H2O is a base and HF is its conjugate acid
   b. H2O is an acid and HF is the conjugate base
   c. HF is an acid and F- is its conjugate base
   d. HF is a base and H3O+ is its conjugate acid

161. The term ph was introduced by
   a. Willams
   b. Sorensen
   c. Bronsted
   d. Rodwell

162. The pka of carboxylic acid _____ by adding ethanol
   a. Increases
   b. Decreases
   c. Remains same
   d. None of these

163. Buffers usually contain ________with its conjugate ________
   a. Weak base, base
   b. Strong base, acid
   c. Weak acid, base
   d. Weak acid, acid

164. Weak acids dissociates only partially in ______ solution.
   a. Acidic
   b. Basic
   c. Neutral
   d. Both a and b

165. Dielectric constant of water

a. 65.4 b. 78.5

c. 85.4 d. 94.8

166. Range of pH scale is

a. 7 to 10 b. 0 to 10

c. 0 to 14 d. 7 to 14

167. What happens to the pH of a solution when a strong acid is added to a buffer solution?

a. The pH increases significantly. b. The pH decreases significantly.

c. The pH remains relatively constant. d. The pH becomes neutral.

168. Which of the following is a characteristic of a weak base?

a. It completely dissociates in water

b. It partially dissociates in water

c. It has a very low pH in solution

d. It has no effect on the pH of a solution

169. In a buffer solution, which component reacts with added acids?

a. The weak acid b. The strong base

c. The strong acid d. The weak base

170. Which of the following statements about water is correct?

a. Water has a pH of 14 in its pure form

b. Water can act as both an acid and a base

c. Water is a strong electrolyte

d. Water does not ionize to any extent

171. A solution with a pH of 3 is considered to be:

a. Basic b. Neutral

c. Acidic d. Buffer

172. Which pH change would likely result in enzyme denaturation?

a. A shift from pH 7.4 to pH 6.5 b. A shift from pH 7.4 to pH 8.0

c. A shift from pH 6.5 to pH 7.0 d. A shift from pH 7.0 to pH 7.4

173. Which of the following statements about amino acids is true in relation to pH?

a. Amino acids always act as strong acids at physiological pH.

b. The side chain of amino acids does not affect their pH behavior.

c. Amino acids can act as buffers due to their ability to accept or donate protons.

d. Amino acids do not change their charge with pH variations

174. What is the typical pH range of the human blood?

a. 6.8 to 7.2 b. 7.35 to 7.45

c. 7.0 to 7.5 d. 6.5 to 7.5

175. The Henderson Hasselbalch equation explains the relationship between-

a. ph and poh b. ph and logKa

c. ph and pka d. poh and ka

176. Which of the following properties of water is most important for its role as a solvent in biological systems?
   a. High specific heat
   b. Cohesion and adhesion
   c. Ability to form hydrogen bonds
   d. Low vapor pressure

177. What is the pH of a solution with a hydrogen ion concentration $[H^+]$ of 1×10^{-5} M?
   a. 5
   b. 7
   c. 9
   d. 10

178. Which of the following solutions would be considered a strong acid?
   a. pH 2
   b. pH 5
   c. pH 7
   d. pH 9

179. Water is often referred to as a "universal solvent." Which of the following best explains why?
   a. Water can dissolve both polar and non-polar substances.
   b. Water can dissolve polar substances due to its polarity and ability to form hydrogen bonds.
   c. Water has a high heat of vaporization.
   d. Water is less dense as a solid than as a liquid

180. Which of the following statements correctly describes the relationship between pH and hydrogen ion concentration $[H^+]$?
   a. As $[H^+]$ increases, pH decreases
   b. As $[H^+]$ increases, pH increases
   c. pH is independent of $[H^+]$
   d. pH and $[H^+]$ are directly proportional

181. A buffer solution typically contains which of the following components?
   a. A strong acid and its conjugate base
   b. A weak acid and its conjugate base
   c. A strong base and its conjugate acid
   d. A weak base and its conjugate acid

182. What is the primary reason why water has a high specific heat capacity?
   a. The low molecular weight of water
   b. The hydrogen bonding between water molecules
   c. The polar nature of water molecules
   d. The presence of dissolved salts in water

183. Which of the following is true regarding the ionization of water?
   a. Pure water at 25°C has an equal concentration of H^+ and OH^-.
   b. Ionization of water increases with a decrease in temperature.
   c. The ionization of water produces H_3O^+ and OH^- ions in unequal concentrations.
   d. The ionization constant of water (Kw) is 1×10^{-7} at 25°C

184. What is the pH of a 0.01 M solution of HCl, a strong acid?

a. 1 b. 2

c. 3 d. 4

185. Which of the following describes the effect of adding a strong acid to water?

a. The pH of the solution will increase

b. The pH of the solution will decrease

c. The concentration of \(OH^-\) will increase

d. The solution will become more basic

186. Which of the following best describes hydrophobic interactions?

a. Attraction between polar molecules in the presence of water.

b. Repulsion between nonpolar molecules and water.

c. Attraction between nonpolar molecules in an aqueous environment.

d. Attraction between charged molecules in the presence of water.

187. Electrostatic interactions between two molecules in water are typically weaker than in a vacuum. What is the primary reason for this difference?

a. Water decreases the distance between charged molecules.

b. Water forms hydrogen bonds with charged molecules, weakening their interactions.

c. The high dielectric constant of water reduces the strength of electrostatic interactions.

d. Water's polarity strengthens electrostatic interactions.

188. Van der Waals forces are crucial for molecular interactions. Which of the following best describes the origin of van der Waals forces?

a. Permanent dipole-dipole attractions between polar molecules.

b. Temporary dipole interactions due to fluctuations in electron distribution.

c. Ionic interactions between charged molecules.

d. Hydrogen bonding between water molecules.

189. How do hydrophobic interactions contribute to the stability of a protein's tertiary structure in an aqueous environment?

a. They increase the solubility of the protein in water.

b. They cause hydrophobic side chains to be exposed to the water.

c. They cause hydrophobic side chains to cluster together inside the protein, away from water.

d. They cause hydrophilic side chains to cluster together inside the protein.

190. In water, why are van der Waals forces considered weaker than in nonpolar solvents?

a. Water's polarity disrupts temporary dipoles.

b. Water forms strong hydrogen bonds that overshadow van der Waals forces.

c. Van der Waals forces are dependent on the presence of ions.

d. Water decreases the distance between interacting molecules, reducing van der Waals forces.

191. Which type of interaction is most likely responsible for the aggregation of nonpolar molecules in an aqueous solution?
   a. Hydrogen bonding.
   b. Electrostatic interactions.
   c. Van der Waals forces.
   d. Hydrophobic interactions.

192. Why is water considered a good nucleophile?
   a. It is highly polar
   b. It has a lone pair of electrons on oxygen
   c. It can easily donate protons
   d. It is amphoteric in nature

193. Which of the following reactions demonstrates the nucleophilicity of water?
   a. The hydrolysis of esters to form carboxylic acids and alcohols
   b. The neutralization of an acid by a base
   c. The formation of a hydrogen bond between water molecules
   d. The dissociation of water into H^+ and OH^-

194. In a nucleophilic substitution reaction, water acts as a nucleophile to attack an electrophile. What role does the oxygen atom in water play in this reaction?
   a. It donates a proton to the electrophile.
   b. It accepts a proton from the electrophile.
   c. It donates a pair of electrons to form a new bond with the electrophile.
   d. It breaks an existing bond in the electrophile.

195. Which of the following factors contributes to water being a better nucleophile in polar protic solvents?
   a. The high dielectric constant of water.
   b. Hydrogen bonding that stabilizes the nucleophile.
   c. Solvent polarity that decreases the nucleophilicity.
   d. The ability of water to act as both a nucleophile and an electrophile.

196. Water is generally a weaker nucleophile compared to other species like hydroxide ion (OH^-). Why is this the case?
   a. Water has fewer lone pairs of electrons compared to OH^-.
   b. Water is less polar than OH^-.
   c. Water is neutral, while OH^- carries a negative charge.
   d. Water is less basic than OH^-.

197. Which of the following best describes the Henderson-Hasselbalch equation?
   a. $pH = pKa + \log\left(\dfrac{\text{[base]}}{\text{[acid]}}\right)$
   b. $pH = pKa - \log\left(\dfrac{\text{[acid]}}{\text{[base]}}\right)$
   c. $pH = pKa + \log\left(\dfrac{\text{[acid]}}{\text{[base]}}\right)$
   d. $pH = pKa - \log\left(\dfrac{\text{[base]}}{\text{[acid]}}\right)$

198. What is the primary application of the Henderson-Hasselbalch equation?
   a. To calculate the pH of a strong acid or base solution.
   b. To determine the pH of a buffer solution.
   c. To find the molarity of a solution.
   d. To predict the solubility of a compound

199. If the concentration of the conjugate base \([A^-]\) is equal to the concentration of the weak acid \([HA]\), what is the pH of the solution relative to the pKa?
   a. pH = pKa + 1 b. pH = pKa - 1
   c. pH = pKa d. pH = 2 × pKa

200. Which of the following changes would increase the pH of a buffer solution containing a weak acid and its conjugate base?
   a. Adding more of the weak acid
   b. Adding more of the conjugate base
   c. Diluting the solution with water
   d. Adding a strong acid

201. Bond angle of H – O – H bond in water molecules
   a. 90° b. 120°
   c. 180° d. 104.5°

202. Intermolecular association between 2 water molecules
   a. Covalent bond b. Ionic bond
   c. Hydrogen bond d. Vander Waals force

203. Each water molecule is surrounded by ________ nearest water molecules
   a. 4 b. 6
   c. 3 d. 2

204. Nature of bond between oxygen and hydrogen in water molecule
   a. Ionic b. Non polar covalent
   c. Polar covalent d. Metallic

205. Density of liquid water is
   a. 1.00g/ml b. 10.0 g/ml
   c. 0.92 g/ml d. 9.2 g/ml

206. Density of ice is
   a. 9.2 g/ml b. 0.92 g/ ml
   c. 9.2 mg/ml d. 0.92 mg/ml

207. Freezing temperature of water
   a. 0°C b. 4°C
   c. -4°C d. -10°C

208. Water ________ on freezing
   a. Contract b. Constrict
   c. No changes d. Expand

209. Intermolecular distance between liquid water
   a. 4.2 Å b. 3.5 Å
   c. 2.4 Å d. 5.3 Å
210. Heat of sublimation of ice at 0°C
   a. 46.9 kJ/mol b. 26.9 kJ/mol
   c. 36.9 kJ/mol d. 56.9 kJ/mol
211. Heat of fusion of ice
   a. 8 kJ/mol b. 4 kJ/mol
   c. 2 kJ/mol d. 6 kJ/mol
212. Physical properties of Ice and liquid water largely result from
   a. Non polar covalent bonding b. Ionic bonding
   c. Polar covalent bonding d. Intermolecular H bonding
213. Energy of hydrogen bond in water
   a. 46.5 kJ/mol b. 40 kJ/mol
   c. 20 kJ/mol d. 26.5 kJ/mol
214. Energy of covalent bond
   a. 46 kJ/mol b. 460 kJ/mol
   c. 4.6 kJ/mol d. 40. kJ/mol
215. ________ has a rapidly fluctuating structure
   a. Ice b. Water at -20° C
   c. Liquid water d. All are same
216. O-H bond distance of water molecule
   a. 9.58 Å b. 0.958 Å
   c. 104.5 Å d. 120 Å
217. Polar and ionic material which are soluble in water
   a. Hydrophobic b. Hydrophilic
   c. Aerophobic d. Aaerophilic
218. Non polar substances which are virtually insoluble in water
   a. Aerophobic b. Hydrophilic
   c. Hydrophobic d. Aerophilic
219. What is the measure of solvent's ability to keep opposite charges apart
   a. Dielectric constant b. Faraday's constant
   c. Rydberg constant d. Planks constant
220. Dielectric constant of water
   a. 65.4 b. 78.5
   c. 85.4 d. 94.8

221. Solubility depends on
   a. Interaction between solute particles
   b. Interaction between solvent particles
   c. Interaction between solvent and solute particles
   d. None of the above
222. As the dielectric constant of medium increases force Between it's embedded charges _________
   a. Increases
   b. Decreases
   c. Remain same
   d. Vary according to medium
223. In the absence of intermolecular association, substances with equal molecular masses have ________ boiling point
   a. Different
   b. Depends on substances
   c. Similar
   d. None
224. Non polar substances dissolve in
   a. Polar solvents
   b. Non polar solvents
   c. Both
   d. None
225. Which of the following is true about density of water?
   a. Ice floats on water because it is less dense
   b. Ice is denser than liquid water
   c. Liquid water is most dense at 0°C
   d. Water is least dense at 4°C
226. Which of the following best describes the molecular geometry of a water molecule?
   a. Linear with a bond angle of 180°
   b. Bent with a bond angle of 104.5°
   c. Trigonal planar with a bond angle of 120°
   d. Tetrahedral with a bond angle of 109.5°
227. What percentage of ionic character is present in the O-H bond of a water molecule?
   a. 50%
   b. 25%
   c. 33%
   d. 75%
228. Which property of water is primarily responsible for its high internal cohesiveness?
   a. High dipole moment
   b. Bent molecular geometry
   c. Low electronegativity difference between H and O
   d. van der Waals forces
229. The dipole moment of water is an indicator of its:
   a. Ability to dissolve non polar substances
   b. Polar nature
   c. Weak internal cohesiveness
   d. Tendency to form non-polar bonds

230. Which of the following statements about water is true?
   a. Water has a linear molecular structure.
   b. Water's physical properties are similar to most other solvents.
   c. Water has a van der Waals radius of 1.44 Å for oxygen.
   d. Water's ability to form hydrogen bonds is not significant for biological processes.
231. What type of bond is primarily responsible for the association between water molecules?
   a. Covalent bond
   b. Ionic bond
   c. Hydrogen bond
   d. van der Waals bond
232. Which of the following best explains why hydrogen atoms are crucial in forming hydrogen bonds?
   a. Their large size allows for close approach to other atoms.
   b. They are highly electronegative.
   c. They carry a partial positive charge and are small, allowing them to approach lone pair electrons closely.
   d. They are highly reactive.
233. What is the approximate energy of a hydrogen bond between water molecules?
   a. 460 kJ/mol
   b. 20 kJ/mol
   c. 10 kJ/mol
   d. 5 kJ/mol
234. Why does ice float on water?
   a. Ice is denser than liquid water.
   b. Ice has a more open structure due to hydrogen bonding, making it less dense than liquid water.
   c. Ice is a different compound than liquid water.
   d. Water expands when it freezes, causing it to sink.
235. What would be the consequence if water contracted upon freezing instead of expanding?
   a. Ice would still float on water, but at a lower level.
   b. Water would boil at a higher temperature.
   c. Oceans and lakes would freeze solid from the bottom up, leading to a permanent ice age on Earth.
   d. The density of water would decrease at 4°C
236. What percentage of hydrogen bonds are estimated to be disrupted in liquid water at 0°C compared to ice?
   a. 5%
   b. 10%
   c. 15%
   d. 25%

237. Why does water have a much higher boiling point than methane (CH_4), despite having nearly the same molecular mass?
   a. Water molecules are larger.
   b. Water molecules form hydrogen bonds, leading to higher internal cohesiveness.
   c. Methane has a stronger molecular structure.
   d. Methane forms more hydrogen bonds than water.

238. Which of the following best describes the structure of liquid water?
   a. It is a stable and rigid tetrahedral structure similar to ice.
   b. It is a rapidly fluctuating, irregular network of hydrogen-bonded molecules.
   c. It consists of separate, non-interacting water molecules.
   d. It has a linear molecular structure due to strong covalent bonds.

239. What is the role of the dielectric constant in the solubility of salts in water?
   a. A higher dielectric constant increases the force between ions, making salts less soluble.
   b. A higher dielectric constant decreases the force between ions, making salts more soluble.
   c. The dielectric constant has no effect on solubility.
   d. The dielectric constant decreases in water, making it a poor solvent for salts.

240. Why are polar substances generally soluble in water?
   a. Water can form hydrogen bonds with nonpolar substances.
   b. Water's polar nature allows it to interact more strongly with polar and ionic materials than they do with each other.
   c. Polar substances can only dissolve in nonpolar solvents.
   d. Water's low dielectric constant makes it ideal for dissolving polar substances.

241. Which definition of acids and bases does not account for ammonia (NH_3) having basic properties?
   a. Arrhenius definition
   b. Bronsted-Lowry definition
   c. Lewis definition
   d. None of the above

242. In the Bronsted-Lowry definition of acid-base reactions, what does a Bronsted acid do?
   a. Accepts a proton
   b. Donates a proton
   c. Accepts an electron pair
   d. Donates an electron pair

243. Which of the following represents the conjugate base in the acid dissociation reaction of acetic acid (CH_3COOH)?
   a. H_3O^-
   b. OH^-
   c. CH_3COO^-
   d. NH_4^+

244. What does the dissociation constant (K_a) of an acid measure?
   a. The relative concentration of the acid in solution
   b. The strength of the base in the reaction
   c. The relative proton affinities of the acid and its conjugate base
   d. The pH of the solution

245. What is the mechanism that accounts for the anomalously high ionic mobility of the H_3O^+ ion in water?

a. Direct physical migration of the ion b. Proton-jump mechanism

c. Electron-pair donation d. Ionic dissociation

246. What is the value of the ion product constant for water (K_e) at 25°C?

a. 10^{-14} M^2 b. 10^{-15} M^2

c. 10^{-13} M^2 d. 10^{-12} M^2

247. If the concentration of [H^+] in a solution is 10^{-15} M, what is the pH of the solution?

a. 5 b. 7

c. 9 d. 10

248. According to the Henderson-Hasselbalch equation, what happens to the pH of a solution when the concentrations of an acid (HA and its conjugate base (A^-) are equal?

a. The pH is equal to the pK_a of the acid

b. The pH is equal to the pH of pure water.

c. The pH is zero.

d. The pH is equal to the concentration of the acid

249. What is the purpose of a buffer solution?

a. To drastically change the pH of a solution.

b. To maintain the pH of a solution relatively constant despite the addition of acids or bases.

c. To neutralize strong acids and bases completely.

d. To alter the concentration of hydrogen ions.

250. In a titration curve of acetic acid with a strong base, where is the pH approximately equal to the pK_a of the acetic acid?

a. At the beginning of the titration

b. At the midpoint of the titration

c. At the end point of the titration

d. At the equivalence point of the titration

251. Water content in the living cell,

a. 80% b. 70%

c. 90% d. 60%

252. The H-O-H bond angle of water molecule is

a. 104.5° b. 103.4°

c. 100.5° d. 102.4°

253. The polarity in water molecule is due to

a. Bond angle

b. Electronegativity difference of H and O

c. Free electron pairs on O

d. None

254. Intermolecular bond present in H2O (liquid).

a. Van der walls
b. Hydrogen bond
c. Covalent bond
d. Ionic bond

255. The density of H2O at O°C is

a. 1g/ml
b. 3g/ml
c. 4 g/ml
d. 2 g/ml

256. Acid generates _____ in aqueous solution.

a. Electron
b. H-
c. Proton
d. OH +

257. The substance which function both as acid and base

a. Ampholyte
b. Electrolyte
c. Neucleophile
d. Conjugate

258. PH is

a. Log[OH-]
b. Log[H+]
c. -Log[OH-]
d. -Log[H+]

259. Range of PH scale is

a. 0-7
b. 0-14
c. -7 to 7
d. -14 to 14

260. PH of pure H2O

a. 7.0
b. 14.0
c. 6.8
d. 7.2

261. If [H+] of a solution increase,

a. PH increase
b. PH decrease
c. PH remains constant
d. Increase followed by decrease

262. Normal PH of blood

a. 7.4
b. 7.2
c. 6.8
d. 7.0

263. Normal PH of urine

a. 5.0-7.5
b. 5.0-5.5
c. 5.0-6.0
d. 5.0-6.5

264. The solution which resist the change in PH by the addition of small amount of acid or base.

a. Acidic solution
b. Basic solution
c. Concentration
d. Buffer

265. Particle size of solute in solution is

a. <1 nm
b. 1 nm
c. 2 nm
d. >2 nm

266. No. of moles of solute per litre of solution is

a. Molality
b. Molarity
c. Normality
d. Polarity

267. Father of colloidal chemistry
   a. Thomas Graham b. Ernst Heckel
   c. Rudolf virchow d. T. H Morgan
268. Partical size of colloidal state
   a. 2-100 nm b. 1-100nm
   c. 5-20nm d. 10-100 nm
269. Lyophobic means
   a. Solvent hating b. Solvent loving
   c. Water loving d. Water hating
270. Emulsifying agent of milk is
   a. Streptokinase b. Kinase
   c. Casein d. Rennin
271. Aggregates of colloidal particles are known as
   a. Micelles b. Conjugation
   c. Emulsion d. Solution
272. Which of the following is not a property of a colloidal solution.
   a. Brownian movement b. Optical property
   c. Electrical property d. Electronegativity
273. Scattering of light is when passed through colloidal solution is known as
   a. Brownian effect b. Tyndall affect
   c. Placebo effect d. None
274. The movement of solute molecules from a higher concentration to lower concentration is known as
   a. Diffusion b. Osmosis
   c. Dialysis d. Transport
275. The rate of diffusion increases when
   a. Temperature ↑ b. Temperature ↓
   c. Remains same d. None.
276. ________ is the movement of solvent through semipermeable membrane.
   a. Diffusion b. Osmosis
   c. Pinocytosis d. None
277. Osmosis is a _____ property of solute particles.
   a. Colligative b. Qualitative
   c. Both A & B d. None
278. The solutions that exert the same osmotic pressure are called as.
   a. Isoosmotic b. Hypoosmotic
   c. Isotonic d. Hypotonic
279. _______ term used to represent the osmotic pressure of colloidal substances
   a. Hydrostatic b. Hypertonic
   c. Oncotic pressure d. None

280. What is the osmotic pressure of plasma (milliosmoles per litre).

a. 280-300 b. 300-400

c. 500-550 d. 1000-2000

281. What is the unit of osmotic pressure.

a. Osmole b. Pascal

c. Barr d. None

282. What happened if RBC are kept in hypotonic solution (0.4%NaCl)

a. Bulging of RBC b. Shrinkage of RBC

c. Normal RBC d. Both A & B

283. What is the name of phenomenon if water flows out of RBC and cytoplasm shrinks.

a. Crenation b. Red tide

c. Chloride shift d. None

284. The mechanism of action of purgatives is mainly due to_______.

a. Red tide phenomenon b. Osmotic phenomenon

c. Both A &B d. None

285. What type of concentration solutions of salts are use to reduce the pressure of cerebrospinal fluid.

a. Isotonic solutions b. Hypotonic solutions

c. Hypertonic solutions d. All of above

286. What is the application of Donnan membrane equilibrium concept.

a. Membrane hydrolysis b. Lower pH of RBC

c. Osmotic imbalance d. All of above

287. Osmotic pressure of biological fluids is frequently expressed as_____

a. Milliosmoles b. Osmole

c. Pascal d. None

288. Unit of viscosity ______

a. Dyne b. Both c & d

c. Poise d. Dynes/cm^2

289. ________ defined as the internal resistance by a liquid or gas to flow.

a. Osmosis b. Tension

c. Viscosity d Both a & c

290. The property of viscosity is due to ___________

a. Gravitational force b. Frictional force

c. Centrifugal force d. None

291. What is the viscosity of blood

a. Lower than water b. More than water

c. Equal to water d. 4 times more than water

292. The term viscosity applied for ____

a. Liquid b. Gas

c. Solid d. Both a & b

293. Which of the following has highest viscosity
   a. Saturated salt solution b. 0.9% Nacl solution
   c. Clean water d. Colloidal solutions

294. What is the effect of excitation of muscles on the viscosity of muscle fibres
   a. Increase b. Decrease
   c. No effect d. Both a & b

295. Blood viscosity is increased in_______
   a. Polycythemia b. Anemia
   c. Nephritis d. None

296. What is the effect of dehydration on viscosity of blood.
   a. Increase b. Decrease
   c. No effect d. None of above

297. As the blood flows through capillaries the viscosity __________ to facilitate free flow of blood.
   a. Increase b. Decrease
   c. Remains constant d. None of above

298. Vitreous body rich in ________
   a. Globulin and glutamic acid b. Albumin and hyaluronic acid
   c. Alanine and aspartic acid d. Both b & c

299. Non diffusible anion in Donnan membrane equilibrium is mostly _______.
   a. Carbohydrates b. Proteins
   c. Fatty acids d. Both a & c

300. For checking the fragility of RBC _____ is done in laboratory.
   a. Haemocytometry b. Osmotic fragility test
   c. Viscosity test d. None

Answer Key

1	c	2	c	3	a	4	a	5	b	6	a	7	d
8	b	9	a	10	c	11	c	12	b	13	d	14	a
15	b	16	c	17	a	18	d	19	b	20	a	21	c
22	d	23	d	24	b	25	a	26	d	27	c	28	a
29	b	30	c	31	b	32	d	33	a	34	a	35	c
36	b	37	b	38	a	39	a	40	b	41	d	42	d
43	d	44	c	45	a	46	b	47	d	48	c	49	b
50	c	51	a	52	c	53	a	54	d	55	d	56	a
57	b	58	c	59	d	60	a	61	b	62	c	63	b
64	c	65	c	66	d	67	c	68	d	69	a	70	d
71	a	72	a	73	c	74	a	75	a	76	a	77	c
78	d	79	a	80	a	81	a	82	d	83	b	84	a

85	b	86	a	87	b	88	a	89	b	90	c	91	d
92	b	93	b	94	b	95	b	96	c	97	b	98	c
99	a	100	b	101	b	102	a	103	d	104	c	105	d
106	b	107	a	108	c	109	a	110	c	111	b	112	c
113	c	114	a	115	d	116	b	117	c	118	a	119	c
120	c	121	a	122	b	123	a	124	c	125	a	126	b
127	c	128	b	129	b	130	c	131	d	132	c	133	b
134	b	135	b	136	d	137	a	138	c	139	c	140	c
141	d	142	a	143	c	144	b	145	a	146	c	147	d
148	c	149	d	150	b	151	a	152	b	153	a	154	b
155	b	156	d	157	b	158	d	159	d	160	c	161	b
162	a	163	c	164	a	165	b	166	c	167	c	168	b
169	d	170	b	171	c	172	a	173	c	174	b	175	c
176	c	177	a	178	a	179	b	180	a	181	b	182	b
183	a	184	b	185	b	186	c	187	c	188	b	189	c
190	b	191	d	192	b	193	a	194	c	195	a	196	c
197	a	198	b	199	c	200	b	201	d	202	c	203	a
204	c	205	a	206	b	207	a	208	d	209	b	210	a
211	d	212	d	213	c	214	b	215	c	216	b	217	b
218	c	219	a	220	b	221	c	222	b	223	c	224	b
225	a	226	b	227	c	228	a	229	b	230	c	231	c
232	d	233	b	234	b	235	c	236	c	237	b	238	b
239	b	240	b	241	a	242	b	243	c	244	c	245	b
246	a	247	a	248	a	249	b	250	b	251	b	252	a
253	b	254	b	255	a	256	c	257	a	258	c	259	b
260	a	261	b	262	a	263	a	264	d	265	a	266	b
267	a	268	b	269	a	270	c	271	a	272	d	273	b
274	a	275	a	276	b	277	a	278	a	279	c	280	a
281	a	282	a	283	a	284	b	285	c	286	d	287	a
288	b	289	c	290	b	291	d	292	d	293	d	294	a
295	a	296	a	297	b	298	b	299	b	300	b		

3

Cellular Structure and Function

Ramesh D.[1] and Barkha Gupta[2]

[1]*Department of Veterinary Physiology and Biochemistry, Veterinary College, Hassan (KVAFSU), Karnataka-573202*

[2]*Department of Veterinary Physiology and Biochemistry, Post Graduate Institute of Veterinary Education and Research (PGIVER), Jaipur (RAJUVAS), Rajasthan-302031*

Introduction

The smallest, most basic, most primitive organisms are known as prokaryotic (Greek: pro= primitive or prior, and karyon = nucleus). Likely, they originated around 3.5 billion years ago. Bacteria, such as Mycoplasma and Cyanobacteria, are known to contain these cells. A prokaryotic cell is a deeply organized single-enveloped system. Its constituent nuclear parts are encased in a plasma membrane, with the cytoplasmic ground substance encircling the center. Prokaryotic cells' cytoplasm lacks distinct cytoplasmic organelles, the nuclear envelope, and any other cytoplasmic membrane.

Despite being incredibly thin and delicate structures, in Eukaryotes plasma membranes are essential to many of a cell's most vital processes. Membranes are lipid-protein assemblages where non-covalent linkages hold the constituents in place in a thin sheet. Both integral protein and phospholipid lateral mobility are significantly impacted by the physical condition of the lipid bilayer. The plasma membrane is a selectively permeable barrier that permits solute passage via assisted diffusion, active transport, and simple diffusion via membrane channels or the lipid bilayer. A system of membrane organelles, such as the endoplasmic reticulum, Golgi complex, and lysosomes, is found in the cytoplasm of eukaryotic cells. These organelles are physically and functionally connected to the plasma membrane and one another. The cytoplasm is separated into a luminal region inside the ER membranes and a cytosolic space outside the membranes by the endoplasmic reticulum (ER), a network of tubules, cisternae, and vesicles. Additionally, the ER is where the majority of a cell's membrane lipids are generated and transported to different locations. Proteins' asparagine residues are added with sugars (a process known as glycosylation), which starts in the rough ER and continues in the Golgi complex. Before the cargo and membrane components created in the ER are sent to their final location, the Golgi complex acts as a processing plant. The complex polysaccharides that comprise the matrix of the plant cell wall are likewise synthesized at the Golgi complex. Specific proteins in the membrane of vesicles that bud from donor compartments are able to identify proteins in the target (acceptor) com. Membrane-bound, lysosomes are diverse-looking organelles with a wide range of acid hydrolases that can break down almost any kind of biological macromolecule. Endocytosis plays a crucial role in the recycling of membrane between the cytoplasm and cell surface, as well as in the uptake of fluid and suspended macromolecules and the internalization of membrane receptors and their attached ligands. The uptake of particulate materials is known as phagocytosis.

Nuclear genes encoding proteins found in peroxisomes, mitochondria, or chloroplasts need to be transported into the organelle through post-translation. Three different types of fibrous structures make up the cytoskeleton: microtubules, intermediate filaments, and microfilaments, or actin filaments. These structures are involved in a variety of cellular processes. Together with the cytoskeleton, microtubules—hollow, tubular structures 25 nm in diameter—are composed of the protein tubulin. They are a component of the mitotic spindle, centrioles, and the center of cilia and flagella. It has been possible to identify and characterize three groups of motor proteins: myosin, which moves along microfilaments, kinesins and dyneins, which move along microtubules. Materials are often moved along microtubules in opposite directions by cytoplasmic dynein and kinesins. Numerous MTOCs (microtubule organizing centers) are involved in the nucleation of microtubules in vivo.

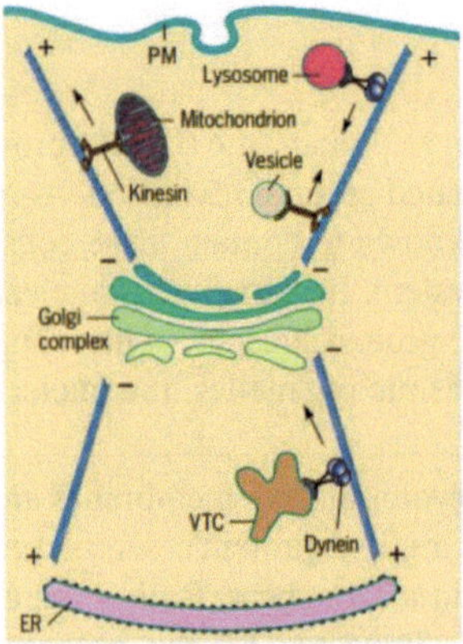

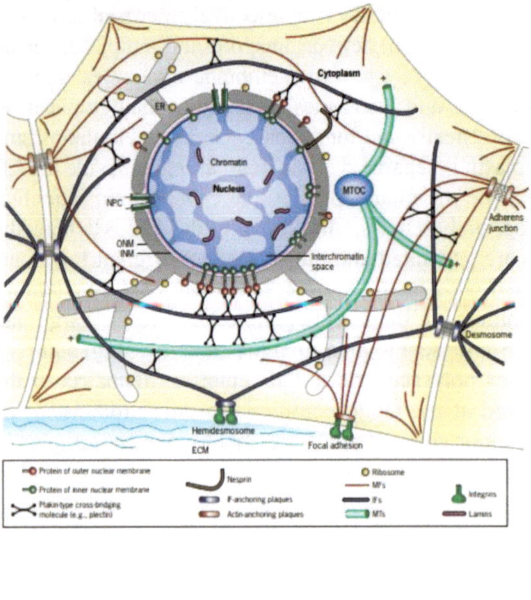

The axoneme, the central component of flagella and cilia, comprises a variety of microtubules that support the organelle as it protrudes from the cell surface and supplies the machinery needed to produce the forces needed for movement. Depending on the kind of cell, intermediate filaments (IFs) are rope-like cytoskeletal structures with a diameter of around 10 nm. They can be made of a range of different protein subunits that can assemble into filaments that resemble one another. Actin filaments, also known as microfilaments, are 8 nm in diameter and are made of the protein actin in a double-helical polymer. They are essential for almost all forms of cellular movement and contractility. Actin filament assembly or, more frequently, interaction with the motor protein myosin can produce forces that are responsible for microfilament-dependent activities. Forces produced in the myosin cross-bridges that stretch outward from the thick filaments drive the sliding of actin-containing thin filaments toward the center of each myofibril's sarcomere, which causes a skeletal muscle fiber to contract. Some of the same proteins that are present in muscle cells are also involved in non-muscle motility and contractility. Although, they are arrayed in less predictable, more labile, and transitory configurations. Cells crawling over a substratum and axonal extension are two examples of non-muscle motility and contractility.

1. The longitudinal rows of globular proteins that make up a microtubule's wall are known as

   a. Actin filaments b. Protofilaments

   c. Microtubules d. None

2. Usually, extra proteins are present in microtubules made from living tissue. These proteins are known as

   a. Kinase proteins

   b. Myosin proteins

   c. Microtubule-Associated Proteins-MAPs

   d. Cyclins

3. Name the protein that holds two sister chromatids

   a. Dyenins b. Cohesin

   c. Myoglo b. Indactin

4. Intracellular Motility was assisted by

   a. Microtubules b. Myoglobin

   c. Hemoglobin d. None

5. What kind of biological cargo are the cytoskeletal proteins responsible for transporting?

   a. Ribo nucleo-protein particles b. Vesicles

   c. Chromosomes d. All of these

6. A motor protein that used microtubules as its track was identified by Ronald Vale and colleagues from the cytoplasm of giant squid axons is called

   a. Dyenins b. Actin

   c. Kinesins d. Myosin

7. Imaging unstained tissues and living cells to provide contrast between variations in the thickness and refractive index of biological components is known as
   a. Phase-contrast microscopy b. Light microscopy
   c. Fluorescent microscopy d. Microscopy
8. Which of the following statement about kinesins is true
   a. Kinesins are not protein
   b. Kinesin is a tetramer constructed from two identical heavy chains and two identical light chains
   c. Kinesin is a Pentamer constructed from two identical heavy chains and two identical light chains
   d. Kinesin is a Dimer constructed from two identical heavy chains and two identical light chains
9. The Resolution of the Light Microscope is About
   a. 0.9 μm b. 0.1 μm
   c. 1.5 μm d. 0.2 μm
10. The first identified motor protein associated with microtubules that drives the motion of cilia and flagella is known as
   a. Dynein b. Actin
   c. Myosin d. Tubulin
11. Which cellular organelles in Eukaryotes are thought to have developed from symbiotic bacteria?
   a. Mitochondria and chloroplast b. Golgi complex
   c. Endoplasmic reticulum d. Lysosome
12. Which of the following does not describe a cell's cytoskeleton's function?
   a. Transport within cells
   b. Preservation of cell morphology and architecture
   c. Movement of cells
   d. Organelle support
13. Which of the following dyes works best for chromosomal staining?
   a. Basic Fuchsin b. Carmine
   c. Methylene blue d. Safranin
14. Within a cell, microtubule nucleation happens quickly and is associated with a range of specialized structures known as
   a. Myosin centers
   b. Actin centers
   c. Microtubule organizing centers (MTOCs)
   d. Titin
15. The term for tiny molecules that start and manage intracellular signaling pathways is
   a. Agonist b. Second messengers
   c. Primary messengers d. Antagonist

16. Ribosomes were first discovered by
    a. Claude in 1945 b. Palade in 1955
    c. Menton in 1970 d. Claude in 1965
17. Which of them was the first to identify the Golgi complex?
    a. Liver Cell b. Nerve cell
    c. Kidney cell d. Skeletal muscle cell
18. The microtubules of a structure, which is located at the base of a cilium or flagellum, give rise to the outer microtubules of that structure called
    a. Cytoplasm b. Basal body
    c. Lysosome d. Cell projections
19. In animal cells, the microtubules of the cytoskeleton are typically nucleated by
    a. Centrioles b. Nucleosome
    c. Spindle fibers d. Centrosome
20. What kind of changes are necessary for mRNA in eukaryotes to produce mature mRNA
    a. RNA splicing b. RNA degradation
    c. RNA duplex formation d. RNA Cyclization
21. The endoplasmic reticulum arises from
    a. Golgi complex b. Lysosome
    c. Chloroplast d. Pre-existing reticulum
22. Golgi complex plays a major role in the following function in the cell
    a. Lipid and protein glycosylation
    b. Protein synthesis
    c. Sulfur is eliminated from the glycolipids' carbohydrate moiety
    d. Secondary lysosome formation
23. Which of the following is the best-studied cytoskeletal microtubule organizing centers in animal cells is
    a. Nucleosome b. Actin
    c. Desmosome d. Centrosome
24. Identify the organelle that breaks down proteins, carbohydrates, lipids, and nucleic acids and has a high concentration of hydrolases.
    a. Mitochondria b. Cell membrane
    c. Golgi complex d. Lysosomes
25. There is no Golgi apparatus in
    a. Eukaryotes b. Yeast
    c. Bacteria and Blue-green algae d. None
26. The type of plastid that stores starch is called
    a. Leucoplast b. Aleuroplast
    c. Amyloplast d. Elaioplast

27. Cristae represent
    a. The inner membrane of chloroplast
    b. The outer membrane of mitochondria
    c. The inner membrane of mitochondria
    d. The outer membrane of chloroplast
28. What keeps DNA apart from the cytoplasmic protein translation machinery in a eukaryotic cell?
    a. Nuclear envelope b. Lysosome
    c. Mitochondria d. Endoplasmic reticulum
29. Ribosomes are present in
    a. Mitochondria b. Chloroplast
    c. Endoplasmic reticulum d. All of the above
30. Which kinds of proteins are involved in the condensing and packaging of DNA into a chromosome's tightly wrapped nucleosome structures?
    a. Actin b. Histones
    c. Hemoglobin d. Myosin
31. The stain used to visualize mitochondria is
    a. Janus green b. Safranin
    c. Acetocarmine d. Fast green
32. Which of the following claims about the plasma membrane is untrue
    a. It is found in both plant and animal cells
    b. It never contains carbohydrates
    c. Lipid is present in it in the form of a bilayer
    d. Proteins are present in it both integrated and loosely connected with the lipid bilayer; and
33. Golgi bodies in cells arise from
    a. Endoplasmic reticulum b. Nuclear membrane
    c. Plasma membrane d. None
34. Is an organelle that acts as the main location for molecules to be packaged before they are disseminated throughout the cell.
    a. Mitochondria b. Chloroplast
    c. Golgi apparatus d. Lysosome
35. The chloroplast thylakoids are in the form of
    a. Interconnected tubule b. Stacked discs
    c. Interconnected sacs d. Independent discs
36. What occupies 70% of the space inside cells?
    a. Water b. O_2
    c. NH_3 d. CO_2

37. The Golgi apparatus's closed, saucer-shaped compartments, the most basic unit, are referred to as

a. Vesicles b. Tubules

c. Cisternae d. Cristae

38. The motile, hair-like organelles that protrude from the surface of different eukaryotic cells are known as

a. Cilia and flagella b. Cytoplasmic structure

c. Cristae d. Cisternae

39. The Golgi apparatus's functions in animal cells include

a. Sorting and packing b. Thyroxine hormone exocytosis

c. Melanin granule exocytosis d. All of these

40. An array of microtubules that runs longitudinally through the entire organelle is found in the cilium's core, which is known as

a. Axoneme b. Sarcolemma

c. Sarcomere d. Vacuole

41. Cytoskeletal proteins that appear as solid, unbranched filaments with a diameter of 10–12 nm under an electron microscope is called

a. Myoglobin b. Tubulin

c. Intermediate filaments d. Titin

42. The monomeric form of actin is called

a. G-actin (globular actin) b. F-actin

c. N-actin d. Z-actin

43. The crucial roles of the cytoskeleton are

a. It gives the cell guidance and structure

b. It facilitates the development of vacuoles

c. It secures several cell organelles in position

d. All of these

44. Which of the following explains the muscle contraction

a. Fluid Mosaic Theory b. Induced Fit Theory

c. Sliding Filament Theory d. Concerted Model

45. The smooth ER is involved in which of the following function

a. Synthesis of lipids b. Synthesis of cholesterol

c. Synthesis of phospholipids d. All of these

46. The point at which an axon's terminus comes into contact with a muscle fiber is known as

a. Tight junction b. Desmosome

c. Neural junction d. Neuromuscular Junction

47. A cavity that is fluid-filled, membrane-lined, and devoid of cytoplasm inside a cell is called

a. Vacuole b. Golgi complex

c. Endoplasmic reticulum d. Nucleus

48. Components of the Electron transport chain proteins are arranged on the inner mitochondrial membrane based on
    a. Increasing Size
    b. Decreasing Size
    c. Decreasing redox potential
    d. Increasing redox potential
49. During muscle contraction which of the following evident
    a. Shortening of sarcomere
    b. Shortening of size
    c. Shortening of shape
    d. None
50. Muscle cells are encircled by a network of specialized tubules and cisterns that store and release calcium ions is called
    a. Endoplasmic reticulum
    b. Sarcoplasmic reticulum
    c. Golgi complex
    d. Lysosome
51. Significant functions of the Vacuole include
    a. Discharge of extra water
    b. Storage, intake of water
    c. Digestion, excretion of extra water
    d. All of these
52. Characteristic features of sarcomere include
    a. It contains several dark bands and light zones
    b. Each sarcomere extends from one Z line to the next Z line
    c. Both a & b
    d. Sarcomere present in the liver
53. Which of the following is considered as the molecular motor of the actin filament
    a. Myoglobin
    b. Titin
    c. Myosin
    d. Hemoglobin
54. How many tubulin molecules join together to form a single tube
    a. 13
    b. 20
    c. 24
    d. 15
55. Actin-binding proteins include
    a. Nucleating protein
    b. Monomer-sequestering proteins
    c. End-blocking (capping) proteins
    d. All of these
56. Spindle fiber joined to the chromosome through a procedure called
    a. Congression
    b. Search and capture
    c. Binding
    d. Alignment
57. Which cells do not have centrosomes and astral microtubules at their poles during cell division?
    a. Plant cells
    b. Kidney cells
    c. Liver cells
    d. Skin cells
58. A process by which a cell uses to get rid of outdated organelles and broken-down cell components
    a. Cytokinesis
    b. Auto-phagocytosis
    c. Cytorhexis
    d. None

59. Which of the following is an example of Type-IV intermediate filaments
    a. Neurofilaments
    b. Nestin
    c. both a & b
    d. Vimentin
60. Microtubules are made up of monomeric proteins called
    a. Actin
    b. Tubulin
    c. Myosin
    d. Myoglobin
61. What is congression
    a. The microtubule's attachment to the chromosomes
    b. The midpoint between the two spindle poles
    c. The spindle pole's terminal
    d. The attachment of the two sister chromatids
62. Which of these proteins causes the microtubules to depolymerize?
    a. CENP-E
    b. Actin
    c. Dynein
    d. Kin I kinesin
63. Thymosins are also called as
    a. G-actin
    b. F-actin
    c. N-actin
    d. Z-actin
64. What is the cycle duration of the M phase in hours?
    a. 3 hr.
    b. 1 hr.
    c. 5 hr.
    d. 8 hr.
65. Which of these triggers the activation of cyclin-dependent kinases?
    a Binding of Cyclins
    b. Tyrosine kinase-mediated phosphorylation
    c Cyclin and CDK-activating protein kinases binding
    d. Using CDK activating kinase to phosphorylate
66. Which of the following is an example of Type-III intermediate filaments
    a. Vimentin
    b. Desmin
    c. Peripherin
    d. All of these
67. Name the cyclin which takes part in the M phase
    a. Cyclin E
    b. Cyclin B
    c. Cyclin D
    d. Cyclin A
68. Which cytoskeletal protein polymerization directly behind the Listeria bacterium propels the bacteria through the cytoplasm of an infected cell like a rocket?
    a. Myosin Filament
    b. Intermediate Filament
    c. Actin filament
    d. Tubulin filament
69. The broad, flattened, veil-like protrusion of fibroblast cells responsible for the locomotion of cells is known as
    a. Cilia
    b. Antenna
    c. Flagella
    d. lamellipodium

70. Identify the enzyme responsible for cyclin's ubiquitylation and degradation.
    a. Hyaluronidase b. Ubiquitin ligase
    c. Phosphatase d. Acid hydrolases
71. Characteristics of Microtubules structure include
    a. Diameter of 24 nm b. Small and spherical
    c. Hallow tubes d. All of these
72. Major functions of Kinesins include
    a. They pull the organelles along the cell membrane
    b. They pull the organelles outside the cell membrane
    c. They pull the organelles toward the nucleus
    d. They pull the organelles toward Mitochondria
73. Cytoskeletal Motor proteins include
    a. Kinesin b. Dyneins
    c. Myosin d. All of these
74. Characteristics of Intermediate filaments include
    a. Provide mechanical strength to cells that are subjected to physical stress
    b. They are strong
    c. Flexible ropelike fibers
    d. All of these
75. Which of the following is an example of Type-I intermediate filaments?
    a. Collagen b. Elastin
    c. Keratin (acidic) d. Myoglobin
76. O-glycosylation of proteins occurs in which of the cell organelles
    a. Golgi complex b. Lysosome
    c. Mitochondria d. Peroxisome
77. Marker enzyme for Endoplasmic reticulum includes
    a. glucose-6-phosphatase b. NADPH cytochrome c reductase
    c. Both a & b d. Enolase
78. Which protein in the cytoskeleton is responsible for cytokinesis, contraction, and gliding in cells?
    a. Microfilaments b. Intermediate filament
    c. Myoglobin d. Tubulin
79. Major functions of Dyneins include
    a. Cell organelles are drawn toward Lysosome
    b. Cell organelles are drawn toward EPR
    c. Cell organelles are drawn toward the Golgi complex
    d. Cell organelles are drawn toward the nucleus
80. Marker enzyme for lysosomes is
    a. Acid phosphatase b. Glucosyl transferase
    c. Alanine transaminases d. DNA polymerase

81. N-glycosylation of proteins occurs in which of the cellular organelle
    a. Golgi complex   b. Endoplasmic reticulum
    c. Mitochondria   d. Nucleus
82. characteristic features of microfilaments include
    a. Composed of globular subunits of the protein actin
    b. Approximately 8 nm in diameter
    c. Microfilaments have polarity
    d. All of the above
83. Which of the following describes an organelle that is double membrane-bound?
    a. Nucleus   b. Mitochondria
    c. Chloroplast   d. All of these
84. Intermediate filaments are identified only in
    a. Plant cells   b. Animal cells
    c. Bacteria   d. Algae
85. Which actin monomers polymerize to create a pliable, helical thread when present?
    a. In the presence of ATP   b. In the presence of UTP
    c. In the presence of CTP   d. In the presence of GTP
86. What specific bicyclic peptide is utilized to stain Actin so that it may be seen fluorescently labeled under a light microscope?
    a. Phalloidin   b. Myosin
    c. Globulin   d. Titin
87. Which gene mutation causes desmin-related myopathy, a hereditary human disease?
    a. Mutation in the Desmin gene   b. Mutation in Keratin gene
    c. Mutation in Lamin gene   d. Mutation in Vimentin gene
88. A powerful cell-permeable and actin polymerization inhibitor is referred to as
    a. Vinblastine   b. Gentamicin
    c. Colchicine   d. Cytochalasin -D
89. Which of the following is an example of Type-V intermediate filaments
    a. Lamin protein   b. Keratin
    c. Vimentin   d. Desmin
90. Every myofibril is made up of a linear array of contractile units that repeats itself, known as
    a. Intermediate filaments   b. Sarcomere
    c. Cytokinesis   d. Sarcolemma
91. Which of the following describes the secretory proteins that guide the ribosome and emerging polypeptide to the ER membrane?
    a. N-terminal signal sequence   b. C-terminal signal sequence
    c. P-terminal signal sequence   d. All of these

92. The region of Nucleolus Organizing Region (NOR) is located in

a. Telomere
b. Centromere
c. Secondary constriction
d. Primary constriction

93. Which of the following is that cells store energy from oxidative processes for use later rather than utilizing it all at once?

a. FMN
b. ATP and NADH
c. Co-Q
d. Acetyl Co-A

94. The location within the mitochondria where, during aerobic respiration, pH is lowest

a. Matrix
b. Cytosol
c. Mitochondria ribosome
d. Intermembrane space

95. The nature of DNA molecules within mitochondria and chloroplast have

a. Only linear form
b. DNA having covalently sealed end
c. Linear dsDNA with single chain breaks
d. Covalently closed circular form

96. during rapid polymerization of the microtubule which is the energy source utilized

a. UTP
b. GTP
c. ATP
d. TTP

97. Which of the following about Intermediate filaments are true

a. Resistant to tensile forces
b. Relatively insoluble
c. Both a & b
d. None

98. Which are the polypeptides found on ribosomes connected to the RER membrane's cytosolic surface

a. Secreted proteins
b. Integral membrane proteins,
c. Soluble proteins that reside within the compartments of the endomembrane system
d. All of these

99. Photosynthetic reactions in chloroplasts occur in

a. Stroma
b. Thylakoid lumen
c. Thylakoid membrane
d. Inner chloroplast membrane

100. Disassembly of the microtubular cytoskeleton can be induced by

a. Cold temperature
b. Colchicine
c. Elevated $Ca2^{+}$ concentration
d. All of these

Answer Key

1	b	2	c	3	a	4	a	5	d	6	c	7	a
8	b	9	d	10	a	11	a	12	a	13	b	14	c
15	b	16	b	17	b	18	b	19	d	20	a	21	d
22	a	23	d	24	d	25	c	26	c	27	c	28	a
29	d	30	b	31	a	32	b	33	a	34	c	35	b
36	a	37	c	38	a	39	d	40	a	41	c	42	a
43	d	44	c	45	d	46	d	47	a	48	d	49	a
50	b	51	d	52	c	53	c	54	a	55	d	56	b
57	a	58	b	59	c	60	d	61	b	62	d	63	a
64	b	65	c	66	d	67	b	68	c	69	d	70	b
71	d	72	a	73	d	74	d	75	c	76	a	77	c
78	a	79	d	80	a	81	b	82	d	83	d	84	b
85	a	86	a	87	a	88	d	89	a	90	b	91	a
92	c	93	b	94	d	95	d	96	b	97	c	98	d
99	c	100	d										

4

Biochemistry of Carbohydrate

Barkha Gupta[1] and Ramesh D.[2]

[1]Department of Veterinary Physiology and Biochemistry, Post Graduate Institute of Veterinary Education and Research (PGIVER), Jaipur (RAJUVAS), Rajasthan-302031

[2]Department of Veterinary Physiology and Biochemistry, Veterinary College, Hassan (KVAFSU), Karnataka-573202

Introduction

Carbohydrates are essential organic biomolecules/macromolecules composed of carbon c., hydrogen (H), and oxygen (O) atoms, typically in a 1:2:1 ratio. They are one of the four major classes of biomolecules, alongside proteins, lipids, and nucleic acids. Carbohydrates play critical roles in energy storage, structural integrity and cell signaling. Carbohydrates with an aldehyde as their functional group are called **Aldoses.** Those with keto as a functional group are called **Ketoses.**

Classification of Carbohydrates: They are broadly classified into three major groups:

1. **Monosaccharides**: The simplest form of carbohydrates, consisting of a single sugar unit. They cannot be hydrolyzed to yield simpler forms of sugar. They can be subdivided into trioses, tetroses, pentoses, hexoses, heptoses and octoses etc., depending upon the number of carbon atoms they possess. Important monosaccharides are:
   - **Glycerose** / Glyceraldehyde (Aldotriose): Glyceraldehyde 6-phosphate is an intermediate in Glycolysis.
   - **Ribose** (Aldopentose): found in Nucleic acids.
   - **Glucose** (Aldohexose): The primary energy source for cells, known as blood sugar.
   - **Fructose** (Ketohexose): Found in fruits (fruit sugar), a major component of sucrose.
   - **Galactose** (Aldohexose): Known as brain sugar. It is a part of lactose sugar.
2. **Oligosaccharides**: Short chains of monosaccharide units (typically 2-10). Based on the number of monosaccharide units, oligosaccharides are further subdivided into disaccharides, trisaccharides, etc.

   Disaccharides: Formed by the condensation reaction between two monosaccharide units by glycosidic linkage. Examples include:

- **Sucrose** (glucose + fructose): Common table sugar/ cane sugar. It is a non-reducing disaccharide.
- **Lactose** (glucose + galactose): Found in milk (milk sugar)
- **Maltose** (glucose + glucose): Formed during starch digestion.
- **Trehalose** (glucose + glucose): A natural, non-reducing disaccharide that's found in many organisms, including bacteria, fungi, yeast, plants, and insects:
- **Trisaccharides:** Raffinose is a trisaccharide consisting of fructose, glucose, and galactose and it is found in some vegetables and whole grains.

3. **Polysaccharides**: They are polymers of monosaccharide units with high molecular weight (up to a million). They are usually tasteless (non-sugars) and form colloids with water. Polysaccharides (or simply Glycans) consist of repeat units of monosaccharides (more than ten to thousand monosaccharide units) or their derivatives, held together by glycosidic bonds. Polysaccharides are linear as well as branched polymers. This contrasts with the structure of proteins and nucleic acids which are only linear polymers. The occurrence of branches in polysaccharides is due to the fact that glycosidic linkages can be formed at any one of the hydroxyl groups of a monosaccharide. They are primarily concerned with two important functions i.e. structural and storage of energy. They are classified into homopolysaccharides and heteropolysaccharides based on the structure.
   - **Homopolysaccharides/Homoglycans** on hydrolysis yield only a single type of monosaccharide. They are named based on the nature of the monosaccharide. Thus, Glucans are polymers of glucose eg. cellulose, starch and glycogen whereas Fructosans are polymers of fructose eg. Inulin.

     Inulin found in dahlia bulbs, garlic, onion etc. It is not utilized by the body. It is used for assessing kidney function through measurement of **glomerular filtration rate (GFR).**
   - **Heteropolysaccharides/ Mucopolysaccharides/ Heteroglycans** on hydrolysis yield a mixture of a few monosaccharides or their derivatives. e.g. Hyaluronic acid, heparin and chondroitin sulphate. They provide extracellular support for organisms of all kingdoms.

Polysaccharides are generally classified based on their functions into two major types:

1. **Storage Polysaccharides:** These polysaccharides serve as energy reserves and can be broken down into simpler sugars when needed.
   - **Starch**: Found in plants, starch is the main storage polysaccharide, made up of alpha glycosidic bonds. It consists of two components i.e. water-soluble **amylose** (a linear chain of glucose units) and water-insoluble amylopectin (a branched chain of glucose units). Starch is a major source of dietary carbohydrates for humans, found in foods like potatoes, rice, and wheat.
   - **Glycogen:** The storage polysaccharide in animals, glycogen is stored primarily in the liver and muscle tissues. It is a highly branched carbohydrate, composed of alpha glycosidic bonds, allowing rapid release of glucose when energy is needed. The structure of glycogen is similar to that of amylopectin with a greater number of branches. Glycogen plays a crucial role in maintaining blood glucose levels and providing energy during physical activity.

2. **Structural Polysaccharides:** These polysaccharides provide structural support to cells and tissues, especially in plants, fungi, and some animals.
   - **Cellulose:** A linear polysaccharide composed of β-glucose units linked by (1→4) glycosidic bonds. Cellulose is the primary structural component of plant cell walls, providing rigidity and strength. It is the most abundant organic molecule on Earth. Humans cannot digest cellulose due to the lack of an enzyme to break the β(1→4) linkages, but it serves as dietary fibre.
   - **Chitin:** Similar in structure to cellulose but made from N-acetylglucosamine units. It is found in the exoskeletons of arthropods (e.g., insects, crabs) and in the cell walls of fungi. It provides toughness and protection.

Biochemical Roles of Carbohydrates

Carbohydrates are versatile molecules that are fundamental to many biological processes.

1. **Energy Production:**
   - **Glycolysis**: Glucose is broken down into pyruvate, producing ATP.
   - **Krebs Cycle and Oxidative Phosphorylation**: Further oxidation of carbohydrates generates additional ATP.
2. **Energy Storage**:
   - **Glycogen** in animals (animal starch) and **starch** in plants serve as storage forms of glucose, providing energy when needed.
3. **Structural Roles**:
   - **Cellulose** provides rigidity to plant cell walls.
   - **Chitin** gives structural support in arthropods and fungi.
4. **Cell Signaling and Recognition**:
   - **Glycoproteins** and **glycolipids** are involved in cell-cell recognition, signaling, and immune responses.

1. The potential number of glucose isomers is:

   a. 2 b. 8

   c. 12 d. 16

2. The carbon atoms involved in osazone formation:

   a. C_1 and C_2 b. C_3 and C_4

   c. C_5 and C_6 d. C_2 and C_3

3. Sucrose is:

   a. Reducing sugar b. Non-reducing sugar

   c. Both d. None

4. Naturally occurring glucose is a member of:

   a. L- series b. D- series

   c. Both d. None of them

5. Dulcitol are obtained by the reduction of:

   a. Mannose b. Galactose

   c. Fructose d. Ribose

6. Anomers are the compounds which differ in configuration only at:
   a. C_1 b. C_2
   c. C_3 d. C_4
7. What type of reaction occurs when a monosaccharide forms a cyclic structure from its open-chain form?
   a. Hydrolysis b. Oxidation
   c. Condensation d. Hemiacetal formation
8. During the oxidation of glucose, which functional group is primarily affected?
   a. Hydroxyl group b. Carboxyl group
   c. Aldehyde group d. Ketone group
9. What type of isomerism is shown by D- glucose and D- fructose?
   a. Enantiomerism b. Diastereomerism
   c. Anomerism d. Functional group isomerism
10. Which monosaccharide is known to form a furanose ring structure?
   a. Mannose b. Fructose
   c. Galactose d. Glucose
11. What is the product when glucose undergoes oxidation with nitric acid?
   a. Gluconic acid b. Glucuronic acid
   c. Glucaric acid d. Gluconolactone
12. One of the following is not an aldose:
   a. Glucose b. Galactose
   c. Mannose d. Fructose
13. What are the functions of carbohydrates?
   a. Source of energy b. Cell Signaling and Recognition
   c. Structural component d. All of the Above
14. Raffinose sugar is present in:
   a. Vegetables b. Whole grain
   c. Both a and b d. None
15. Oligosaccharides have monosaccharide molecules/units in numbers:
   a. 2-10 b. 2-8
   c. 10 d. 2-3
16. Which sugar is Pentoses?
   a. Ribose b. Xylose
   c. Xylulose d. All of the above
17. The glycosidic bond found at the branching point in the starch is:
   a. α- 1,4 glycosidic bond b. α- 1,6 glycosidic bond
   c. Both a and b d. None
18. Which sugar belongs to the tetrose class?
   a. Galactose b. Fructose
   c. Idose d. Erythose

19. Liver alcohol dehydrogenase contains:
    a. Sodium b. Copper
    c. Potassium d. Zinc
20. Barfoed solution is not reduced by;
    a. Ribose b. Sucrose
    c. Glucose d. Mannose
21. A carbohydrate found in DNA is;
    a. Ribose b. Deoxyribose
    c. Ribulose d. All of these
22. A positive Seliwanoff's test is obtained with:
    a. Glucose b. Fructose
    c. Lactose d. Maltose
23. Osazones are not formed with the:
    c. Glucose b. Fructose
    c. Sucrose d. Lactose
24. Which of the following is a common reaction used to distinguish between aldoses and ketoses?
    a. Oxidation with bromine water b. Fehling's test
    c. Benedict's test d. Tollen's test
25. Which of the following monosaccharides is a reducing sugar?
    a. Sucrose b. Glucose
    c. Fructose d. Both b and c
26. Which reagent is used to test for the presence of starch?
    a. Fehling's solution b. Iodine solution
    c. Benedict's solution d. Barfoed's solution
27. What is the chemical formula of maltose?
    a. $C_6H_{12}O_6$ b. $C_{12}H_{22}O_{11}$
    c. $C_6H_{10}O_5$ d. $C_{12}H_{24}O_{12}$
28. Maltose is composed of which two monosaccharides?
    a. Glucose and fructose b. Fructose and galactose
    c. Glucose and galactose d. Glucose and glucose
29. Which enzyme catalyzes the hydrolysis of maltose into glucose?
    a. Lactase b. Maltase
    b. Sucrase d. Amylase
30. Maltose is classified as which type of carbohydrate:
    a. Monosaccharide b. Polysaccharide
    c. Disaccharide d. Oligosaccharide
31. In what process is maltose most commonly produced?
    a. Photosynthesis b. Glycolysis
    c. Fermentation d. Starch digestion

32. What is the glycosidic bond type in maltose?
    a. α (1→4) b. β (1→6)
    c. α (1→6) d. β (1→4)
33. Which of the following statements about maltose is correct?
    a. Maltose is sweeter than sucrose
    b. Maltose is not reducing sugar
    c. Maltose is found naturally in some grains
    d. Maltose cannot be fermented by yeast
34. Which of the following is not a property of maltose?
    a. It is a reducing sugar
    b. It can be hydrolyzed by maltase
    c. It is less sweet than glucose
    d. It contains a β (1→4) glycosidic bond
35. Which food product is most likely to contain maltose?
    a. Honey b. Barley malt
    c. Table sugar d. Milk
36. What type of sugar is lactose?
    a. Monosaccharide b. Polysaccharide
    c. Oligosaccharide d. Disaccharide
37. Which two monosaccharides make up lactose?
    a. Glucose and fructose b. Glucose and maltose
    c. Glucose and galactose d. Glucose and sucrose
38. What enzyme is required to digest lactose sugar?
    a. Amylase b. Sucrose
    c. Lactase d. Maltase
39. What condition is caused by the inability to digest lactose?
    a. Diabetes b. Celiac disease
    c. Lactose intolerance d. Hypoglycemia
40. Erythromycin has:
    a. Trimethyl amino sugars b. Diethyl amino sugars
    c. Dimethyl amino sugars d. Triethyl amino sugars
41. Glycosides are found in:
    a. Drugs b. Vitamins
    c. Minerals d. None
42. A racemic mixture is:
    a. Optically active b. Optically inactive
    c. Both d. None
43. Which of the following is sugar alcohol?
    a. Maltose b. Mannitol
    c. Gluconic acid d. All of the above

44. Which of the following is a characteristic of galactose?
   a. It is a monosaccharide
   b. It is a disaccharide
   c. It is a polysaccharide
   d. It is a lipid
45. Galactose is commonly found in which of the following:
   a. Table sugar
   b. Cellulose
   c. Starch
   d. Lactose
46. Which enzyme is responsible for converting galactose to glucose?
   a. Lactase
   b. Galactose-1-phosphate uridyltransferase (GALT)
   c. Amylase
   d. Glucose-6-phosphate
47. Galactose is an epimer of which of the following sugars:
   a. Fructose
   b. Sucrose
   c. Ribose
   d. Glucose
48. What is the consequence of the deficiency of enzyme galactose-1-phosphate uridyltransferase (GALT)?
   a. Lactose intolerance
   b. Diabetes
   c. Galactosemia
   d. Fructose intolerance
49. In the Leloir pathway, what is the first step involving galactose:
   a. Galactose is phosphorylated to galactose-1-phosphate
   b. Galactose is converted directly to glucose.
   c. Galactose is dephosphorylated to galactose-6-phosphate.
   d. Galactose is broken down to pyruvate.
50. Which of the following statements is true about galactose?
   a. It is sweeter than glucose
   b. It is a component of maltose
   c. It is primarily found in fruits
   d. It is a C-4 epimer of glucose
51. Which organ is primarily responsible for glycogen storage?
   a. Heart
   b. Brain
   c. Liver
   d. Kidney
52. What is the building block of glycogen?
   a. Fructose
   b. Galactose
   c. Glucose
   d. Lactose
53. What is the name of the process by which glycogen is broken down into glucose?
   a. Glycolysis
   b. Glycogenesis
   c. Gluconeogenesis
   d. Glycogenolysis
54. Glycogen is broken down to release glucose during which condition:
   a. During digestion
   b. After a meal
   c. During fasting
   d. None

55. Which hormone stimulates glycogen breakdown in the liver?
    a. Insulin b. Cortisol
    c. Glucagon d. None
56. What type of bond links glucose molecules in glycogen?
    a. Hydrogen bond b. Glycosidic bond
    c. Peptide bond d. All of the above
57. What is the function of glycogen in muscles?
    a. Provide energy during prolonged fasting
    b. Provide immediate energy during physical activity
    c. Regulate blood sugar levels
    d. None
58. What enzyme is crucial for the synthesis of glycogen?
    a. Glycogen synthase b. Phosphofructokinase
    c. Hexokinase d. None
59. What condition results from the inability to metabolize glycogen properly?
    a. Diabetes mellitus b. Hyperglycemia
    c. Glycogen storage disease d. All of the above
60. Mucopolysaccharides are also known as:
    a. Glycolipids b. Glycosaminoglycans
    c. Proteoglycans d. All of the above
61. Which of the following is not a mucopolysaccharide?
    a. Hyaluronic acid b. Chondroitin sulfate
    c. Heparin d. Collagen
62. The primary function of mucopolysaccharides is to:
    a. Provide energy
    b. Store genetic information
    c. Maintain the structural integrity of tissues
    d. None
63. Which of the following diseases is associated with a deficiency of enzymes that degrade Mucopolysaccharide?
    a. Marfan syndrome b. Tay-Sachs disease
    c. Hunter syndrome d. None
64. Which mucopolysaccharide is abundant in the vitreous humor of the eye?
    a. Dermatan sulfate b. Hyaluronic acid
    b. Keratan sulfate d. None
65. Hyaluronic acid is commonly used as:
    a. Antibiotics b. Cosmetics and joint supplements
    c. Anti-inflammatory drugs d. None

66. Which enzyme is deficient in Hurler syndrome?
   a. Alpha-L-iduronidase
   b. Beta-glucuronidase
   c. N-acetylgalactosamine-4-sulfatase
   d. Both a and b
67. Mucopolysaccharidosis can be diagnosed through:
   a. Blood glucose levels
   b. Urine tests for glycosaminoglycans
   c. Cholesterol levels
   d. Both b and c
68. Which mucopolysaccharides are involved in the formation of cartilage?
   a. Hyaluronic acid
   b. Dermatan sulfate
   c. Heparin
   d. Chondroitin sulfate
69. Which mucopolysaccharide is known for its anticoagulant properties?
   a. Hyaluronic acid
   b. Dermatan sulfate
   c. Heparin
   d. None
70. dermatan sulfate is found in:
   a. Blood vessel valves
   b. Skin
   c. Heart valves
   d. All of the above
71. Mucopolysaccharides are mainly composed of:
   a. Amino acids
   b. Fatty acid
   c. Monosaccharides
   d. Nucleotides
72. Which glycosaminoglycan is used as a lubricant in joint fluid?
   a. chondroitin sulfate
   b. Heparan sulfate
   c. Hyaluronic acid
   d. All of the above
73. Hunter syndrome is also known as:
   a. Mucopolysaccharidosis I
   b. Mucopolysaccharidosis II
   c. Mucopolysaccharidosis III
   d. Mucopolysaccharidosis IV
74. Which mucopolysaccharide is commonly found in connective tissues?
   a. Heparin
   b. Hyaluronic acid
   c. Chondroitin sulfate
   d. None
75. Which of the following is not a function of mucopolysaccharides?
   a. Structural support
   b. Energy storage
   c. Lubrication
   d. Shock absorption
76. Mucopolysaccharides are:
   a. Homopolysaccharide
   b. Heteropolysaccharide
   c. Both a and b
   d. None
77. Which enzyme breaks down heparin?
   a. Heparinase
   b. Elastase
   c. Hyaluronidase
   d. All of the above

78. Sanfilippo syndrome affects the degradation of:
    a. Dermatan sulfate b. Keratan sulfate
    c. Heparan sulfate d. All of the above
79. What is the major function of intrinsic factor glycoprotein?
    a. Transport b. Antigens
    c. Blood clotting d. Absorption of Vit. B_{12}
80. Agarose of polymer of:
    a. Galactose and anhydrogalactose b. Glucose and anhydroglucose
    c. Glucose and galactose d. None
81. Dextrans are polymers of:
    a. Glucose b. Galactose
    c. Fructose d. None
82. Sucralose is:
    a. Dichlorosucrose b. Trichlorosucrose
    c. Tetrachlorosucrose d. None
83. Inulin is a polymer of:
    a. Glucose b. Mannose
    c. Maltose d. Fructose
84. Which sugars are used as plasma volume expanders?
    a. Dextrans b. Inulin
    c. Mannose d. All of the above
85. Which sugar is useful for the treatment of hepatic encephalopathy?
    a. Inulin b. Lactulose
    c. Mannose d. None
86. Repeating units of hyaluronic acid are:
    a. N-acetyl glucosamine and D-glucuronic acid
    b. N-acetyl galactosamine and D-glucuronic acid
    c. N-acetyl glucosamine and Glucose
    d. None
87. Which carbohydrate, known commonly as invert sugar is:
    a. Fructose b. Sucrose
    c. Glucose d. Lactose
88. A heteropolysaccharide among the following is:
    a. Inulin b. Cellulose
    c. Heparin d. Dextrin
89. The smallest monosaccharide that has a furanose ring structure is:
    a. Erythrose b. Ribose
    c. Glucose d. Fructose

90. Which of the following is an epimer pair:
   a. Glucose and fructose
   b. Glucose and galactose
   c. Galactose and mannose
   d. Lactose and maltose

91. α-Glycosidic bond is present in:
   a. Lactose
   b. Maltose
   c. Sucrose
   d. Both b and c

92. Glucose has a total no. of chiral centers:
   a. 2
   b. 3
   c. 4
   d. 5

93. Two sugars that differ only in the configuration around a single specific carbon atom (other than anomeric carbon) are known as:
   a. Epimer
   b. Anomer
   c. Hemiacetal
   d. None

94. The α and β anomers of D-glucose interconvert in aqueous solution by a process:
   a. Mutarotation
   b. Racemization
   c. Electrophoresis
   d. None

95. The highest concentrations of fructose are found in:
   a. Aqueous humor
   b. Vitreous humor
   c. CSF
   d. Seminal fluid

96. The renal threshold for glucose is decreased in:
   a. Diabetes mellitus
   b. Insulinoma
   c. Renal glycosuria
   d. Alimentary glycosuria

97. Gluconeogenesis is decreased by which hormone?
   a. Glucagon
   b. Epinephrine
   c. Glucocorticoids
   d. Insulin

98. In essential pentosuria, urine contains:
   a. D-Ribose
   b. D-Xylulose
   c. L-Xylulose
   d. D-Xylose

99. What is the "sugar code" in biology?
   a. The genetic code in DNA
   b. The sequence of amino acids in proteins
   c. The diverse structures of carbohydrates and their roles in cell signaling
   d. All of the above

100. Which of the following molecules is primarily related to the sugar code?
   a. DNA
   b. Glycans
   c. RNA
   d. Lipid

101. Glycosylation is the process of attaching sugars to which types of molecules:
   a. Proteins and lipids
   b. Carbohydrates and lipids
   c. DNA and RNA
   d. None

102. What is the main function of the sugar code in cellular processes?
   a. Providing energy for cellular activities
   b. Encoding genetic information
   c. Mediating cell-cell communication and recognition
   d. All
103. Which type of glycan is most commonly found on the surface of animal cells?
   a. Cellulose b. Starch
   c. Glycosaminoglycans d. N-glycans
104. Which of the following is a key enzyme involved in the synthesis of glycans?
   a. Polymerase b. Protease
   c. Glycosyltransferase d. Ligase
105. In which organelle does the initial glycosylation of proteins typically occur:
   a. Nucleus b. Endoplasmic reticulum
   c. Mitochondria d. None
106. Lectins are proteins that bind specifically to:
   a. Lipids b. Carbohydrates
   c. Proteins d. None
107. Which cellular process is directly influenced by the sugar code?
   a. DNA replication b. RNA transcription
   c. Protein translation d. Immune response
108. Lactose sugar gives osazone:
   a. Powder puff-shaped b. Sunflower- shaped
   c. Needle-shaped d. Cone-shaped
109. Which product is given by pentose sugar on dehydration?
   a. Furfural b. Hydroxymethyl furfural
   c. Pentonic acid d. None
110. Which test is useful for the detection of xylose in urine in essential pentosuria?
   a. Mucic acid test b. Molisch test
   c. Bial's test d. None
111. Which sugar is the sweetener used in sugarless gums and candies?
   a. Amino sugar b. Polyols
   c. L-ascorbic acid d. Alditols
112. Trehalose sugar is:
   a. Reducing sugar b. Non-reducing sugar
   c. Both d. None
113. Which sugar is used in chromatography?
   a. Dextrins b. Dextrans
   c. Inulin d. None

114. Cellulose is made up of the molecules of:
   a. α-glucose b. β-glucose
   c. Both of the above d. None
115. Iodine solution produces no color with:
   a. Cellulose b. Starch
   c. Dextrin d. Glycogen
116. The general test for the detection of carbohydrates is:
   a. Iodine test b. Molisch test
   c. Barfoed test d. None
117. N-acetylneuraminic acid (NANA) is an example of:
   a. Sialic acid b. Mucic acid
   c. Glucuronic acid d. Hippuric acid
118. A carbohydrate commonly known as dextrose is:
   a. Dextrin b. D-fructose
   c. D-Glucose d. Glycogen
119. A homopolymer of glucose is:
   a. Starch b. Dextrin
   c. Glycogen d. All of the above

Answer Key

1	d	2	a	3	b	4	d	5	b	6	a	7	d
8	c	9	d	10	b	11	c	12	d	13	d	14	c
15	a	16	d	17	b	18	d	19	d	20	b	21	b
22	b	23	c	24	c	25	d	26	b	27	b	28	d
29	b	30	c	31	d	32	a	33	c	34	d	35	b
36	d	37	c	38	c	39	c	40	c	41	a	42	b
43	b	44	a	45	d	46	b	47	d	48	c	49	a
50	d	51	c	52	c	53	d	54	c	55	c	56	b
57	b	58	a	59	c	60	b	61	d	62	c	63	c
64	b	65	b	66	a	67	b	68	d	69	c	70	d
71	c	72	c	73	b	74	c	75	b	76	b	77	a
78	c	79	d	80	a	81	a	82	b	83	d	84	a
85	b	86	a	87	b	88	c	89	b	90	b	91	d
92	c	93	a	94	a	95	d	96	c	97	d	98	d
99	c	100	b	101	a	102	c	103	d	104	c	105	b
106	b	107	d	108	a	109	a	110	c	111	d	112	b
113	b	114	b	115	a	116	b	117	a	118	c	119	d

5

Biochemistry of Lipids

***Ramesh D.*[1] *and Barkha Gupta*[2]**

[1]*Department of Veterinary Physiology and Biochemistry, Veterinary College, Hassan (KVAFSU), Karnataka-573202*

[2]*Department of Veterinary Physiology and Biochemistry, Post Graduate Institute of Veterinary Education and Research (PGIVER), (RAJUVAS) Jaipur-302031 Rajasthan*

Introduction

Lipids may be regarded as organic substances relatively insoluble in water, soluble in organic solvents (chloroform, ether, benzene, ethanol and other non-polar solvents, etc.), actually or potentially related to fatty acids and utilized by living cells. Lipids are a diverse group of hydrophobic or amphipathic biomolecules that play crucial roles in energy storage, cell membrane structure, and signaling. Unlike carbohydrates and proteins, lipids are not defined by a specific polymer structure but rather by their solubility in non-polar solvents.

Broadly lipids are classified based on their function as 'Storage lipids' and 'Structural lipids'. Some of them are co-factors, hormones, electron carriers, light-absorbing pigments and hydrophobic anchors of proteins.

Fatty Acids: Fatty acids are straight aliphatic chains with a methyl group at one end and a carboxyl group (-COOH) at the other end. They are the simplest form of lipids.

- **Saturated Fatty Acids** have no double bonds between carbon atoms, leading to straight chains (e.g., palmitic acid).
- **Unsaturated Fatty Acids** contain one or more double bonds, causing kinks in the chain (e.g., oleic acid). Fatty acids containing more than one double bond (polyunsaturated fatty acids/PUFA) are found in relatively minor amounts.

Functions of Fatty Acids

- They are the constituents of phospholipids and glycolipids (components of biological membranes).
- Fatty acids are fuel molecules. They are stored as triacylglycerols, which are uncharged esters of glycerol. They provide physical protection for the organs of the body.
- Fatty acid derivatives such as prostaglandins, leukotrienes and thromboxanes serve as local hormones and an intracellular messenger in cell signaling mechanisms.

Essential Fatty Acids

Those polyunsaturated fatty acids that cannot be synthesized and must be supplied through the diet are called essential fatty acids.

- Essential fatty acids for many species including man are
  - Linoleic (ω6) acid
  - Linolenic(ω3) acid
  - Arachidonic acid is also an essential fatty acid and it can be formed from linoleic acid in most mammals but not in the cat family.

Classification of Lipids

Lipids can be classified according to their hydrolysis products and according to similarities in their molecular structures. Three major subclasses are recognized:

1. Simple lipids

a) **Fats and oils (Triglycerides/TG):** Triacylglycerols yield fatty acids and glycerol upon hydrolysis.
   - The difference between fats and oils is based on their physical states at room temperature. It is customary to call a lipid a fat if it is solid at 25°C and oil if it is a liquid at the same temperature.
   - These differences in melting points reflect differences in the degree of unsaturation of the constituent fatty acids.

b) **Waxes:** Waxes yield fatty acids and long-chain alcohols (Cetyl alcohol) upon hydrolysis.

2. Compound lipids

a) **Phospholipids** are composed of fatty acids, glycerol or amino alcohol sphingosine, phosphoric acid and nitrogenous base. They may be **glycerophospholipids** or **sphingophospholipid** depending upon the alcohol group present (glycerol or sphingosine).

   The phospholipids containing glycerol as the backbone:
   - Phosphatidic acid and phosphatidyl glycerol
   - Phosphatidyl choline (Lecithin)
   - Phosphatidyl ethanolamine (Cephalin)
   - Phosphatidyl inositol
   - Phosphatidyl serine
   - Lysophospholipids
   - Plasmalogens
   - Cardiolipins

   The phospholipids containing sphingosine as the backbone:
   - **Sphingomyelins:** It contains amino alcohol, sphingosine (synthesized from serine and palmitic acid) rather than glycerol. A fatty acid is attached to the amino group of sphingosines by an amide linkage, producing a ceramide. The alcohol group at carbon 1 of sphingosine is esterified to phosphorylcholine,

producing sphingomyelin, an important constituent of myelin of nerve fibers, which insulates and protects the nerve fibres of CNS.

b) **Glycolipids** The sugar-containing sphingolipids are also called "glycosphingolipids" eg. cerebrosides.

   Gangliosides are most complex glycosphingolipids, which contain ceramide and one or more molecules of sialic acid (N- acetyl neuraminic acid)

c) **Lipoproteins**: Complex of lipids and proteins. Based on the density lipoproteins are classified in:
   - Chylomicrons
   - VLDL (pre-beta lipoprotein)
   - LDL (beta-lipoprotein)
   - HDL (alpha–lipoprotein)

3. Derived lipids:

Hydrolysis products of simple and compound lipids are called derived lipids. They include fatty acid, glycerol, sphingosine and steroid derivatives.

Steroid derivatives are phenanthrene structures. Cholesterol has a steroid nucleus i.e. cyclopentanoperhydrophenanthrene (CPPP).

Functions of Lipids

1. **Energy Storage**:
   - **Triglycerides** store more energy per gram than carbohydrates or proteins, making them an efficient energy reserve.
2. **Cell Membrane Structure**:
   - **Phospholipids** and **cholesterol** are key components of cell membranes, providing structural integrity and fluidity.
   - The lipid bilayer serves as a barrier, regulating the movement of substances in and out of cells.
3. **Signaling Molecules**:
   - **Steroid hormones** (e.g., cortisol, estrogen) regulate various physiological processes, including metabolism, immune response, and reproduction.
   - **Eicosanoids** (derived from arachidonic acid) are involved in inflammation and other cellular functions.
4. **Insulation and Protection**:
   - **Adipose tissue** provides thermal insulation and protects vital organs by cushioning them.
5. **Vitamins and Pigments**:
   - **Lipid-soluble vitamins** (A, D, E, K) are essential for various biological functions, including vision, calcium metabolism, and antioxidant activity.
   - **Carotenoids** are pigments involved in photosynthesis and also serve as precursors for vitamin A.
6. **Lung surfactant** is **dipalmitoyl phosphatidylcholine/ dipalmitoyl lecithin** which prevents adherence of the inner surface of the lungs. **Respiratory distress**

syndrome in premature infants is due to the lack of surfactant production in the lungs.

7. **Choline** acts as a **lipotropic factor** and prevents the accumulation of fats in the liver.
8. **Cephalins** are involved in the process of **blood coagulation/ clotting**.
9. **Phosphatidylinositol** (PI) is a precursor for the **second messenger**, involved in the action of some hormones.
10. **Cardiolipin** is the only phospholipids that possess **antigenic properties**.

1. The number of double bonds in Arachidonic acid (A A) is:

a. 1 b. 2

c. 4 d. 6

2. Lipids are soluble in:

a. Organic solvents b. Water

c. both d. None

3. Which of the following is a type of lipid?

a. Triglycerides b. Steroids

c. Phospholipids d. All of the above

4. Lipids are primarily composed of which elements?

a. Carbon, hydrogen, and oxygen

b. Nitrogen, hydrogen and oxygen

c. Carbon, nitrogen and sulphur

d. Hydrogen, oxygen and phosphorus

5. What is the *main* function of triglycerides in the body?

a. Structural support b. Genetic information storage

c. Energy storage d. Catalyzing biochemical reactions

6. Which of the following is a characteristic feature of phospholipids?

a. They have a hydrophilic head and a hydrophobic tail

b. They are completely hydrophilic

c. They are completely hydrophobic

d. They have a hydrophobic head and a hydrophilic tail

7. Steroids are a type of lipid characterized by:

a. Long hydrocarbon chains b. Glycerol backbone

c. Four fused carbon rings d. Peptide bonds

8. Which lipid is a major component of cell membranes?

a. Triglycerides b. Phospholipids

c. Cholesterol d. Glycolipids

9. Which process breaks down lipids into fatty acids and glycerol?

a. Dehydration synthesis b. Fermentation

c. Hydrolysis d. None

10. The body cannot synthesize essential fatty acids which must be obtained from the diet. Which of the following is an essential fatty acid?
    a. Palmitic acid b. Linoleic acid
    c. Stearic acid d. Oleic acid
11. What is the primary role of cholesterol in the body?
    a. Energy storage b. Insulation and protection
    c. Precursor for steroid hormones d. Enzyme activation
12. Which type of lipoprotein is considered "good" cholesterol?
    a. Low-density lipoprotein (LDL)
    b. High-density lipoprotein (HDL)
    c. Very low-density lipoprotein (VLDL)
    d. Intermediate-density lipoprotein (IDL)
13. Lipids are soluble in:
    a. Water b. Non-polar solvents
    c. Polar solvents d. None
14. Fatty acids are classified based on the presence of double bonds. What type of fatty acid has *no* double bond:
    a. Saturated fatty acids b. Monounsaturated fatty acids
    c. Polyunsaturated fatty acids d. Trans fatty acids
15. Which of the following is an example of saturated fat?
    a. Olive oil b. Fish oil
    c. butter d. Sunflower oil
16. Trans fats are primarily produced by:
    a. Natural fermentation
    b. Partial hydrogenation of vegetable oils
    c. Full hydrogenation of animal fats
    d. Dehydration synthesis
17. Which of the following is *not* a function of lipids in the body?
    a. Energy storage b. Hormone production
    c. Insulation d. Transport of oxygen
18. Omega-3 and omega-6 fatty acids are examples of:
    a. Saturated fats b. Essential fatty acids
    c. Trans fats d. Non-essential fatty acid
19. Which of the following is a lipid that acts as a hormone?
    a. Estrogen b. Insulin
    c. Hemoglobin d. None
20. The process of lipid metabolism primarily occurs in which organ?
    a. Heart b. Brain
    c. Liver d. Kidney

21. Adipose tissue primarily stores:

a. Proteins b. Lipids
c. Carbohydrates d. Minerals

22. Which of the following lipid types is involved in the formation of myelin sheaths around nerve fibre?

a. Triglycerides b. Sphingolipids
c. Phospholipids d. Steroids

23. A lipid containing alcoholic amine residue is:

a. Phosphatidic acid b. Cephalin
c. Cholesterol d. Sphingomyelin

24. Cephalin consists of:

a. Glycerol, fatty acids, phosphoric acid and choline
b. Glycerol, fatty acids, phosphoric acid and ethanolamine
c. Glycerol, fatty acids, phosphoric acid and inositol
d. Glycerol, fatty acids, phosphoric acid and serine

25. An example of a saturated fatty acid is:

a. Palmitic acid b. Oleic acid
c. Linoleic acid d. All of the above

26. If the fatty acid is esterified with an alcohol of high molecular weight instead of glycerol, the resulting compound known is:

a. Lecithin b. Plasmalogen
c. Wax d. Cephalin

27. A fatty acid **not** synthesized in the body and supplied in the diet is?

a. Palmitic acid b. Lauric acid
c. Linolenic acid d. Palmitoleic acid

28. Essential fatty acid:

a. Linoleic acid b. Linolenic acid
c. arachidonic acid d. All of the above

29. Gangliosides derived from glucosylceramide contain in addition one or more molecules of:

a. Sialic acid b. Glycerol
c. Diacylglycerol d. Fatty acid

30. 'Drying oil', oxidized spontaneously by atmospheric oxygen at ordinary temperature and forms a hard water waterproof material:

a. Coconut oil b. Peanut oil
c. Rape seed oil d. Linseed oil

31. Deterioration of food (rancidity) is due to the presence of:

a. Cholesterol b. Vitamin E
c. Peroxidation of lipids d. All of the above

32. The number of ml of N/10 KOH required to neutralize the fatty acids in the distillate from 5 gm of fat is called:
    a. Reichert-Meissl number
    b. Iodine number
    c. Acetyl number
    d. Non-volatile fatty acid number
33. What is the primary role of phospholipids in biological membranes?
    a. Energy storage
    b. Catalyzing chemical reactions
    c. Forming a barrier to protect cells
    d. Storing genetic information
34. Which of the following is a key structural feature of phospholipids that contributes to membrane fluidity?
    a. The phosphate group
    b. The glycerol backbone
    c. The fatty acid chains
    d. The carbohydrate group
35. Phospholipids are amphipathic molecules. What does this mean?
    a. They have only hydrophobic properties
    b. They can only form solid structures
    c. They have both hydrophilic and hydrophobic regions
    d. They do not interact with water at all
36. Which part of the phospholipid is hydrophilic?
    a. The fatty acid tails
    b. The phosphate head group
    c. The glycerol backbone
    d. The entire molecule
37. Phospholipids are crucial for which of the following cellular processes?
    a. DNA replication
    b. ATP production
    c. Protein synthesis
    d. Membrane transport
38. Which of the following is true about the bilayer formation of phospholipids?
    a. It requires energy to form
    b. It forms spontaneously in an aqueous environment
    c. It is held together by covalent bonds
    d. It is impermeable to all molecules
39. Phospholipids contribute to the fluidity of cell membranes by:
    a. Forming a rigid structure
    b. Allowing lateral movement within the bilayer
    c. Acting as enzymes to break down other molecules
    d. Binding tightly to adjacent cells
40. The ability of phospholipids to form liposomes is primarily used in which application?
    a. Genetic engineering
    b. Protein synthesis
    c. Drug delivery
    d. Energy production
41. Which function of phospholipids helps in signal transduction across cell membranes?
    a. Energy storage
    b. Acting as enzymes
    c. Forming lipid rafts
    d. Serving as precursors for signaling molecules

42. What is the role of phospholipids in the formation of the myelin sheath around nerve Cells?
    a. They provide energy for nerve impulse transmission
    b. They insulate axons to speed up signal transmission
    c. They directly interact with neurotransmitters
    d. They control the synthesis of neurotransmitters
43. The cholesterol molecule is:
    a. Benzene derivative
    b. Quinoline derivative
    c. Steroid
    d. None
44. The Salkowski test is performed to detect:
    a. Glycerol
    b. Cholesterol
    c. Fatty acids
    d. Vitamin A
45. Palmitic, oleic, or stearic acid ester of cholesterol used in the manufacture of cosmetic creams are:
    a. Elaidic oil
    b. Lanoline
    c. Spermaceti
    d. Chaulmoogric oil
46. What is the primary function of glycolipids in the cell membrane?
    a. Energy storage
    b. Protein synthesis
    c. Cell recognition and communication
    d. DNA replication
47. Glycolipids are composed of which two main components?
    a. Amino acids and fatty acids
    b. Carbohydrates and lipids
    c. Proteins and nucleic acids
    d. Carbohydrates and phospholipids
48. In which part of the cell are glycolipids primarily found?
    a. Cytoplasm
    b. Mitochondria
    c. Nucleus
    d. Cell membrane
49. Glycolipids are particularly abundant in which type of tissue?
    a. Muscle tissue
    b. Bone tissue
    c. Nervous tissue
    d. Connective tissue
50. Ergosterol is an important precursor of:
    a. Vitamin D
    b. Vitamin A
    c. Vitamin C
    d. Vitamin E
51. Dietary fats after absorption appear in the circulation as:
    a. HDL
    b. VLDL
    c. LDL
    d. Chylomicron
52. Free fatty acids are transported in the blood:
    a. Combined with albumin
    b. Combined with fatty acid binding protein
    c. Combined with β -lipoprotein
    d. None

53. Long-chain fatty acids are first activated to acetyl-CoA in:
   a. Cytosol b. Microsomes
   c. Nucleus d. Mitochondria
54. The enzyme acyl-CoA synthase catalyses the conversion of a fatty acid into an active fatty acid in the presence of:
   a. AMP b. ADP
   c. ATP d. GTP
55. Carnitine is synthesized from:
   a. Lysine and methionine b. Glycine and valine
   c. Aspartate and glutamate d. Proline and hydroxyproline
56. The enzymes of β-oxidation proper are found in:
   a. Mitochondri A b. Cytosol
   c. Golgi apparatus d. Ribosome
57. Prostaglandins are synthesized from:
   a. Oleic acid b. Arachidonic acid
   c. Linoleic acid d. Linolenic acid
58. Protein molecule of lipoprotein is:
   a. Preprotein b. Pseudo protein
   c. Post protein d. Apoprotein
59. Gangliosides are glycolipids occurring in:
   a. Kidney b. Brain
   c. Muscle d. Liver
60. In sphingomyelins the alcohol moiety is:
   a. Glycol b. Glycerol
   c. Sphingosine d. All of the above
61. Esterification of cholesterol occurs at carbon position:
   a. 1 b. 2
   c. 3 d. 4
62. One of the following is an amphipathic lipid:
   a. Fatty acid b. Phospholipid
   c. Bile salts d. All of the above
63. The smell of fat turns rancid due to the presence of:
   a. Volatile fatty acid b. Vitamin E
   c. Cholesterol d. Quinone
64. Which of the following is considered "bad" cholesterol?
   a. HDL b. VLDL
   c. LDL d. All of the above

65. What is the main function of cholesterol in the body?
    a. To produce energy
    b. To build and maintain cell membranes
    c. To store fat
    d. To eliminate toxins
66. Which of the following is a healthy level of total cholesterol?
    a. Less than 200 mg/dL
    b. 200-239 mg/dL
    c. 240-279 mg/dL
    d. 280 mg/dL or more
67. Which of the following factors does NOT typically raise cholesterol levels?
    a. Saturated fats
    b. Trans fats
    c. Physical activity
    d. Genetic predisposition
68. Which organ is primarily responsible for producing cholesterol in the body?
    a. Heart
    b. Pancreas
    c. Liver
    d. Kidneys
69. High levels of which type of cholesterol are associated with a lower risk of heart disease?
    a. HDL
    b. VLDL
    c. LDL
    d. None
70. Which of the following lifestyle changes can help lower LDL cholesterol levels?
    a. Increasing intake of trans fats
    b. Smoking more
    c. Regular physical exercise
    d. Eating more red meat
71. Which medication is commonly prescribed to lower cholesterol levels?
    a. Antibiotics
    b. Diuretics
    c. Statins
    d. Beta-block
72. Which of the following is a characteristic of trans fatty acids?
    a. They have a cis configuration of the double bond
    b. They are typically found in high amounts in fruits and vegetables
    c. They increase LDL ("bad") cholesterol levels in the blood
    d. They are essential fatty acids needed by the human body
73. Trans fatty acids are most commonly found in:
    a. Fresh fruits
    b. Partially hydrogenated oils
    c. Whole grains
    d. Lean meats
74. What is the primary source of artificial trans fatty acids in the diet?
    a. Naturally occurring in meat and dairy
    b. Full-fat yogurt
    c. Processed foods like margarine and baked goods
    d. Olive oil

75. Which of the following is a health risk associated with the consumption of trans fatty acids?
   a. Reduced risk of heart disease
   b. Increased risk of developing diabetes and heart attacks
   c. Improved immune function
   d. Reduced cholesterol levels

76. Trans fatty acids have been shown to:
   a. Decrease the risk of stroke
   b. Decrease levels of HDL ("good") cholesterol
   c. Improve the body's response to insulin
   d. Have no impact on health

77. Which of the following is an essential fatty acid?
   a. Oleic acid
   b. Stearic acid
   c. Palmitic acid
   d. Linolenic acid

78. Which of the following foods is the richest source of omega-3 fatty acids, an essential fatty acid?
   a. Olive oil
   b. Butter
   c. Flaxseed
   d. None

79. Which essential fatty acid is primarily found in fish oil?
   a. Linoleic acid
   b. Arachidonic acid
   c. Alpha-linolenic acid (ALA)
   d. Eicosapentaenoic acid (EPA)

80. deficiency in essential fatty acids may lead to which of the following symptoms:
   a. Hair loss and scaly skin
   b. Increased blood pressure
   c. Reduced cholesterol levels
   d. Improved immune function

81. The molecular size of fatty acid can be determined from:
   a. Iodine number
   b. Acid number
   c. RM value
   d. Saponification value

82. N-acetylneuraminic acid (NANA is present in:
   a. Phospholipids
   b. cerebrosides
   c. Gangliosides
   d. Triglycerides

83. Which of the following is Glycerophospholipid?
   a. Lecithin
   b. Plasmalogens
   c. cardiolipin
   d. All of the above

84. Sphingosine is not present in:
   a. Cephalin
   b. Sphingomyelin
   c. Cerebrosides
   d. Sulphatides

85. Free fatty acids are transported in circulation by:
   a. Albumin
   b. HDL
   c. LDL
   d. VLDL

86. Which of the following is an amphipathic lipid?
    a. Phospholipids b. Fatty acids
    c. Bile salts d. All of the above
87. Degree of unsaturation of fatty acid can be determined from:
    a. Iodine number b. Acid number
    c. RM value d. Saponification value
88. Which of the following is Glycerophospholipid except?
    a. Lecithin b. Cephalin
    c. Cardiolipin d. Sphingomyelin
89. The highest phospholipid content is found in
    a. Chylomicrons b. HDL
    c. LDL d. VLDL
90. Cholesterol is the precursor of:
    a. Vitamin D b. Sex hormones
    c. Bile acids d. All of the above
91. The major lipids in chylomicrons are:
    a. Triglycerides b. Phospholipids
    c. Cholesterol d. Free fatty acids
92. Phrynoderma is a deficiency of:
    a. Essential fatty acids b. Proteins
    c. Amino acids d. None of these
93. Acylsphingosine is also known as:
    a. Sphingomyelin b. Cerebroside
    c. Ceramide d. Sulphatide
94. HDL is synthesized in:
    a. adipose tissue b. Liver
    c. Intestine d. Liver and intestine
95. All the following are omega-6 fatty acids except:
    a. Linoleic acid b. α-Linolenic acid
    c. γ-Linolenic acid d. Arachidonic acid
96. The major storage form of lipids:
    a. Triglycerides b. Phospholipids
    c. Esterified cholesterol d. Sphingolipids
97. The nitrogen base in lecithin is:
    a. Choline b. Ethanolamine
    c. Serine d. Betaine
98. All the following contain nitrogen except:
    a. Cephalin b. Cephalin
    c. Phosphatidyl inositol d. Phosphatidyl serine

99. Sphingosine is not found in:
   a. Sulphatides
   b. Gangliosides
   c. Cerebrosides
   d. Plasmalogens

100. Hexosamine are present in:
   a. Cerebrosides
   b. Gangliosides
   c. Sulphatides
   d. Sphingosine

Answer Key

1	c	2	a	3	d	4	a	5	c	6	a	7	c
8	b	9	c	10	b	11	c	12	b	13	b	14	a
15	c	16	b	17	d	18	b	19	a	20	b	21	b
22	b	23	d	24	b	25	a	26	c	27	c	28	d
29	a	30	d	31	c	32	a	33	c	34	c	35	c
36	b	37	d	38	b	39	b	40	c	41	d	42	b
43	c	44	b	45	b	46	c	47	b	48	d	49	c
50	a	51	d	52	a	53	a	54	c	55	a	56	a
57	b	58	d	59	b	60	c	61	c	62	d	63	a
64	c	65	b	66	a	67	c	68	c	69	a	70	c
71	c	72	c	73	b	74	c	75	b	76	b	77	d
78	c	79	d	80	a	81	d	82	c	83	d	84	a
85	a	86	d	87	a	88	d	89	b	90	d	91	a
92	a	93		94	d	95	b	96	a	97	b	98	c
99	d	100	b										

6

Biochemistry of Protein

Barkha Gupta[1] and Ramesh D.[2]

[1]Department of Veterinary Physiology and Biochemistry, Post Graduate Institute of Veterinary Education and Research (PGIVER), Jaipur (RAJUVAS), Rajasthan-302031

[2]Department of Veterinary Physiology and Biochemistry, Veterinary College, Hassan (KVAFSU), Karnataka-573202

Introduction

Proteins are complex biomolecules composed of amino acids, playing crucial roles in virtually all biological processes. They serve as enzymes, hormones, structural components, signaling molecules etc.

Structure/ Levels of Organization of Proteins

Generally, Proteins are polymers of L-alpha amino acids, linked by peptide bonds. The sequence and structure of these amino acids determine the protein's function. Protein structure is hierarchically organized into four levels:

1. **Primary Structure**
   - The linear sequence of amino acids in a polypeptide chain, determined by the genetic code.
2. **Secondary Structure**
   - Local folding of the polypeptide chain into structures such as α-helices and β-pleated sheets, stabilized by hydrogen bonds.
3. **Tertiary Structure**
   - The three-dimensional conformation of a single polypeptide chain, stabilized by various interactions including hydrogen bonds, ionic bonds, hydrophobic interactions, and disulfide bridges.
4. **Quaternary Structure**
   - The arrangement of multiple polypeptide chains (subunits) into a functional protein complex. Examples include hemoglobin, composed of four subunits.

Classification of Proteins

Proteins are broadly classified into 3 major groups based on chemical nature and solubility

1. **Simple proteins:** They are composed of only amino acid residues. They are further classified into (a) **Globular proteins** eg. Albumins, Globulins, Globins, Lectins etc.

b. **Fibrous proteins** eg. Collagens, Elastins, Keratins etc.

2. **Conjugated proteins:** Besides the amino acids, these proteins contain a non-protein moiety is known as the prosthetic group or conjugating group eg. Glycoproteins, Nucleoproteins, Lipoproteins, Metalloproteins, Chromoproteins etc.
3. **Derived proteins:** These are the denatured or degraded products of simple and conjugated proteins eg. Proteans, Proteoses, Peptones, Polypeptides, Peptides etc.

Functions of Proteins

1. **Enzymatic Catalysis**
   - Enzymes are proteins that accelerate biochemical reactions by lowering the activation energy. Example: Amylase, which breaks down starch.
2. **Structural Support**
   - Proteins provide structure and support to cells and tissues. Example: Collagen in connective tissue.
3. **Transport and Storage**
   - Proteins transport molecules across membranes or within the body. Example: Hemoglobin transports oxygen in the blood.
4. **Cell Signaling**
   - Proteins are involved in cell communication and signal transduction. Example: Insulin, a hormone that regulates blood glucose levels.
5. **Immune Response**:
   - Antibodies are proteins that recognize and neutralize foreign substances like pathogens.
6. **Movement**
   - Proteins are essential for muscle contraction and movement. Example: Actin and myosin in muscle fibers.

Amino Acids

- Amino acids are organic acids containing an amino group and a carboxyl group attached to the a – carbon atom. In addition to the amino and carboxyl groups, each amino acid contains a side chain, called R group, which is also attached to α- carbon atom. The side chain differs for each of the 20 amino acids.
- All the amino acids found in protein are of L configuration. The functions of the amino acids and their roles in protein structure are related mainly to the chemical properties of their side chain.
- The α-carbon atom of all the amino acids except glycine is attached to four different chemical groups and is therefore asymmetric in nature.

There are 20 standard amino acids, classified based on the characteristics of their side chains (R groups):

- Nonpolar (hydrophobic): e.g., Alanine, Valine, Leucine.
- Polar uncharged: e.g., Serine, Threonine, Asparagine.
- Positively charged (basic): e.g., Lysine, Arginine.
- Negatively charged (acidic): e.g., Aspartic acid, Glutamic acid.

Essential amino acids

- They cannot be synthesized in the body. They must be supplied in the diet.
- Eg: methionine, arginine, threonine, tryptophan, valine, isoleucine, leucine, phenylalanine, histidine and lysine. Out of these ten amino acids, two amino acids namely arginine and histidine can be partly synthesized by adult humans – hence called Semi-essential amino acids.

Non-essential amino acids

- The other ten amino acids can be synthesized in the body – hence called as non-essential amino acids. Eg: glycine, alanine, serine, tyrosine, cysteine, glutamic acid, aspartic acid, asparagine, glutamine and proline.

Zwitterion or dipolar ion and pI

The name zwitter is derived from the German word which means hybrid Zwitterion (or dipolar ion) is a hybrid molecule containing positive and negative ionic groups. The amino acids rarely exist in a neutral form with free carboxylic (COOH) and free amino (NH_2) groups. Isoelectric pH (pI) is defined as the pH at which a molecule exists as a zwitterion or dipolar ion and carries no net charge. Thus, the molecule is electrically neutral.

1. What is the primary structure of a protein?
   a. The sequence of amino acids in a polypeptide chain
   b. The folding and coiling of the polypeptide chain into α-helices and β-sheets
   c. The overall 3D shape of the protein
   d. The association of multiple polypeptide chains into a functional protein
2. Which of the following is a function of proteins in the body?
   a. Energy storage
   b. Catalyzing biochemical reactions
   c. Genetic information storage
   d. Insulation
3. What type of bond connects amino acids in a protein?
   a. Ionic bond b. Peptide bond
   c. Hydrogen bond d. covalent bond
4. Which level of protein structure is stabilized by hydrogen bonds between the backbone of the polypeptide chain?
   a. Primary structure b. Secondary structure
   c. Tertiary structure d. Quaternary structure
5. Which of the following is an example of a fibrous protein?
   a. Hemoglobin b. Insulin
   c. Myoglobin d. Keratin
6. Which of the following amino acids is essential in the human diet?
   a. Glycine b. Proline
   c. Alanine d. Lysine

7. Which amino acid has a sulfur-containing side chain?
   a. Serine b. Tyrosine
   c. Methionine d. Glutamine
8. What is the primary function of tryptophan in the human body?
   a. Protein synthesis b. Precursor to serotonin
   c. Antioxidant production d. Formation of bile salts
9. Which of the following amino acids is polar and uncharged at physiological pH?
   a. Glutamic acid b. Asparagine
   c. Arginine d. Phenylalanine
10. Which amino acid is involved in the formation of disulfide bonds in proteins?
   a. Histidine b. Leucine
   c. Cysteine d. Threonine
11. Which of the following is a primary structure of a protein?
   a. Alpha-helix b. Beta-pleated sheet
   c. Sequence of amino acids d. Tertiary structure
12. Proteins are classified into fibrous and globular based on their:
   a. Function b. Structure
   c. Molecular weight d. Amino acid composition
13. Which of the following proteins is a fibrous protein?
   a. Hemoglobin b. Insulin
   c. Myoglobin d. Collagen
14. Enzymes are a class of proteins that are primarily classified based on their:
   a. Structure b. Size
   c. Catalytic function d. Solubility
15. Which of the following is an example of a conjugated protein?
   a. Actin b. Glycoprotein
   c. Keratin d. Albumin
16. Which one of the following is a semi-essential amino acid for humans?
   a. Valine b. Arginine
   c. Lysine d. Tyrosine
17. An example of a polar amino acid is:
   a. Alanine b. Leucine
   c. Arginine d. Valine
18. The amino acid with a non-polar side chain is:
   a. Serine b. Valine
   c. Asparagine d. Threonine
19. A ketogenic amino acid is:
   a. Valine b. Cysteine
   c. Leucine d. Threonine

20. An example of phosphoprotein is:
   a. Casein b. Ferritin
   c. Albumin d. None
21. Which of the following is a dipeptide?
   a. Anserine b. Glutathione
   c. Glucagon d. β -Lipoprotein
22. Which of the following is a tripeptide?
   a. Anserine b. Oxytocin
   c. Kallidin d. Glutathione
23. All the following are branched-chain amino acids except:
   a. Isoleucine b. Alanine
   c. Leucine d. Valine
24. Plasma proteins which contain more than 4% hexosamine are:
   a. Microglobulins b. Glycoproteins
   c. Mucoproteins d. Orosomucoids
25. Carbonic anhydrase is an example of:
   a. Lipoprotein b. Phosphoprotein
   c. Metalloprotein d. Chromoprotein
26. An example of chromoprotein is:
   a. Haemoglobin b. Sturine
   c. Nuclein d. None
27. An example of scleroprotein is:
   a. Zein b. Keratin
   c. Glutenin d. All of the above
28. Casein, the milk protein is:
   a. Nucleoprotein b. Chromoprotein
   c. Phosphoprotein d. Glycoprotein
29. An example of phosphoprotein present in egg yolk is
   a. Ovoalbumin b. Ovoglobulin
   c. Ovovitellin d. Avidin
30. Which level of protein structure involves interactions between multiple polypeptides Chains?
   a. Primary b. Tertiary
   c. Secondary d. Quaternary
31. Which interaction is NOT involved in stabilizing the tertiary structure of a protein?
   a. Hydrogen bonds b. Peptide bonds
   c. Hydrophobic interactions d. Van der Waals forces
32. Ultraviolet light is absorbed by:
   a. Histidine b. Proline
   c. Phenylalanine d. All of the above

33. The example of globulins:
 a. Legunelin b. Leucosin
 c. Tuberin d. Oryzenin
34. An amino acid having no asymmetrical carbon atom is:
 a. Alanine b. Leucine
 c. Glycine d. Arginine
35. Each turn of the α-helix contains the amino acid residues (number):
 a. 3.6 b. 3.0
 c. 4.2 d. 4.5
36. Distance travelled per turn of α–helix in nm is:
 a. 0.53b. 0.54
 c. 0.44d. 0.48
37. Sanger's reagent contains:
 a. Phenylisothiocyanate b. Dansyl chloride
 c. 1-fluoro-2,4- dinitrobenzene d. Ninhydrin
38. Fibrous proteins have an axial ratio of more than:
 a. 3 b. 6
 c. 9 d. 10 or more
39. The number of helices present in a collagen molecule is:
 a. 1 b. 2
 c. 3 d. 4
40. In proteins the α-helix and β-pleated sheet are examples of:
 a. Primary structure b. Secondary structure
 c. Tertiary structure d. Quaternary structure
41. Which of the following is true about amino acids?
 a. All amino acids are essential
 b. All amino acids have at least one amino group and one carboxyl group
 c. Amino acids cannot form peptide bonds
 d. Amino acids do not have stereoisomers
42. Which of the following amino acids has a sulfur-containing side chain?
 a. Lysine b. Valine
 c. Serine d. Methionine
43. Which of the following amino acids is acidic?
 a. Glutamic acid b. Histidine
 c. Alanine d. All of the above
44. What type of bond forms between the carboxyl group of one amino acid and the amino group of another?
 a. Hydrogen bond b. Peptide bone
 c. Ionic bond d. None

45. Which amino acid has the simplest side chain, consisting only of a hydrogen atom?
    a. Glycine b. Proline
    c. Valine d. None
46. Which amino acid has a cyclic structure?
    a. Proline b. Serine
    c. Leucine d. All of the above
47. Which of the following amino acids is aromatic?
    a. Tryptophan b. Threonine
    c. Lysine d. All of the above
48. Where does the translation process that leads to the synthesis of polypeptide chains, in Eukaryotic cells?
    a. Nucleus b. Mitochondria
    c. Cytoplasm d. None
49. Which molecule brings the correct amino acid to the ribosome during protein synthesis?
    a. mRNA b. tRNA
    c. rRNA d. None
50. What is the role of the ribosome during polypeptide synthesis?
    a. It synthesizes mRNA from DNA
    b. It transports amino acids to the tRNA
    c. It catalyzes the formation of peptide bonds between amino acids
    d. It degrades proteins into amino acids.
51. Which of the following matches the first step of translation initiation in eukaryotes?
    a. The ribosome binds to the tRNA carrying methionine
    b. The ribosome binds to the 5' cap of mRNA
    c. The ribosome binds directly to the mRNA stop codon
    d. None
52. Which of the following codons serves as the start codon in mRNA and initiates the synthesis of a polypeptide chain?
    a. UAG b. AUG
    c. UGA d. AUU
53. What happens to a protein when it undergoes denaturation?
    a. Its primary structure is destroyed
    b. Its secondary and tertiary structures are disrupted
    c. It is completely hydrolyzed into amino acids
    d. It becomes more active as an enzyme
54. Which of the following can cause protein denaturation?
    a. High temperature b. Extreme pH levels
    c. Organic solvents d. All of the above

55. Which method is commonly used to purify proteins based on their size?
    a. Ion-exchange chromatography b. Gel-filtration chromatography
    c. Affinity chromatography d. None
56. In protein purification, which technique is based on the specific binding of a protein to a ligand attached to a chromatography column:
    a. Size-exclusion chromatography b. Affinity chromatography
    c. Ultracentrifugation d. Dialysis
57. What is the effect of SDS (sodium dodecyl sulfate) on proteins during SDS-PAGE?
    a. SDS enhances the enzymatic activity of proteins
    b. SDS denatures proteins and gives them a uniform negative charge
    c. SDS increases the native structure of proteins
    d. SDS breaks peptide bonds between amino acids
58. Which of the following is not a primary function of proteins in living organisms?
    a. Catalyzing biochemical reactions
    b. Storing genetic information
    c. Providing structural support
    d. Transporting molecules across membranes
59. Which type of protein is responsible for speeding up chemical reactions in the body?
    a. Structural proteins b. Hormone
    c. Enzymes d. None
60. Hemoglobin, a protein in red blood cells, is crucial for which of the following functions?
    a. Immune defense b. Oxygen transport
    c. DNA replication d. Muscle contraction
61. Which protein is primarily involved in muscle contraction?
    a. Myoglobin b. Collagen
    c. Hemoglobin d. Actin and Myosin
62. Proteins are made up of which type of building blocks?
    a. Fatty acids b. Nucleotides
    c. Amino acids d. Monosaccharides
63. What causes a protein to exhibit optical activity?
    a. The presence of peptide bonds
    b. The asymmetry of its amino acid residues
    c. Its ability to form hydrogen bonds
    d. None
64. Which instrument is commonly used to measure the optical activity of proteins?
    a. Spectrophotometer b. Fluorometer
    c. Polarimeter d. None

65. What type of optical rotation is exhibited by a solution of proteins that rotate plane-polarized light to the right (clockwise)?
    a. Dextrorotatory (+) b. Levorotatory (-)
    c. Achiral d. Racemic
66. α -helix is stabilized by:
    a. H – bond b. Disulphide bond
    c. Salt bond d. Non polar bond
67. The H-bond between peptide linkages is interfered by:
    a. Uric acid b. Guanidine
    c. Oxalic acid d. None
68. The hydrogen bonds in the secondary and tertiary structure of proteins are directly attacked by:
    a. Alkalies b. Detergents
    c. Salts d. All of the above
69. The following is a non-protein amino acid:
    a. Ornithine b. Histamine
    c. Homocysteine d. All of the above
70. The reaction given by two or more peptide linkages is:
    a. Ninhydrin test b. Xanthoproteic reaction
    c. Pauley test d. Biuret test
71. Which bonds in protein structure that are not broken on denaturation?
    a. H- bond b. Peptide bond
    c. Ionic bond d. None
72. The reagent used in the sequenator automatic machine is:
    a. Edman reagent b. Trypsin
    c. Sanger reagent d. None
73. The average nitrogen content of protein is:
    a. 16% b. 18%
    c. 20% d. 22%
74. Protein was first described by:
    a. Linus Pauling b. Gerardus Mulder
    c. Frederick Banting d. Michel Chevreul
75. Which amino acid has a sweet taste?
    a. Glycine b. Alanine
    c. Both d. None
76. Which amino acid is used as a flavoring agent in the food industry?
    a. Valine b. Proline
    c. Monosodium glutamate d. None

77. Which reaction is effectively used for the quantitative determination of amino acids and proteins?
    a. Ninhydrin reaction b. Oxidative deamination
    c. Transamination d. None
78. Azaserine is
    a. Antituberculosis drug b. Anticancer drug
    c. Antioxidant d. All of the above
79. Which amino acid is used for the therapy of Wilson's disease?
    a. N- Acetylcysteine b. Gabapentin
    c. Histidine d. D-Penicillamine
80. The lipoprotein with the fastest electrophoretic mobility and the lowest triglyceride content is:
    a. Chylomicron b. VLDL
    c. IDL d. HDL
81. The lipoprotein associated with the activation of LCAT is:
    a. HDL b. LDL
    c. VLDL d. IDL
82. The presence of Arginine can be detected by:
    a. Millon's reaction b. Hopkins Cole reaction
    c. Sakaguchi reaction d. Pauly's test
83. The presence of Tyrosine can be detected by:
    a. Millon's reaction b. Hopkins Cole reaction
    c. Sakaguchi reaction d. Pauly's test
84. HDL2 has a density in the range of:
    a. 1.008–1.019 b. 1.019–1.035
    c. 1.035–1.063 d. 1.063–1.125
85. Renin converts casein to paracasein in presence of:
    a. ca++ b. Mg++
    c. Na+ d. K+
86. Millon's test is used for:
    a. Phenolic group b. Indole ring
    c. Guanidino group d. All of the above
87. Hopkins-Cole reaction is used for:
    a. Phenolic group b. Indole ring
    c. Guanidino group d. All of the above
88. An example of a globular protein is:
    a. Albumin b. Hemoglobin
    c. Insulin d. All of the above

89. Source of complete protein is
a. Egg
b. Milk
c. Both
d. None

90. Which techniques are used to measure proteins quantitatively?
a. Nephelometry
b. Turbidimetry
c. both
d. None

91. Edman's reagent contains:
a. Phenylisothiocyanate
b. Dansyl chloride
c. 1-fluoro-2,4- dinitrobenzene
d. Ninhydrin

92. Which of the following is an imino acid?
a. Serine
b. Alanine
c. Glycine
d. Proline

93. Which among the following is a non-essential amino acid?
a. Serine
b. Threonine
c. Lysine
d. Histidine

94. Proteins are polymers of:
a. α-amino acids
b. β-amino acids
c. γ-amino acids
d. δ-amino acids

95. What is the one-letter code for tyrosine?
a. T
b. Y
c. R
d. S

96. Two amino groups are present in:
a. Leucine
b. Threonine
c. Lysine
d. Glutamate

97. What is the symbol for lysine?
a. T
b. K
c. L
d. S

98. Which of these techniques are used for the characterization of proteins?
a. Chromatography
b. Salting out
c. Dialysis
d. Electrophoresis

99. An amino acid that does not participate in alpha helix formation is:
a. Histidine
b. Tyrosine
c. Tryptophan
d. Proline

100. The number of peptide bonds in glutathione is:
a. Two
b. One
c. Three
d. Four

101. Both alpha helix and beta pleated sheet conformation of proteins were proposed by:
a. Watson and Crick
b. Pauling and Corey
c. Waugh and King
d. Y.S. Rao

Answer Key

1	a	2	b	3	b	4	b	5	d	6	d	7	c
8	b	9	b	10	c	11	c	12	b	13	d	14	c
15	b	16	b	17	c	18	b	19	c	20	a	21	a
22	d	23	b	24	c	25	c	26	a	27	b	28	c
29	c	30	d	31	b	32	c	33	c	34	c	35	a
36	b	37	c	38	d	39	c	40	b	41	b	42	d
43	a	44	b	45	a	46	a	47	a	48	c	49	b
50	c	51	b	52	b	53	b	54	d	55	b	56	b
57	b	58	b	59	c	60	b	61	d	62	c	63	b
64	c	65	a	66	a	67	b	68	a	69	d	70	d
71	b	72	a	73	a	74	b	75	c	76	c	77	a
78	b	79	d	80	d	81	a	82	c	83	a	84	d
85	a	86	a	87	b	88	d	89	c	90	c	91	d
92	d	93	a	94	a	95	b	96	c	97	b	98	d
99	d	100	a	101	b								

7

Biochemistry of Nucleic Acid

Ramesh D.[1] and Barkha Gupta[2]

[1]*Department of Veterinary Physiology and Biochemistry, Veterinary College, Hassan (KVAFSU), Karnataka-573202*

[2]*Department of Veterinary Physiology and Biochemistry, Post Graduate Institute of Veterinary Education and Research (PGIVER), Jaipur (RAJUVAS), Rajasthan-302031*

Introduction

A pentose sugar, one or more phosphate groups, and a nitrogenous base (purine or pyrimidine) make up a nucleotide. Phosphodiester bonds, which connect the 5'-hydroxyl group of one pentose to the 3'-hydroxyl group of the next, bind nucleic acids together as polymers of nucleotides. RNA and DNA are the two different forms of nucleic acids. RNA nucleotides contain ribose, while uracil and cytosine are typical pyrimidine bases. Thymine and cytosine are common pyrimidine bases, and DNA contains 2'-deoxyribose in its nucleotides. In both RNA and DNA, adenine and guanine are the main purines. There is ample evidence to suggest that genetic information is encoded in DNA The Avery MacLeod-McCarty experiment, in particular, demonstrated how DNA obtained from one bacterial strain may infiltrate and change the cells of another strain, giving it some of the genes from the donor. The Hershey-Chase experiment demonstrated that a bacterial virus's DNA contains the genetic instructions needed for the virus to replicate in a host cell, but not its protein coat. Watson and Crick proposed that native DNA is made up of two antiparallel chains arranged in a right-handed double helical configuration based on a compilation of numerous published data points. A-T and G-C, two complementary base pairs, are created by hydrogen bonds inside the helix. 10.5 base pairs are stacked per turn, perpendicular to the double helix's long axis, at a distance of 3.4 Å. There are various structural configurations for DNA A- and Z-DNA are two variants of the Watson-Crick form or B-DNA The DNA molecule bends as a result of certain sequence-dependent structural differences. Sequences that are suitable for forming hairpin or cruciform structures, triplex, or tetraplex DNA can be formed by DNA strands. Messenger RNA helps ribosomes synthesize proteins by transferring genetic information from DNA Protein synthesis also involves ribosomal and transfer RNA Single strands of RNA can fold into complicated loops, double-stranded sections, or hairpins due to the structural complexity of RNA When native DNA is heated or exposed to pH extremes, it can irreversibly unwind and separate its strands, a process known as melting. The melting temperatures (Tm) of DNAs rich in G-C pairs are higher than those of DNAs rich in A-T pairs. Two species' denatured single-stranded DNAs can combine to form a hybrid duplex; the degree of hybridization depends on how similar the sequences are. The key method used to examine and separate particular genes and RNAs is hybridization. The polymer DNA is comparatively stable. Because cells have a very low tolerance for genetic material alterations, spontaneous processes such as oxidative damage, radiation-induced pyrimidine dimer formation, hydrolysis of base-sugar N-glycosyl bonds, and deamination of certain bases occur at very low rates but are nonetheless significant. Chemical and enzymatic techniques can be used in straightforward, automated approaches to determine DNA sequences and create DNA polymers. The main source of chemical energy in cells is ATP. The presence of an adenosine moiety in different cofactors of enzymes might be connected to the energy required for binding. Adenylyl cyclase catalyzes the formation of cyclic AMP from ATP, which is a frequent second messenger produced in response to hormones and other biological signals.

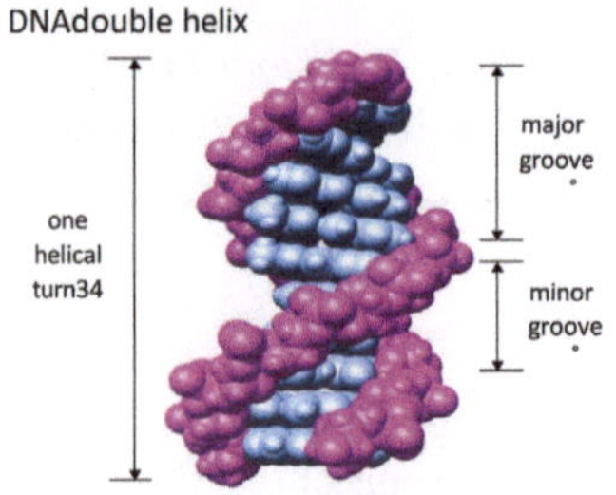

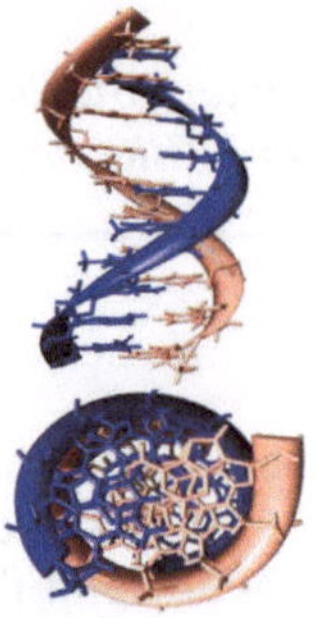

Backbone: deoxyribose and phosphodiester linkage

1. What is the correct statement regarding phosphodiester linkage?
   a. The 3'-hydroxyl group of the subsequent nucleotide is connected to the 3'-phosphate group of the preceding nucleotide unit.
   b. The 3'-phosphate group of one nucleotide unit is connected to the following nucleotide's 5'-hydroxyl group.
   c. One nucleotide unit's 5'-phosphate group is connected to the subsequent nucleotide's 5'-hydroxyl group.
   d. One nucleotide unit's 5'-phosphate group is connected to the subsequent nucleotide's 3'-hydroxyl group
2. Approximately 5% of the cytidine residues in DNA in eukaryotic cells are methylated to
   a. 5-methylcytidine b. 3-Methyl adenine
   c. 4-Methyl thymidine d. 2-Methyl guanidine
3. Permanent alterations in genetic information resulting from modifications in the structure of DNA are referred to as
   a. Mutation b. Carcinogenic
   c. Epigenetic alteration d. Genetic change
4. Under alkaline conditions, the hydrolysis of RNA yields
   a. No hydrolysis occurs
   b. Only 5' Monophosphate
   c. The mixture of 2'- and 3'-monophosphates
   d. None

5. Which of the following reagents is considered a dsDNA alkylating agent
   a. Methionine
   b. S-adenosylmethionine
   c. Uric acid
   d. Ornithine
6. DNA pairs known as Hoogsteen base pairs enable the creation of
   a. Triplex DNAs
   b. Double DNA
   c. Multiplex DNA
   d. None
7. Nucleic acids absorb UV light at a wavelength of
   a. 200 nm
   b. 280 nm
   c. 220 nm
   d. 260 nm
8. 40 nucleotides make up a single-stranded DNA molecule, which bears the sequence 5'-(GA)20-3. When a complementary DNA strand attaches to this single strand
   a. A cruciform structure may form if the complementary strand, which contains the sequence 5'-(CT)20-3', is use^D
   b. An H-DNA structure may arise if the complementary strand has the sequence 5'-(TC)20-3'
   c. A hairpin structure may arise if the complementary strand has the sequence 5'-(TC)20-3'.
   d. A Z-DNA structure might arise if the complementary strand bears the sequence 5'-(CT)20-3'.
9. DNA double helical structure was discovered by
   a. Craig C Melow
   b. Arther Z fire
   c. Linus Pauling
   d. Watson and Crick
10. The secondary structure of RNA includes
    a. Bulge
    b. Internal loop
    c. Hairpin loop
    d. All of the above
11. The number of base pairs per turn in B-DNA is
    a. 10.5 base pairs per turn
    b. 11.5 base pairs per turn
    c. 9.5 base pairs per turn
    d. 12.5 base pairs per turn
12. The temperature at which 50% denaturation of dsDNA occurs is called
    a. Denaturation temperature
    b. Annealing temperature
    c. Melting temperature (Tm)
    d. None
13. The discovery made by Oswald T. Avery, Colin MacLeod, and Maclyn McCarty using the strain of the bacterium Streptococcus pneumonia suggestive of
    a. DNA as genetic material
    b. RNA is the genetic material
    c. Protein is genetic material
    d. None
14. X-ray diffraction of the dsDNA in the 1950s was carried out by
    a. Linus Pauling
    b. Rosalind Franklin and Maurice Wilkins
    c. Arther Nirenberg
    d. HG Khorana

15. Each strand's self-complementary DNA sequences are referred to as
    a. Palindrome b. Hairpin or Cruciform
    c. Tetraplex d. Mirror repeats
16. Which of the following reagents causes deamination of dsDNA
    a. Nitrous acid b. Formic acid
    c. Acetic acid d. Carbonic acid
17. DNA sequencing by enzymatic method or di-deoxy method is also called as
    a. Maxam Gilbert method b. Sanger method
    c. Anionic method d. None
18. ddNTPs lack which of the following
    a. 3'-OH group b. 3'-NH2 group
    c. 5'-OH group d. 5'-COO group
19. The formation of pyrimidine dimers in the dsDNA was induced by.
    a. Salt solution b. UV light
    c. Buffer d. Air
20. The dsDNA undergoes denaturation when it is exposed to
    a. Extreme pH b. Extreme temperature
    c. Both a & b d. None
21. The depth of the major groove and Minor groove in B-DNA is
    a. 12 Å and 6 Å respectively b. 12 Å and 10 Å respectively
    c. 18 Å and 6 Å respectively d. 6 Å and 12 Å respectively
22. In Prokaryotes the nature of mRNA is
    a. Acistronic b. Polycistronic
    c. No transcription d. None
23. Hydrolysis of each anhydride bond in ATP yields
    a. 40 kJ/mol. b. 30 kJ/mol.
    c. 20 kJ/mol. d. 60 kJ/mol.
24. A dsDNA molecule's renaturation is a
    a. Slow and multiple process b. Rapid one-step process
    c. Very slow and time-consuming d. None
25. The chemical methods for synthesizing nucleic acids were developed by
    a. Watson and crick b. Ramachandran
    c. Bruce Merrifield d. H. Gobind Khorana
26. Which of the following was produced using ATP in a process that was aided by the enzyme adenylyl cyclase, which is connected to the plasma membrane's inner face
    a. Adenosine 3', 5'-cyclic monophosphate
    b. Guanosine 3', 5'-cyclic monophosphate
    c. Cytosine 3', 5'-cyclic monophosphate
    d. All of the above

27. Maxam Gilbert's Method of DNA sequencing is also called as
    a. Enzymatic method
    b. Chemical method
    c. Ionic method
    d. Amino method
28. In eukaryotes the nature of mRNA is
    a. Cistron
    b. Monocistronic
    c. Polycistronic
    d. None
29. DNA segments with inverted base sequence repeats with twofold symmetry over two strands are referred to as
    a. Palindrome
    b. Cruciform
    c. Hairpin
    d. None
30. Find the accurate statement regarding the phosphodiester bonding in nucleic acids between neighboring nucleotides.
    a. The next nucleotide's 3'-hydroxyl joins the 3'-phosphate of the previous nucleotide.
    b. The next nucleotide's 5'-hydroxyl joins the 5'-phosphate of the previous nucleotide.
    c. The 3'-hydroxyl of one nucleotide links the 5'-phosphate of the subsequent nucleotide.
    d. The 5'-hydroxyl of one nucleotide links the 3'-phosphate of the subsequent nucleotide.
31. Which of the following nucleotides does not contain deoxyribose but solely ribose sugar?
    a. Pentose sugar-phosphate uracil
    b. Pentose sugar-phosphate thymine
    c. Pentose sugar-phosphate thymine
    d. Phosphate, pentose, and cytosine
32. Which characteristic does this double-stranded molecule possess when it forms a B-DNA structure
    a. The two strands will have parallel orientations and identical sequences.
    b. Every base pair will contain one purine and one pyrimidine.
    c. The helix will be right-handed with 12 base pairs per turn
    d. There are both covalent and non-covalent bonds between the two chains
33. Determine which strand of the below-mentioned is the complimentary sequence of DNA with ATGCCGATC.
    a. TACGGCUAG
    b. TTCGGCTAG
    c. UTCGGCUAG
    d. TACGGCTAG
34. Which way does the basic structure of DNA and RNA synthesis proceed in?
    a. 5' —> 3'
    b. 3' —> 5"
    c. 4' —> 6'
    d. 3' > 6'

35. It is a feature of genetic material that is eukaryotic
    a. The supercoiled circular DNA molecules that make up eukaryotic genetic material are complexed with proteins to form chromosomes.
    b. To compress eukaryotic genetic material, the double helix is wrapped around histone proteins to create nucleosomes.
    c. To create a scaffold, linker sections are folded around non-histone proteins to compress the genetic material of eukaryotes
    d. Relaxed linear DNA molecules complexed with RNA into a 30 nm fiber make up the genetic material of eukaryotes
36. A type of soil bacterium known as a crown gall is capable of transforming neighboring cells and causing them to grow into a tumor
    a. Salmonella
    b. Pseudomonas
    c. Streptococcus
    d. Agrobacterium tumefaciens
37. When a double-stranded nucleic acid is denatured, it increases its ability to absorb UV radiation and is known as
    a. Hypochromic effect.b. Melting temperature
    c. Hyperchromic effect.d.annealing temperature
38. The sequence of inverted repeats that appears within every single strand of DNA is known as
    a. Mirror repeat
    b. Palindrome
    c. Hairpin
    d. None
39. This explains a eukaryotic chromosome's structural characteristics
    a. A double helix made up of nucleosomes, each with four million base pairs, is present.
    b. It is organized into a fiber that is 30 nm in diameter and affixed to the cell membrane.
    c. It has linker sections that are wound into a helix and placed into loops
    d. For compaction, a single double-stranded linear DNA molecule is attached to proteins.
40. Which characteristic does each of the five histone proteins share?
    a. These proteins have comparatively large molecular weights and are acidi C
    b. They are positively charged globular proteins.
    c. These proteins are fibrous and include a lot of α-helix
    d. They are multimeric proteins that contain large amounts of Lys and Arg
41. It is a characteristic shared by the genetic material of bacteria and viruses
    a. Plasmids can be formed by compacting both
    b. both may be linear, single-stranded RNA
    c. It is possible to compress both into inverted repeats
    d. Double-stranded, circular DNA is possible for both.

42. In eukaryotic cells, characteristics of histones are
    a. Are globular proteins that carry a negative charge.
    b. Include a significant quantity of basic amino acids
    c. Be more than 100,000 molecular weights
    d. Have a β-pleated sheet and an α-helix
43. Which of the following statements about the retroviral genome is true?
    a. Gag, pol, and env genes present in the retroviral genome
    b. Genome is dsDNA
    c. Genome contains introns
    d. Genome contains histones
44. What force can stabilize a typical DNA double helix?-helix
    a. The phosphate groups that join adjacent nucleotides together create N-glycosidic linkages with the deoxyribose rings.
    b. A non-covalent interaction known as "base-stacking" takes place between the comparatively hydrophobic bases inside the helix.
    c. A non-covalent contact known as base-pairing takes place between adjacent bases on the same strand of DNA
    d. The hydrophilic sugar-phosphate groups can interact with one another because they are outside of the helix
45. Virus X, a novel virus, is isolated and investigate Which chemical is most likely to contain virus X's genetic material?
    a. A linear RNA molecule with plasmids
    b. A nucleosome - containing circular DNA molecule
    c. A 10 billion molecular weight circular RNA molecule
    d. A linear DNA molecule with 10,000 base pairs
46. which are traits of the genetic material found in bacteria
    a. It is joined to a protein scaffold and is linear
    b. It is supercoiled and double-stranded
    c. It is compacted into palindromes and round in shape
    d. It is relaxed and single-stranded
47. Name the double-stranded DNA molecule that would denature at roughly the same temperature as the molecule with a 5'-(GA)20-3' strand
    a. One of two types of molecules is present with (GC)20 strand
    b. A molecule with a (GACT)10 strand inside of it
    c. A molecule with a (GGGA)10 strand inside of it
    d. One of two types of molecules with (TA)20 strands.

48. What trait will the single 5'-(GA)20-3' strand and another single-stranded DNA molecule with the sequence 5'-(AT)20-3' have in common?
    a. A palindromic sequence is present in both.
    b. They might hybridize to form an RNA molecule together.
    c. The same secondary structures may emerge in both cases
    d. The total charge for both will be the same.
49. Assume that the following characteristics of DNA molecules are discovered after research on a range of animals. Which characteristic would be consistent with the theory that DNA makes up genetic material?
    a. All creatures' DNA is made up of the same nucleotides
    b. The base composition of DNA from two distinct creatures is the same
    c. An organism's DNA doesn't change as it gets older
    d. Two distinct cells belonging to the same organism have different DNA
50. Which is a possible sequence and structure for this DNA molecule
    a. If the single-stranded molecule has the sequence 5'-(GATC)10, then its double-stranded form could assume an H-DNA structure.
    b. If the single-stranded molecule has the sequence 5'-(CTGA)10, then its double-stranded form could assume a hairpin structure
    c. If the single-stranded molecule has the sequence 5'-(ATGC)10, then its double-stranded form could assume a Z-DNA structure
    d. If the single-stranded molecule has the sequence 5'-(TGAC)10, then its double-stranded form could assume a cruciform structure.
51. Which force is known to stabilize a DNA double-helix
    a. The interior of the helix contains hydrophobic bases, where each base pair is supported by an equal amount of hydrogen bonds.
    b. In opposing strands of the helix, nitrogenous bases may create non-covalent N-glycosidic bonds
    c. Adjacent bases within the same strand of the helix may interact covalently through base-stacking
    d. The outside of the helix contains hydrophilic sugar-phosphate groups, which are capable of interacting with water.
52. Which of the following double-stranded DNA molecules would denature at a temperature lower than that of the double-stranded molecule with 40 base pairs that were previously described?
    a. A 40-base pair molecule with adenines making up 25% of the bases
    b. A molecule consisting of 10 base pairs, 20% of which are cytosines
    c. A molecule with 20 base pairs, 10% of which are thymines
    d. A molecule consisting of 30 base pairs, 40% of which are guanines

53. What feature of a double-stranded RNA molecule of the same size will this one have in common with it?
    a. There will be a secondary structure in both.
    b. The base will break down both of them
    c. There are four different kinds of base pairs in each.
    d. Inverted repeats will be present in both.
54. 40 nucleotides make up a single-stranded DNA molecule, which bears the sequence 5'-(GA)20-3'. What is the characteristic of this one single strand
    a. There will be several phosphodiester bonds in the single-stranded chain, each connecting a 2'- and a 5'-carbon.
    b. There will be one 5' end and one 3' end in the single-stranded chain.
    c. Purines and pyrimidines will both be present in the single-stranded chain
    d. Both ribose and deoxyribose will be present in the single-stranded chain
55. Which is a general property in both of nucleosides and nucleotides
    a. both contain a hemiacetal or hemiketal bond
    b. Both contain a pentose in the form of a furanose
    c. Both contain at least one 5'-phosphate group
    d. Both contain a nitrogenous base that forms covalent H-bonds
56. Which structural feature is found in the single-stranded DNA molecule
    a. A It can have a negatively charged backbone composed of nitrogenous bases
    b. Each purine and pyrimidine will be paired with a complementary base
    c. It can have one end with a 5'-phosphate group while the other end has A 2'-hydroxyl group
    d. Each 3',5'-phosphodiester bond will contain one phosphate group linking two deoxyribose sugars
57. Which of the following function of DNA is necessary for the purpose of evolution
    a. Transcription b. Replication
    c. Translation d. Mutation
58. Which property is shared commonly by both CTP and dTDP
    a. Both contain the same sugar.
    b. Both contain a planar six-membered ring
    c. Both contain the same charge at cellular pH
    d. Both contain phosphodiester bonds
59. Which characteristic is found similar in both purines and pyrimidines
    a. They both have aromatic rings that undergo substantial tautomerization at neutral pH
    b. They both can form stable N-glycosidic bonds with β D-ribofuranose
    c. They both are weak bases that can be positively charged at neutral pH
    d. They both have multiple pKa values that result in zwitterion forms

60. Which component is commonly found in both guanosine and uridine
   a. Both contain an aldohexose.
   b. Both contain a 1',9 - bond
   c. Both contain a pyranose
   d. Both contain three hydroxyl groups.
61. Which characteristic is commonly shared by both adenine and cytosine
   a. Both contain one methyl group b. Both are heterocyclic
   c. Both contain one keto group d. Both are anomeric
62. How does a nucleoside become made?
   a. A sugar + a phosphate b. A base + a phosphate
   c. A base + a sugar d. A base + a sugar + phosphate
63. Which property is commonly found in nucleosides and nucleotides
   a. Both contain a nitrogenous base, a pentose and at least one phosphate group.
   b. Both contain an anomeric carbon atom that is part of a β-N-glycosidic bond
   c. Both contain an aldose with hydroxyl groups that can tautomerize.
   d. Both contain a covalent phosphodiester bond that is broken in strong acid
64. Which of the following is not promoted by histone tail modification
   a. Nucleosome remodeling
   b. Nucleosome sliding
   c. Gene expression
   d. Formation of repressive structures
65. Which property is commonly shared by both GDP and AMP
   a. Both contain the same charge at neutral pH
   b. Both contain the same furanose
   c. Both contain the same purine
   d Both contain the same number of phosphate groups
66. Which component is found in both adenosine and deoxycytidine
   a. Both contain a pyranose.
   b. Both contain a 3'-OH group
   c. Both contain a pyrimidine.
   d. Both contain a 1,1'-N-glycosidic bond
67. Which characteristic is commonly shared by purines and pyrimidines
   a. Both contain two heterocyclic rings with aromatic character
   b. Both exist as neutral zwitterions under cellular conditions
   c. Both exist in planar configurations with a hemiacetal linkage
   d. Both can form multiple non-covalent hydrogen bonds
68. In the following, identify the purine base of nucleic acids
   a. Cytosine b. Guanine
   c. Thymine d. Uracil

69. What is the correct pair of the four segments (R1, R2, R3, and R4) during recombination of the DNA
   a. R1 and R2, R3 and R4
   b. R1 and R3, R2 and R4
   c. R2 and R1, R3 and R4
   d. R2 and R3, R1 and R4
70. Which histone molecule produces novel binding sites for protein components of the kinetochore
   a. H3
   b. CENP – A
   c. H2A
   d. H4
71. Which of the following describes a Eukaryotic ORF character?
   a. Non – overlapping
   b. Contiguous
   c. Intron
   d. 3 – nucleotide codons
72. How many unusual bases are observed in a tRNA molecule?
   a. 1
   b. 6
   c. 3
   d. 5
73. Which structural feature is commonly shared by both uracil and thymine?
   a. Both contain one methyl group
   b. Both contain two keto groups.
   c. Both contain three nitrogen atoms
   d. Both contain a five-membered ring
74. Which of the following pairs is incorrect?
   a. Phospholipids –phosphor diester linkage
   b. Nucleic acid – hydrophobic bond
   c. Polysaccharide – glycosidic bond
   d. Proteins – peptide bond
75. What is the slowest process out of the following ones?
   a. Splicing
   b. Transcription
   c. Translation
   d. Replication
76. Select the unusual nucleic acid library from the list below
   a. A DNA library
   b. C DNA library
   c. Z DNA library
   d. B DNA library
77. Which chemical bond keeps DNA's double helix stable?
   a. Hydrophobic bond
   b. Covalent bond
   c. Ionic bond
   d. Hydrogen bond
78. Which of the following does not belong to the RNA molecule?
   a. Adenine
   b. Cytosine
   c. Guanine
   d. Thymine
79. Which of the following describes RNA as the genetic material?
   a. Some viruses and prokaryotes
   b. Some prokaryotes only
   c. Some Eukaryotes
   d. Some viruses only

80. Which of these claims, as per Chargaff's guidelines, is INCORRECT?
    a. The molar ratio of A to T or C to G = 1
    b. The composition of DNA remains the same in all the species
    c. The % C+G $\neq$ % A+T
    d. The sum of purine = sum of pyrimidine
81. A leaf sample with its DNA purified has 20.0 mole of guanine. Determine the approximate purine residue percentage.
    a. 20% b. 50%
    c. 40% d. 60%
82. What two molecules of the Uvr component examine the DNA during nucleotide excision repair?
    a. UvrB, UvrC b. UvrA, UvrB
    c. UvrD, UvrA d. UvrC, UvrA
83. In nucleotides, the pentoses are
    a. In α furanose form b. In β furanose form
    c. Both d. None
84. Which of the following compounds has an anticodon?
    a. Messenger RNA b. Transfer RNA
    c. DNA d. Ribosomal RNA
85. A set of neighboring nucleotides is connected by
    a. Peptide bond b. Phosphodiester bond
    c. Ionic bond d. Covalent bond
86. The B-DNA's width is
    a. 340 Å b. 20 Å
    c. 3.4 Å d. 34 Å
87. The genetic material DNA found in which of the following
    a. In Prokaryotes only
    b. Eukaryotes only
    c. Some Viruses, prokaryotes and Eukaryotes
    d. Viruses only
88. Which of the following describes RNA as the genetic material?
    a. Some viruses and prokaryotes b. Some prokaryotes only
    c. Some Eukaryotes d. Some viruses only
89. The length of a B-DNA turn is
    a. 34 Å b. 3.4 Å
    c. 340 Å d. 20 Å

90. DNA can be found in
   a. Nucleus only
   b. Nucleus, Mitochondria and Chloroplast
   c. Nucleus, Mitochondria and Golgi Bodies
   d. Nucleus, Mitochondria and ER

91. There are 60 guanine and 60 thymine residues in a brief segment of DNA The DNA fragment's total nucleotide count is
   a. 240   b. 220
   c. 180   d. 120

92. A nucleotide's sugar molecule is
   a. Hexose   b. Pentose
   c. Triose   d. Tetrose

93. In a DNA double helix, the two strands are connected by
   a. Covalent bond   b. Ionic bond
   c. Hydrogen bond   d. Phosphodiester bond

94. Out of the following claims, which one is false?
   a. Deoxyribose, depending on the situation.
   b. A glycosidic bond binds the bases of nucleotides to a pentose sugar molecule.
   c. The nucleotide's sugar molecule is arranged in a L shape.
   d. A nucleotide's sugar component is either ribose

95. Which of these is NOT a characteristic of DNA?
   a. The nucleoside is the base unit
   b. Base pairs are connected by hydrogen bonds
   c. The antiparallel and complementary strands
   d. The sugar-phosphate backbone

96. Which of the following compounds has a codon on it?
   a. DNA   b. Ribosomal RNA
   c. Transfer RNA   d. Messenger RNA

97. What are nucleotides composed?
   a. A sugar + a phosphate   b. A base + a sugar + phosphate
   c. A base + a phosphate   d. A base + a sugar

98. A five-carbon sugar with a hydrogen atom missing from the second carbon can be found in
   a. RNA   b. rDNA
   c. mRNA   d. dNA

99. Nucleic acid-building components are
   a. Histones   b. Nucleosides
   c. Nucleotides   d. Amino acids

100. Which of the following is present in RNA but absent in DNA?

a. Phosphate b. Deoxyribose

c. Adenine d. Uracil

Answer Key

1	d	2	a	3	a	4	c	5	b	6	a	7	d
8	b	9	d	10	d	11	a	12	c	13	a	14	b
15	b	16	a	17	b	18	a	19	b	20	c	21	a
22		23	b	24	b	25	d	26	a	27	b	28	a
29	a	30	c	31	a	32	b	33	d	34	a	35	b
36	d	37	c	38	a	39	d	40	b	41	d	42	b
43	a	44	b	45	a	46	b	47	b	48	d	49	c
50	c	51	c	52	b	53	d	54	b	55	b	56	d
57	d	58	b	59	b	60	d	61	b	62	c	63	b
64	b	65	b	66	b	67	d	68	b	69	d	70	b
71	c	72	a	73	b	74	b	75	c	76	b	77	d
78	d	79	d	80	b	81	b	82	b	83	b	84	b
85	b	86	b	87	c	88	d	89	a	90	b	91	a
92	b	93	c	94	b	95	a	96	d	97	b	98	d
99	c	100	d										

8

Biochemistry of Enzymes

***Ramesh D.*[1] *and Barkha Gupta*[2]**

[1]*Department of Veterinary Physiology and Biochemistry, Veterinary College, Hassan (KVAFSU), Karnataka-573202*

[2]*Department of Veterinary Physiology and Biochemistry, Post Graduate Institute of Veterinary Education and Research (PGIVER), Jaipur (RAJUVAS), Rajasthan-302031*

Introduction

All enzymes are proteins, except a tiny subset of catalytic RNA molecules. Most of the classical metabolic enzymes are named by adding the suffix -ase to the name of their substrates or to a descriptive term for the reactions they catalyze. For example, urease has urea as a substrate. Alcohol dehydrogenase catalyzes the removal of hydrogen from alcohols (i.e., the oxidation of alcohols). A committee of the International Union of Biochemistry and Molecular Biology (IUBMB maintains a classification scheme that categorizes enzymes according to the general class of organic chemical reaction that is catalyzed The six classes are Oxidoreductases, Transferases, Hydrolases, Lyases, Isomerases, and Ligases.

The integrity of their natural protein structure is necessary for their catalytic activity. Catalytic activity is typically lost when an enzyme denatures or dissociates into its constituent subunits. An enzyme's catalytic activity is always eliminated when it is disassembled into its constituent amino acids. Thus, the catalytic activity of protein enzymes depends on their primary, secondary, tertiary, and quaternary structures. Aside from their amino acid residues, certain enzymes don't need any other chemical groups to function. Others need a cofactor, which is an extra chemical element. Cofactors can be complex organic or metalloorganic molecules called coenzymes, or they can be one or more inorganic ions like Fe^{2+}, Mg^{2+}, Mn^{2+}, or Zn^{2+}.

Charles-Adolphe Wurtz first hypothesized the existence of the enzyme-substrate complex in 1880. The ground state, which is the average molecule's (S or P) contribution to the system's free energy under a specific set of conditions, is the beginning point for either the forward or backward reaction.

The activation energy, ΔG, is the difference between the ground state and transition state energy levels. Catalysts mediated by enzymes reduce activation energies, increasing reaction rates. The step (or steps) having the highest activation energy, known as the rate-limiting step, determines the overall pace of a reaction when multiple stages are involved. In the transition state, weak enzyme-substrate interactions are optimized.

Various catalytic mechanisms encompass entropy reduction, metal ion catalysis, covalent catalysis, and general acid-base catalysis. One can quantitatively express the relationship between substrate concentration and reaction rate. The rate equation for an enzyme-catalyzed reaction involving a single substrate is known as the **Michaelis-Menten equation**. The Michaelis constant Km, which is unique to each enzyme operating on a particular substrate, is the substrate concentration that yields a reaction rate equal to half of Vmax.

- Featuring universal acid-base catalysis, covalent catalysis, and transition-state stabilization, chymotrypsin is a serine protease whose mechanism is well understood.
- One great example of induced fit employing substrate binding energy is seen in hexokinase.
- Metal ion catalysis drives the enolase reaction forward Lysozyme catalyzes two consecutive nucleophilic displacement reactions by means of covalent and general acid catalysis.

Enzyme inhibitors are substances that bind to enzymes and decrease their activity. Two broad classes of enzyme inhibitors are classified as **Reversible enzymes** and **Irreversible enzymes**. Competitive and non-competitive enzyme inhibition is a prevalent form of reversible inhibition. A competitive inhibitor and substrate engage in competition for an enzyme's active site.

An enzyme can be irreversibly inhibited in a competitive, noncompetitive, or mixed manner. Competitive inhibitors do not undergo enzymatic transformation; instead, they bind reversibly to the active site and compete with the substrate. Only the ES complex, and not the active site, is bound by non-competitive inhibitors. Once more, mixed inhibitors bind to E or ES at a location different from the active site. An inhibitor forms a covalent bond or a very stable non-covalent contact with an active site to permanently bind in irreversible inhibition.

Suicide inactivators are irreversible inhibitors. Until they attach to an enzyme's active site, these substances are largely inert. The initial chemical stages of a typical enzymatic reaction are followed by a suicide inactivator, but instead of becoming the typical result, the inactivator becomes a highly reactive substance that irreversibly unites with the enzyme.

In response to specific signals, regulatory enzymes show changes in their catalytic activity. The cell can adapt to changing needs for energy and for the biomolecules needed for growth and repair by modifying the pace of reactions catalyzed by regulatory enzymes and, consequently, the rate of complete metabolic sequences. When a modulator binds, allosteric enzymes undergo conformational changes.

An allosteric enzyme catalyzes the regulatory step in many metabolic pathways. Allosteric enzyme kinetic properties deviate from Michaelis-Menten behavior. Certain regulatory enzymes experience reversible covalent changes. In feedback inhibition, the pathway's final product inhibits the pathway's initial enzyme. Proteolytic cleavage of an enzyme precursor regulates certain enzymes and other proteins. Allosteric enzyme activity is modulated by the reversible binding of a particular modulator to a regulatory site. The substrate itself or another metabolite can act as modulators, and they can have either an inhibitory or stimulatory impact. Allosteric enzymes' kinetic behavior reflects the cooperative interactions between their subunits.

The covalent alteration of a particular functional group required for activity affects other regulating enzymes. One popular method of controlling enzyme activity is the phosphorylation of the amino acid residues. Many proteolytic enzymes are produced as zymogens, which are inactive precursors that are activated by breaking apart short peptide segments.

1. Enzymes that catalyze the transfer of atoms or groups between two molecules are known as
   a. Oxidoreductases b. Transferases
   c. Ligases d. Isomerases
2. Complex organic or metalloorganic molecules necessary for enzymes to function at their best are
   a. Coenzymes b. Iso enzyme
   b. Organic compounds d. Apoenzyme
3. Who concluded that yeast could only convert sugar into alcohol through fermentation in the 1850s?
   a. Emil fisher b. Edward Jenner
   c. Eduard Buchner d. Louis Pasteur
4. Scientist who coined the term Enzyme is
   a. Michaelis–Menten b. Frederick W. Kühne
   c. Robert Corey d. Nirenberg
5. Scientist isolated and crystallized the urease enzyme in 1926
   a. Linus Pauling b. Max Perutz
   c. James Sumner d. Watson and crick
6. Nicotinamide adenine dinucleotide –NAD is a coenzyme which can transfer which of the following group
   a. Amino group b. Hydride ion (H-)
   c. Carboxyl group d. Acyl group
7. Pyridoxal phosphate is involved in the transfer of which of the following group
   a. Carboxyl group b. Acyl group
   c. Amino group d. Phosphoryl group
8. Tetrahydrofolate is involved in the transfer of which of the following group
   a. Carboxyl groupb. One-carbon group
   c. Sulfhydryl groupd. Nitrogen group
9. Thiamine pyrophosphate is involved in the transfer of which of the following group
   a. Carboxyl group b. Amino group
   c. Sulfhydryl group d. Aldehydes group
10. The existence of the enzyme substrate complex was initially hypothesized in 1880 by
   a. Charles-Adolphe Wurtz b. JBS Haldane
   c. Maud Menton d. Michaelis

11. The portion of the enzyme that is responsible for the enzyme-catalyzed reaction is
    a. Coenzyme b. rRNA
    c. Cofactor d. Active site
12. Which of the following best describes how the catalytic efficacy of the two enzymes differed
    a. The Km value of the enzyme b. Protein
    c. Substrate concentration d. Temperature
13. It is a popular enzyme used to tenderize meat
    a. Pepsin b. LDH
    c. Amylase d. Papain
14. Enzymes accelerate the catalytic processes by lowering
    a. Free energy b. Activation energy
    c. Randomness d. Temperature
15. Which of the following coenzyme is derived from riboflavin (B2)
    a. FMN and FAD b. NAD
    c. Co-A d. Lipoamide
16. Which vitamin among these is connected to the coenzyme biocytin?
    a. Thiamine b. Nicotinic acid
    c. Biotin d. Pyridoxine
17. Which classes of enzymes are responsible for catalyzing the reduction-oxidation process?
    a. Oxidoreductase b. Transaminase
    c. Phosphofructokinase d. Glutamine Synthetase
18. Which of the following processes is catalyzed by Lyase?
    a. Bond formation b. Bond breaking
    c. Bond intramolecular rearrangement d. No action on bonds
19. What function does phosphorylase fulfill?
    a. Sulfate group transfer
    b. Inorganic phosphate can be transferred
    c. Amino group transfer
    d. Acyl group transfer
20. An enzyme is responsible for joining the ends of two nucleic acid strands
    a. Oxidoreductase b. Synthetase
    c. Ligase d. Transferase
21. Which of these is an illustration of an enzyme's competitive inhibition?
    a. Papain by phosphorous
    b. Succinic dehydrogenase by malonic acid
    c. Carbonic anhydrase by zinc
    d. cytochrome oxidase by cyanide

22. The model was proposed by Koshland in 1958
    a. Lock and key model
    b. Concerted model
    c. Substrate strain theory
    d. Induced fit model
23. An un-catalyzed reaction involved which of the following
    a. High activation energy
    b. Low activation energy
    c. Balanced activation energy
    d. Binding energy
24. Which of the following statements about the enzymes are true
    a. Enzyme is a biocatalyst
    b. Enzyme increases the rate of reaction
    c. Enzyme decreases the activation energy of the reaction
    d. All of the above
25. Which of these statements regarding enzymes is true
    a. Apoenzyme-Cofactor=Holoenzyme
    b. Apoenzyme + Cofactor = Holoenzyme
    c. Apoenzyme=Cofactor-Holoenzyme
    d. None
26. Structurally an enzyme's competitive inhibitor is
    a. Structural analog of substrate
    b. Functional analog of substrate
    c. Structural analog of Enzyme
    d. Functional analog of enzyme
27. SI Unit of enzymatic activity is called
    a. Kg
    b. Katal
    c. Km
    d. Svedberg
28. Which of the following conditions describes Gout?
    a. Decreased production of CPK
    b. Overproduction of LDH
    c. Overproduction of Xanthine Oxidase
    d. Less production of xanthine oxidase
29. A deficiency of ß-glucocerebrosidase leads to which of the following metabolic disorder
    a. Gaucher's Disease
    b. Faber's disease
    c. Krabbe's disease
    d. Lesh-Nyhan Syndrome
30. The group of enzymes differ in amino acid composition but catalyzing the same reaction is called
    a. Co-enzyme
    b. Apo enzyme
    c. Co-factor
    d. Isoenzyme
31. Which type of enzymes are pepsin and urease examples of the following?
    a. Hydrolases
    b. Lyases
    c. Oxidoreductases
    d. Ligases

32. Of the following enzyme, which is related to molecular biology?
    a. DNA ligase
    b. DNA topoisomerase
    c. Polymerase
    d. All of the above
33. Ribozymes are
    a. Protein acting as an enzyme
    b. RNA acting as an enzyme
    c. DNA acting as an enzyme
    d. None
34. Abzymes are known as
    a. Antigen acting as an enzyme
    b. Protein acting as an enzyme
    c. Antibody acting as an enzyme
    d. Lipid act as antigen
35. Which of the following is an Illustration of a Pro-enzyme?
    a. Trypsin
    b. Pepsinogen
    c. Papain
    d. Amylase
36. Which of the following enzymes do not require co-enzymes for their activity?
    a. Intracellular enzymes
    b. Pro enzymes
    c. Extracellular enzymes
    d. Co enzymes
37. allosteric enzyme activity is affected by
    a. Cofactors
    b. Metal ions
    c. Coenzyme
    d. Allosteric modulators
38. Feedback inhibition entails
    a. End Product inhibition
    b. Suicide inhibition
    c. Non-competitive inhibition
    d. competitive inhibition
39. In competitive inhibition, inhibitors have a structural resemblance to the
    a. Inhibitor
    b. Enzyme
    c. Coenzyme
    d. Substrate
40. Enzyme functions best at a specific temperature called
    a. Melting temperature
    b. Freezing temperature
    c. Optimum temperature
    d. Thermal inactivity
41. Another name for the "Ping-Pong reaction" is
    a. Double-displacement bi-substrate reaction
    b. Single substrate
    c. Competitive reaction
    d. Lineweaver Burk plot
42. Another name for the Lock and Key model is
    a. Template Model
    b. Sequential
    c. Concerted model
    d. Random
43. Which bond does not correspond to the enzyme-substrate complex formation?
    a. Ionic bond
    b. Di-sulfide bonds
    c. Wander walls interaction
    d. Hydrogen bond

44. Which of the following claims is untrue about the nature of enzymes?
    a. Enzymes are proteins in nature
    b. Enzymes are colloidal
    c. Enzymes are thermolabile
    d. Enzymes are the inorganic catalyst
45. Which of the enzymatic inhibitors listed below has a lower Km Value?
    a. Competitive inhibitors b. Un-competitive
    c. Non-competitive d. Irreversible
46. In which condition the apoenzymes separate from coenzymes
    a. Change in substrate b. Change in pH
    c. Change in enzyme d. Change in water
47. Reversible covalent alteration entails
    a. Activation of co-enzyme b. Activation of protein
    c. Activation of pro-enzymes d. Activation of co-factor
48. by adding which of the suffixes, enzyme names are derived from their substrates
    a. -ase b. -in
    c. -ion d. -eos
49. Within the cells enzyme exists as
    a. Solid b. Gaseous
    c. Crystal d. Colloid
50. The enzymes responsible for the hydrolysis of peptides and esters are
    a. Transferases b. Lyases
    c. Hydrolases d. Isomerase
51. Without changing the molecular weight or number of atoms, an enzyme can catalyze the rearrangement of atomic groups
    a. Hydrolase b. Transferase
    c. Isomerase d. Oxidoreductase
52. The enzyme that hydrolyses starch to maltose is called
    a. Amylase b. Pepsin
    c. Chymotrypsin d. Trypsin
53. Effect of pH on the enzyme activity results in
    a. Hyperbola curve b. Bell-shaped curve
    c. Parabola curve d. Rectangular curve
54. Serum amylase is used for the detection of
    a. Nephritis b. Myositis
    c. Acute pancreatitis d. Pruritis
55. Serum glutamate pyruvate transaminase (SGPT)/ALT is used to identify
    a. Kidney disorder b. Liver disorder
    c. Spleen disorder d. Urinary bladder affections

56. Acid phosphatase (ACP) is specific for the detection of
    a. Liver cancer b. Prostate cancer
    c. Kidney cancer d. Skeletal muscle disorder
57. Aldolase is used for the detection of
    a. Liver disorder b. Kidney disorder
    c. Brain affections d. Muscular dystrophy
58. The earliest enzymatic marker of Myocardial infarction is
    a. Creatine phosphokinase (CPK) b. LDH
    c. ALP d. AST
59. Number of Iso enzymes in LDH
    a. 4 b. 5
    c. 6 d. 3
60. Serum Alkaline phosphatase (ALP) is an indicator of the
    a. Rickets and obstructive jaundice b. Kidney disorder
    c. Brain affections d. Liver disorder
61. Early protein marker and cardiac-specific to Myocardial infarction
    a. Cardiac troponin I b. Myosin
    c. Myoglobin d. Actin
62. Enzymes are classified into
    a. Two classes b. Three classes
    c. Six major classes d. Five classes
63. Decreased Glucose 6-phosphate dehydrogenase (G6PD in RBC results in
    a. Fatty liver
    b. Congenital deficiency with hemolytic anemia
    c. Nephritis
    d. Pericarditis
64. γ-Glutamyl transpeptidase (GGT) is a sensitive indicator of
    a. Brain disorders b. Gall bladder affections
    c. Biliary disorder d. Alcoholism
65. The number of Isoenzymes of creatine phosphokinase includes
    a. Three b. Two
    c. four d. One
66. The Isoenzyme of CPK is known to be the earliest reliable indication of myocardial infarction
    a. CPK 1 b. CPK2 (MB)
    c. CPK-3 d. CPK-4

67. Decreased serum Ceruloplasmin results in
    a. Parkinson's Disease
    b. Wilson's disease (hepatolenticular degeneration)
    c. Addison's disease
    d. Cushing's disease
68. Streptokinase enzyme is commercially used to dissolve
    a. Blood clots in circulation
    b. Cells in circulation
    c. Albumin in circulation
    d. Protein in circulation
69. Enzymes like asparaginase are commercially employed in the treatment of
    a. Fever
    b. Multiple ulcers
    c. Leukemias
    d. Diarrhea
70. Which of the following enzymatic reactions is an example of feedback inhibition
    a. Cholesterol inhibits HMG CoA reductase
    b. Hexokinase by G6P
    c. Pyruvate kinase by glucose
    d. PFK by glucose
71. The Isoenzyme of CPK present in the Brain mainly contains which of the following
    a. MM
    b. MB
    c. BR
    d. BB
72. Enzyme Rennin is commercially used for the production of
    a. Mutton
    b. Cheese
    c. Paneer
    d. Khoa
73. Which of the following enzymes is commonly used in ELISA
    a. Horseradish peroxidase
    b. Alkaline phosphatase
    c. Both a & b
    d. None
74. Diisopropyl fluorophosphate (DFP) inhibits which of the following enzymes irreversibly
    a. Acetylcholine esterase (AChE)
    b. Glucose oxidase
    c. Arginase
    d. Hexokinase
75. The regulatory enzyme of Glycolysis
    a. Hexokinase
    b. Phosphofructokinase
    c. Pyruvate Kinase
    d. All of the above
76. The regulatory enzyme of Cholesterol synthesis includes
    a. HMG Co-A synthase
    b. HMG Co-A reductase
    c. HMG Co-A oxidase
    d. None
77. Allopurinol, employed in the treatment of gout, inhibits which enzyme to reduce the formation of uric acid
    a. Mixed function oxidase
    b. Xanthine oxidase
    c. Urease
    d. Allointase

78. The regulatory enzyme of Ketone body synthesis includes
    a. HMG Co-A Synthase
    b. HMG Co-A reductase
    c. HMG Co-A
    d. HMG Co-A lyase
79. The regulatory enzyme of the Urea cycle includes
    a. Arginase
    b. Carbamoyl phosphate synthetase II
    c. Carbamoyl phosphate synthetase I
    d. Arginosuccinase
80. Which of the following enzymes is most sensitive to fluoride ions?
    a. Aldolase
    b. Enolase
    c. Pyruvate kinase
    d. Aconitase
81. Regarding the Active site of an enzyme
    a. Very Rigid
    b. Preformed conformation
    c. Very flexible
    d. Not rigid and not pre-shaped
82. The specificity of the enzyme is mostly dependent on which of the following
    a. Co enzyme
    b. Apoenzyme
    c. Co factor
    d. None
83. The function of the Co-enzyme S – Adenosylmethionine is
    a. Donates sulfhydryl group
    b. Donates ethyl group
    c. Donates methyl group in biosynthetic reactions
    d. Donates hydroxy methyl group
84. Severe combined immunodeficiency (SCID is a serious immunodeficiency disorder that is mainly due to
    a. Adenosine deaminase (ADA)
    b. Sphingomyelinase
    c. Arginase
    d. Hexosaminidase
85. Lesch-Nyhan syndrome is an X-linked recessive disorder, caused by a deficiency of
    a. Adenosine phosphoribosyl transferase (APRT)
    b. Hypoxanthine-guanine phosphoribosyl transferase (HGPRT)
    c. Adenosine deaminase (ADA)
    d. Sphingomyelinase
86. Which of the following enzymes that converts ribonucleotides into deoxyribonucleotides
    a. Ribonucleotide reductase
    b. Sphingomyelinase
    c. Adenosine phosphoribosyl transferase (APRT)
    d. Hexosaminidase

87. Velocity versus Substrate concentration in a single subunit enzyme result in
   a. Hyperbolic curve b. Parabolic
   c. Straight line d. Rectangular

88. A competitive inhibitor of the enzyme Dihydrofolate reductase is
   a. Riboflavin b. Aminopterin
   c. Biotin d. CO_2

89. Coenzyme A (CoA) is derived from the vitamin
   a. Pantothenic acid b. Riboflavin
   c. Thiamine d. Biotin

90. Coenzyme Phosphoadenosine phosphosulfate (PAPS) is involved in which of the following?
   a. Donates sulfate for the synthesis of mucopolysaccharides
   b. Donates methyl group
   c. Donates ethyl group
   d. Donates hydroxy methyl group

91. Allosteric enzymes undergo which of the following in response to modulator binding
   a. Change its active site b. Conformational Changes
   c. Change its composition d. No changes occur

92. Suicide inhibitors are also called
   a. Sequential inhibitor b. Substrate analogue
   c. Ping pong inhibitor d. Mechanism-based inactivators

93. Numerous proteolytic enzymes begin their synthesis as inactive precursors known as
   a. Zymogens b. Trypsin
   c. Papain d. Chymotrypsin

94. Which of the following is true about non-competitive inhibitors?
   a. Affects the Km but not the Vmax b. Affects the Vmax but not the Km
   c. Affect both Km and Vmax d. None

95. The regulatory enzymes of beta-oxidation of fatty acids include
   a. Carnitine acyl transferase 1 b. Carnitine acyl transferase 1I
   c. Arginase d. Acyl Co-A dehydrogenase

96. Enzymes hold the metals rather tightly which are not readily exchanged are called
   a. Metallo enzyme b. Organic enzyme
   c. Pepsin d. Inorganic enzyme

97. When the enzymes are exposed to a temperature above 50°C results in
   a. Coagulation b. Flocculation
   c. Precipitation d. Denaturation

98. The km value of an enzyme is not dependent on the
   a. Concentration of substrate   b. Concentration of enzyme
   c. Concentration of inhibitor   d. None

99. A low Km value indicates the following between enzyme and substrate
   a. Strong affinity   b. High affinity
   c. Moderate affinity   d. None

100. Velocity versus substrate concentration in Allosteric enzymes results in
   a. Hyperbolic curve   b. Straight line
   c. Rectangular curve   d. Sigmoid curve

Answer Key

1	b	2	a	3	d	4	b	5	c	6	c	7	c
8	b	9	d	10	a	11	d	12	a	13	d	14	b
15	a	16	c	17	a	18	b	19	b	20	c	21	b
22	d	23	a	24	d	25	b	26	a	27	b	28	c
29	a	30	d	31	a	32	d	33	b	34	c	35	b
36	c	37	d	38	a	39	d	40	c	41	a	42	a
43	b	44	d	45	a	46	b	47	c	48	a	49	d
50	c	51	c	52	a	53	b	54	c	55	b	56	b
57	d	58	a	59	b	60	a	61	a	62	c	63	b
64	d	65	a	66	b	67	b	68	a	69	c	70	a
71	d	72	b	73	c	74	a	75	d	76	b	77	b
78	a	79	c	80	b	81	d	82	b	83	c	84	a
85	b	86	a	87	a	88	b	89	a	90	a	91	b
92	d	93	a	94	b	95	a	96	a	97	d	98	b
99	a	100	d										

9

Biochemistry of Biological Oxidation

***Sasmita Barik*[1] *and Shiv Kumar Yadav*[2]**

[1]*Department of Veterinary Physiology and Biochemistry, College of Veterinary Sciences and Animal Husbandry, Guru Angad Dev Animal and Veterinary Sciences University, Ludhiana, Punjab*

[2]*KVK, Shahjahanpur, Uttar Pradesh*

Introduction

Energy is the major source required to maintain the structure and function of all living cells. This energy is derived from oxidation of carbohydrates, lipids and proteins that is taken in the form of diet. The energy liberated from the process of oxidation is generally captured in the form of ATP, which is known as energy currency of the living cells. Each gram of carbohydrate and protein gives about 4 Kcal on oxidation, while each gram of fat gives about 9 Kcal. Oxidation means addition of oxygen or removal of hydrogen from a compound or removal of electron from an ion or atom increasing its positive charge. Reduction means removal of oxygen or addition of hydrogen to a compound or addition of electron to an ion or atom decreasing its positive charge. Commonly the oxidation reactions are conjugated with reduction reactions and known as redox reactions. Redox reactions are often associated with release of energy. The redox chain constitutes chain of different compounds of increasing redox potentials between hydrogen and oxygen. The living cells depend on redox reactions for their energy requirements. The reactions start by removal of H2 from the substrate, which is then transferred to different components of redox chain, then finally to oxygen to form water. Components of redox chains have a redox potential higher than hydrogen and lower than oxygen.

The vital redox chain present in inner mitochondrial membrane of a cell meant for energy generation is known as electron transport chain (ETC). It is the final common pathway in every aerobic cell by which electrons derived from various substances are transferred to oxygen to form water. The biomolecules like carbohydrate, amino acids and fatty acids undergoes oxidation process to generate the intermediated that finally pass through respiratory chain as the electrons get oxidized coenzymes NAD^+ and FAD+ to form the energy rich reduced coenzymes, $NADH^+$, FADH2, $NADH^\cdot$, FADH2 give hydrogen and a pair of electrons to electron carriers. Hydrogen and electrons flow through respiratory chain in steps from more electronegative component (low redox potential) to more electropositive substance. Oxygen is the most electropositive component with highest electron affinity (highest redox potential). So, oxygen is the final acceptor of electrons and protons in respiratory chain. As electrons are passed down the respiratory chain, they lose their free energy which is captured and stored by the production of ATP from ADP and inorganic phosphate (Pi). This process is called oxidative phosphorylation. The remainder of the free energy not trapped as ATP is released as heat. The inner mitochondrial membrane contains 5 separate enzyme complexes (I, II, Ill, IV and V). Complex V is responsible for ATP synthesis. Each complex accepts or donates electrons to relatively mobile electron carriers such as coenzyme Q and cytochrome C. Each carrier of electron transport chain can receive electrons from the more electronegative donor and can subsequently donate electrons to the next more electropositive carrier in the chain. Finally, electrons combine with oxygen and protons to form water. All members of the respiratory chain are protein except coenzyme Q. All are embedded in the inner mitochondrial membrane. Complex I contain an enzyme called NADH dehydrogenase with coenzyme FMN and several iron-sulfur atoms. It oxidizes NADH+H' into NADat the same time converts coenzyme FMN into FMNH2.Complex II contain the enzyme flavoprotein dehydrogenase e.g. succinate dehydrogenase of TCA and acyl CoA dehydrogenase of fatty acid oxidation. Its coenzyme is FAD and it contains iron-sulfur atoms. Complex III contains cytochrome b enzyme and cytochrome c. Complex IV contains cytochromes a + a3 (cytochrome c oxidase).

Coenzyme Q is quinine derivative with a long Isoprenoid tall. It accepts hydrogen atoms both from FMNH2, produced by NADH dehydrogenase in complex I and from FADH2, which is produced by succinate dehydrogenase and other similar enzymes in complex II. There are 5 types of cytochromes (b, c1, c, a and a3) present in ETC All cytochromes are conjugated proteins formed of protein conjugated with heme ring. The heme ring contains iron (Fe). And the iron oscillates between ferric ions (Fe3•) when it loses an electron, and ferrous (Fe2•) when it accepts electrons. Cytochrome b is associated with sulfur (S) In addition to iron (Fe). Cytochrome c is the only mobile carrier. It receives electrons from complex Ill (cyto b and cyto C and transfer them to cytochrome c oxidase (cyto a and cyto a3). Cytochrome c oxidase is a complex enzyme that contains two heme, cytochrome a, cytochrome a3, Iron and copper. It is the last enzyme In the respiratory chain and is the only electron carrier that can react directly with molecular oxygen. It receives electrons from cyto c and transfer them to one oxygen molecule.

ETC inhibitors are compounds that prevent passage of electrons at specific sites by binding to a component of the chain, blocking the oxidation - reduction reaction. In complex I it preventing passage of electrons from FMN to coenzyme A like barbiturates, piericidin A antibiotic and Insecticide and fish poison rotenone. In complex III preventing passage of electrons from cytochrome b to cytochrome C like Antimycin A and dimercaprol. In complex IV, preventing passage of electrons from cytochrome a to O2. Like H2S, CN, CO and sodium azide. Because electron transport and oxidative phosphorylation are tightly coupled, inhibition of the respiratory chain also inhibits ATP synthase.Electrons are transferred down the respiratory chain from $NADH^+$ to oxygen. This is because $NADH^+$ is a strong electron donor, while oxygen is a strong electron acceptor. The flow of electrons from $NADH^+$ to oxygen results in ATP synthesis by phosphorylation of ADP by inorganic phosphate. Therefore, there is a coupling between oxidation and phosphorylation. Two theories explain the ATP synthesis, chemiosmotic hypothesis and membrane transport system. Chemiosmotic hypothesis is also known as Mitchell hypothesis. The transport of electrons down the respiratory chain Gives energy which is used to transport H+ from the mitochondrial matrix from Inside to outside the membrane. This process creates across the inner mitochondrial membrane creates an electrical gradient with more positive charges on the outside of the membrane than on the inside. The energy generated by this proton gradient is the source for ATP synthesis. In the inner mitochondrial membrane, there is a phosphorylating enzyme complex known as ATP synthase (or complex V). It has 2 subunits: F1 and F0. F1subunit which protrudes into the matrix and F0 subunit which is present in the membrane. The protons outside the inner mitochondrial membrane renter the mitochondrial matrix by pa ssing F0- F, complex to pass by ATP synthase enzyme which is present in F, subunit. This results in the synthesis of ATP from ADP + Pi. Uncouplers are the compounds that allow oxidation to proceed but prevent phosphorylation. So, energy released by electron transport will be lost in the form of heat. Oligomycin binds to the stalk of the ATP synthase closing the H' channel, and prevent re-entry of protons to the mitochondrial matrix. The compound 2,4 Dinitrophenol increases the permeability of the inner mitochondrial membrane to proton causing decrease proton gradient. Antibiotics valinomycin and Nigericin are lipophilic substances and they have the ability to make a complex with cations as potassium K^{++} and facilitate their transport into mitochondria and other biological membranes. They Inhibit phosphorylation because they decrease both electrical and pH gradient.

1. All of the following electron carriers are components of the mitochondrial ETC except
   a. NAD+ b. FMN
   b. NADP+ d. FAD
2. Electron transport chain carriers are located in the mitochondria
   a. In mitochondrial matrix
   b. In the inner mitochondrial membrane
   c. In the intermembrane space
   d. On the inner surface of outer mitochondrial membrane
3. Electrons from pyruvic acid enter the mitochondrial ETC at
   a. NADH-Q reductase
   b. Cytochrome oxidase
   c. Coenzyme Q
   d. Between CoQ and cyto- chrome b
4. The phosphate: Oxygen ratio is defined as
   a. The moles of phosphate consumed divided by moles of oxygen consumed
   b. The moles of CO2 produced divided by moles of O2 consumed
   c. The moles of ATP synthesized divided by the atom equivalents of O2 consumed
   d. The moles of ATP formed divided by the milligrams of protein
5. Number of ATP molecules produced in oxidative phosphorylation from one molecule NADH is
   a. Zero b. 3
   c. 2 d. 4
6. Number of ATP molecules produced in oxidative phosphorylation from oxidation of one molecule of flavoprotein is
   a. Zero b. 2
   c. 3 d. 4

7. Rotenone causes
   a. FADH2 is oxidized by ETC
   b. Cytochrome a 3 is reduced
   c. NADH is oxidized by ETC
   d. Cytochrome c is reduced
8. Which of the following statement regarding cytochrome oxidase is true?
   a. It is a single cytochrome
   b. It is inhibited by copper
   c. It is also known as cytochrome b
   d. It transfers four electrons and four protons to form water molecule
9. Which one is the inhibitor of complex I in ETC.
   a. BAL
   b. Rotenone
   c. Antimycin
   d. None of these
10. Dinitrophenol causes which of the following biological oxidation?
    a. Increased synthesis of ATP
    b. Increased hydrolysis of ATP
    c. Decreases body heat production
    d. Prevents electron transfer
11. Cyanide is poisonous as it stops respiration because of its
    a. Inhibition of TCA cycle
    b. Inhibition of cytochrome oxidase
    c. Formation of complex with Hb
    d. Inhibition of myoglobin
12. Which of the following is not a component of ETC?
    a. Nicotinamide
    b. Biotin
    c. Riboflavin
    d. Ubiquinone
13. The oxidation and phosphorylation in intact mitochondria is blocked by
    a. Streptomycin
    b. Septran
    c. Oligomycin
    d. Gentamycin
14. Which of the following compound has greatest standard free energy?
    a. ATP
    b. cAMP
    c. Phosphocreatine
    d. Phosphoenol pyruvate
15. Which of the following components of electron transport chain possesses isoprenoid units?
    a. Cytochrome
    b. Coenzyme
    c. Cytochrome b
    d. Iron
16. ATP synthase activity is associated with the mitochondrial enzyme complex
    a. I
    b. III
    c. IV
    d. V
17. The Phosphorus:Oxygen ratio for the oxidation of FADH2 is
    a. 1
    b. 2
    c. 3
    d. 4
18. The enzyme marker of electron transport system is
    a. Fumarase
    b. Malate dehydrogenase
    c. Pyruvate
    d. Cytochrome reductase

19. The total number of ATP molecules synthesized during glycolysis is
    a. 1 b. 2
    c. 3 d. 4
20. The main function of mitochondria is
    a. Oxidation b. Lipid synthesis
    c. Protein synthesis d. Electron transfer
21. Which is the an effect of dinitrophenol on oxidative phosphorylation?
    a. Inhibition of cytochrome b
    b. Inhibition of ATP synthesis with normal electron transport
    c. Inhibition of electron transport but not ATP synthesis
    d. Blockade of both electron transport and ATP synthesis
22. Cytochrome oxidase is inhibited by
    a. Aluminium phosphide b. Carbon mono oxide
    c. Cyanide d. Phenobarbitone
23. The following poisons which act by causing inhibition of complex IV of respiratory chain except
    a. H2S b. Malonate
    c. Cyanide d. CO
24. The NADPH molecule is generated in the reaction catalysed by
    a. Alcohol dehydrogenase b. G-6 PD
    c. LDH d. G-3PD
25. The product of hexos monophosphate shunt are
    a. FADH and pentose phosphate b. FADH2 and pentose phosphate
    c. NADH and pentose phosphate d. NADPH and pentose phosphate
26. A continuous supply of energy to the body is necessary to meet the requirements of
    a. Basal metabolic rate b. Physical activity
    c. Specific dynamic action d. All of the above
27. NADPH is used for
    a. Xenobiotic metabolism b. Formation of reduced glutathione
    c. Fatty acid biosynthesiss d. All of the above
28. NADPH molecule is generated by the action of
    a. Glu-6 phosphatase b. Glu-6 PO4 dehydrogenase
    c. Glu-1,6 diphosphatase d. Myophosphorylase
29. The specialized tissue/organ in which the oxidation of fuel not produces ATP but generate heat?
    a. Heart b. Adrenal gland

30. Carbon monoxide inhibits mitochondrial electron transport by
    a. Combining with Coenzyme Q
    b. Inhibiting the electron transfer of NADH-Q reductase
    c. Blocking electron transport at the level of the cyt.b to cyt.c1
    d. All of the above
31. How many ATP molecules are required for conversion of two molecules of lactic acid to glucose?
    a. 6 b. 4
    c. 8 d. 10
32. Cyanide is poisonous and lethal because it
    a. Combines with RB cells
    b. Forms complex with Hb molecule
    c. Inhibit cytochrome oxide
    d. Binds to ribosomes
33. Cyanide inhibits the following enzyme/s involved in oxidative phosphorylation
    a. NAND dehydrogenase
    b. cytochrome oxidase
    c. Succinate dehydrogenase
    d. All of the above
34. In aerobic glycolysis in brain tissue the NADH formed is oxidized through
    a. Malate aspartatebshuttle b. Glycerol phosphate shuttle
    c. Conversion of pyruvate to lactate d. Conversion of 1.3 BPG to 3PG
35. Thermogenin is a
    a. Molecule required in the functioning of ETC
    b. A protein involved in the synthesis of glycogen
    c. Protein uncoupling oxidation phosphorylation
    d. Molecule concerned with the inhibition of purine synthesis
36. Is a site specific inhibitor of ETC
    a. Antimycin-A b. Atractyloside
    c. 2, 4, DNP d. Oligomycin
37. Cyanide is poisonous as it stops respiration because of its
    a. Inhibition of TCA cycle b. Inhibition of cytochrome oxidase
    c. Formation of complex with Hb d. Inhibition of myoglobin
38. Which of the following components of electron transport chain possesses isoprenoid units?
    a. Cytochrome b. Coenzyme
    c. Cytochrome b d. Iron
39. The Phosphorus:Oxygen ratio for the oxidation of FADH2 is
    a. 1 b. 2
    c. 3 d. 4

40. Which of the following essential dietary factors is a precursor for a compound that can act as carrier of one carbon fragments at different levels of oxidation?
    a. Thiamine
    b. Biotin
    c. Methionine
    d. Folic acid
41. Which of the following oxidation-reduction system has highest redox potential
    a. Fe+3 cytochome a/Fe+2
    b. Fe+3 cytochrome b/Fe+2
    c. NAD+/NADH
    d. Ubiquinone ox/red
42. A more negative redox potential represents a greater tendency to lose ______
    a. Electrons
    b. Proton
    c. Both
    d. None
43. The electron transport chain is located in
    a. Cytosol
    b. Ribosome
    c. Mitochondria
    d. Nucleus
44. The component of ETC which can directly react with molecular oxygen
    a. Monoxygenase
    b. Cytochrome oxidase
    c. Dehydrogenase
    d. Reductase
45. The site of ETC inhibited by cyanide
    a. Monoxygenase
    b. Cytochrome oxidase
    c. Dehydrogenase
    d. Reductase
46. Oxidoreductases functions in biosynthetic processes in mammalian system tend to use which of the following as reductant.
    a. NADP
    b. NADPH
    c. FADP
    d. FDP
47. Oxidoreductases functions in catabolic processes in mammalian system tend to use which of the following as oxidant
    a. NAD+
    b. NADPHa
    c. FADP
    d. FDP
48. If the reaction is exergonic, then the ΔG will be
    a. Negative
    b. Positive
    c. zero
    d. None
49. If the reaction is endergonic, then the ΔG will be
    a. Negative
    b. Positive
    c. Zero
    d. None
50 For spontaneous process the total entropy of a system must
    a. Increase
    b. Decrease
    c. Zero
    d. None
51. No of oxidation/reduction loop in respiratory chain is folded into in the membrane.
    a. Two
    b. Three
    c. Zero
    d. Four

52. The carrier in single oxidation/reduction loop in ETC consists of
    a. Hydrogen b. Electron
    c. Both d. None
53. For conversion of oxaloacetate to phosphoenol pyruvate, high energy molecule is required in the form of
    a. GTP only b. ITP only
    c. GTP (or) ITP d. None of thes
54. If the more negative standard reduction potential of a redox pair, the greater the tendency t
    a. To lose electrons b. To gain electrons
    c. To lose/gain electrons d. To lose and gain electrons
55. Electron transport and phosphorylation can be uncoupled by compounds that increase the permeability of the inner mitochondrial membrane to
    a. Electrons b. Protons
    c. Uncouplers d. All of the above
56. The more positive the E0, the greater the tendency of the oxidant member of that pair to
    a. Lose electrons b. Gain electrons
    c. Lose (or) gain electrons d. Lose and gain electrons
57. The standard free energy of hydrolysis of terminal phosphate group of ATP is
    a. –7,300 cal/mol b. –8,300 cal/mol
    c. 10,000 cal/mol d. +7,300 cal/mol
58. The transport of a pair of electrons from NADH to O2 via the electron transport chain produces
    a. –52,580 cal b. –50,580 cal
    c. 21,900 cal d. +52,580 cal
59. Sufficient energy required to produce 3 ATP from 3 ADP and 3 pi is
    a. –21,900 cal b. 29,900 cal
    c. 31,900 cal d. 39,900 cal
60. The free energy change, ΔG
    a. Is directly proportional to the standard free energy change, Δg
    b. Is equal to zero at equilibrium
    c. Can only be calculated when the reactants and products are present at 1mol/1 concentrations
    d. Is equal to –RT in keq
61. Under standard conditions
    a. The free energy change $\Delta g°$, is equal to 0
    b. The standard free energy change Δg, is equal to 0
    c. The free energy change, $\Delta g°$, is equal to the standard free energy change, $\Delta g°$
    d. Keq is equal to 1t

62. An uncoupler of oxidative phosphorylation such as dinitrophenol
   a. Inhibits electron transport and atp synthesis
   b. Allow electron transport to proceed without atp synthesis
   c. Inhibits electron transport without impairment of atp synthesis
   d. Specially inhibits cytochrome b
63. All of the following statements about the enzymic complex that carries out the synthesis of ATP during oxidative phosphorylation are correct except
   a. It is located on the matrix side of the inner mitochondrial membrane
   b. It is inhibited by oligomycin
   c. It can exhibit ATPase activity
   d. It can bind molecular O2
64. The reaction catalysed by phosphofructokinase
   a. Is activated by high concentrations of atp and citrate
   b. Uses fruitose-1-phosphate as substrate
   c. Is the rate-limiting reaction of the glycolytic pathway
   d. Is inhibited by fructose 2, 6-bisphosphate
65. Compared to the resting state, vigorously contracting muscle shows
   a. An increased conversion of pyruvate to lactate
   b. Decreased oxidation of pyruvate of co2 and water
   c. A decreased nadh/nad+ ratio
   d. Decreased concentration of AMP
66. Which of the following are High-energy phosphates
   a. Phosphoenol pyruvate   b. Carbamoyl phosphate
   c. 1,3-Bisphosphoglycerate   d. All of the above
67. Which of the following are low-energy phosphates
   a. Glucose 1-phosphate   b. Fructose 6-phosphate
   c. Glucose 6-phosphate   d. All of the above
68. Which of the following has high ΔG
   a. 1,3-Bisphosphoglycerate   b. ATP to ADP + Pi
   c. Both   d. None
69. Most of the high-energy compounds contain phosphate group
   a. True   b. False
   c. Both   d. None
70. Which one of the following is a Phosphagens
   a. 1,3-bisphosphoglycerate.   b. Phosphoenol pyruvate
   c. Carbamoyl phosphatc   d. Phosphocrcatinc
71. Which one of the following is the inhibitors of electron transport chain
   a. Rotenone   b. Amytal
   c. Antimycin,   d. All of the above

72. Which one of the following is the inhibitors of oxidative phosphorylation
    a. Oligomycin b. Atractyloside
    c. Both d. None
73. Which one are the substances that delink ETC from oxidative phosphorylation.
    a. Inhibitors b. Uncouplers
    c. Both d. None
74. Which group of enzymes belong to the class oxidoreductases.
    a. Oxidases, b. Aerobic dehydrogenases
    c. Hydroperoxidases d. All of the above
75. Which one of the following components of ETC possesses isoprenoid units
    a. Coenzyme Q b. Complex 1
    c. Cytochrome b d. Non-heme iron.
76. ATP synthase activity is associated with the mitochondrial enzyme complex
    a. V b. III
    c. IV d. I
77. The prosthetic group present in cytochromes is
    a. Copper b. Iron
    c. Heme d. None
78. Superoxide is converted to H2O2 by the enzyme
    a. Catalase b. Peroxidase
    c. Both d. None
79. Which one is NAD+ dependent dehydrogenases
    a. Alcohol dehydrogenase
    b. Glycerol 3-phosphate dehydrogenase
    c. Both
    d. None
80. Which one is NADP+ dependent dehydrogenase
    a. HMG CoA reductase b. Enoyl reductase
    c. Both d. None
81. Which one is FAD dependent dehydrogenases
    a. Succinate dehydrogenase b. Acyl CoA dehydrogenase
    c. Both d. None
82. Which of the following don't belong to cytochromes
    a. B b. C1
    c. c d. a
83. The harmful effects of H2O2 are prevented by
    a. Peroxidase b. Catalase
    c. Both d. None

84. Which one is true oxygenase
    a. Homogentisate oxidase b. L-tryptophan pyrrolase
    c. Both d. None
85. Which one is the reducing equivalents to monooxygenases
    a. NADPH b. NADH
    c. Both d. None
86. Monooxygenases are responsible for the metabolism of many drugs like
    a. Amino pyrine b. Morphine
    c. Aniline d. All of the above
87. Oxidases that are flavoprotein in nature
    a. L-amino acid oxidase b. Xanthine oxidase
    c. Both d. None
88. L-amino acid oxidase contain which flavoprotein
    a. FMN b. FAD
    c. Both d. None
89. Xanthine oxidase contain which flavoprotein
    a. FMN b. FAD
    c. Both d. None
90. Uncouplers increase the permeability of inner mitochondrial membrane to
    a. Protons b. Electrons
    c. Both d. None
91. Uncouplers causes which one of the following
    a. ATP synthesis b. Heat generation
    c. Both d. None
92. The uncouplers may cause
    a. Oxidation of substrates b. NADH or FADH2generation
    c. Both d. None
93. Which one of the following is an uncoupler
    a. 2,4-dinitrophenol (DNP)
    b. Pentachlorophenol
    c. Trifluorocarbonylcyanide phenylhydrazone
    d. All of the above
94. Which one of the following is more toxic
    a. 2,4-dinitrophenol (DNP)
    b. Pentachlorophenol
    c. Trifluorocarbonylcyanide phenylhydrazone
    d. All of the above

95. The physiological substances which act as uncouplers are
    a. Thermogenin b. Thyroxine
    c. Long chainfree fatty acids d. All of the above
96. Ionophores are
    a. Lipophilic b. Hydrophilic
    c. Amphiphilic d. None
97. Cyanide binds to
    a. Fe b. Heme
    c. Both d. None
98. Which one of the following are inhibitors of cytochrome oxidase
    a. Carbon monoxide b. Cyanide
    c. Hydrogen sulphide d. All of the above
99. Antimycin A inhibits
    a. b b. C1
    c. Both d. None
100. Leber's hereditary optic neuropathyis an inherited disorder of
    a. Mitochondris b. Ribosome
    c. Nucleus d. All of the above

Answer Key

1	b	2	b	3	a	4	c	5	b	6	b	7	a
8	d	9	b	10	b	11	b	12	b	13	c	14	d
15	b	16	d	17	b	18	d	19	d	20	d	21	b
22	b	23	b	24	b	25	d	26	d	27	d	28	b
29	b	30	c	31	a	32	c	33	b	34	b	35	c
36	a	37	b	38	b	39	b	40	d	41	a	42	a
43	c	44	b	45	b	46	a	47	a	48	a	49	b
50	a	51	b	52	c	53	a	54	a	55	b	56	b
57	a	58	d	59	a	60	b	61	c	62	b	63	d
64	c	65	a	66	d	67	d	68	b	69	a	70	d
71	d	72	c	73	d	74	d	75	a	76	a	77	c
78	a	79	c	80	c	81	c	82	d	83	c	84	c
85	a	86	d	87	c	88	a	89	b	90	a	91	b
92	c	93	d	94	c	95	d	96	a	97	a	98	d
99	c	100	a										

10

Biochemistry of Carbohydrate Metabolism

Shabnam Akhtar

Department of Veterinary Pharmacology and Toxicology, Institute of Veterinary Science and Animal Husbandry (IVS&AH), Siksha 'O' Anusandhan Deemed-to be-University (SOA-DU), Campus-4, Bhubaneswar-751030, Odisha

Introduction

Carbohydrates, the aldehyde/ ketone derivatives of the higher polyhydric alcohols, or compounds that yield these derivatives on hydrolysis, constitute of mainly four groups viz. monosaccharides, disaccharides, oligosaccharides and polysaccharides. Energy comes mostly from carbohydrates, and products of their degradation are also used for the synthesis of other substances including fatty acids, cholesterol, amino acids etc They are also components of compound lipids, conjugated proteins, and some of their derivatives can even function as medications (e.g., cardiac glycosides, etc). Disorders such as glycogen storage disorders (GSDs) and galactosemia can be brought on by an inherited lack of certain enzymes in the metabolic pathways of various carbohydrates. Diabetes mellitus is characterized by disruption of the metabolism of glucose.

In ruminants, the end products of digestion are largely volatile fatty acids viz. acetic acid, propionic acid and butyric acid and some monosaccharides. As they pass through the ruminal epithelium, they undergo different degrees of metabolism. The fate of volatile fatty acids are as follows: Acetate as precursor to Acetyl CoA (TCA cycle; fat synthesis); Propionate as precursor to glucose (glycolysis; milk lactose) and Butyrate as precursor to Acetyl CoA (TCA cycle). All the digested and absorbed monosaccharides and volatile fatty acids enter into the liver, where two mechanisms operate such as withdrawal of carbohydrates from blood (e.g. glycogenesis; glycolysis etc) and release of glucose by liver to blood (e.g. glycogenolysis, gluconeogenesis etc). In case of monogastrics, the processes of digestion/ fermentation of carbohydrates especially occur in the small intestine. The fate of absorbed glucose and metabolic conversions in the animal body mainly comprise of storage as glycogen in liver and muscle (small amount); oxidation of glucose for providing energy (via Glycolysis pathway; other alternative pathways such as **Hexose Monophosphate Pathway (HMP)**/ HMP Shunt and **Uronic acid pathway** etc) and fat synthesis as well as storage in the form of fat in adipose tissue.

The major pathways of glucose catabolism include Glycolysis and Kreb's Cycle. While anaerobic catabolism mostly includes Glycolysis pathway or Embden-Meyerhof pathway, the aerobic catabolism includes pathways namely, Hexose Monophosphate Pathway

(HMP) or Pentose Phosphate Pathway or Phosphogluconate Pathway and Tricarboxylic Acid Cycle (TCA or Kreb's Cycle. On the other hand, the anabolic processes include Glycogenesis (process of glycogen synthesis) in liver/ muscle, Glucogenesis, Synthesis of fat from carbohydrates as well as Gluconeogenesis.

The ***Glycolysis*** or ***Embden Meyerhof pathway*** includes aerobic and anaerobic phases and the enzymes involved in glycolysis are extramitochondrial (located in the cytosol). There is breakdown of 6 C glucose to 3 C end products i.e. pyruvate in aerobic metabolism and lactic acid in anaerobic metabolism. It is also the pathway by which other sugars like fructose or galactose are catabolized by converting them to intermediates of glycolysis.

In the aerobic phase of glycolysis, there is a net gain of 8 ATP per mole of glucose. For each mole of glucose, 2 ATP were used (preparatory phase) and 2 NADH, 4 ATP and 2 pyruvate molecules (payoff phase) were generated that equals a net production of 2 NADH, 2 ATP and 2 pyruvate molecules resulting in net gain of 8 ATP. On the other hand, the anaerobic metabolism of glucose produces 2 ATP per glucose molecule.

The fate of pyruvate generated through glycolysis depends on the conditions of the animal and the cell type viz. lactic acid production or acetyl CoA production (serves as the main precursor for the TCA Cycle, lipogenesis and ketogenesis (during negative balance)). Pyruvate dehydrogenase links glycolysis with the TCA Cycle by converting pyruvate into acetyl CoA.

The ***TCA Cycle*** constitute the central metabolic hub of the cell occurring in the mitochondri A Here, 24 ATPs are produced from one mole of glucose. This cycle is the final common pathway for oxidation of carbohydrates, fats and proteins thereby providing energy. The whole process is aerobic, requiring oxygen as the final oxidant of the reducing equivalents. Absence of O2 (anoxi A or partial deficiency of O2 (hypoxi A causes total or partial inhibition of the cycle. The H atoms removed in the successive dehydrogenations are accepted by corresponding coenzymes. Reduced coenzymes transfer the reducing equivalents to electron-transport system, where oxidative phosphorylation produces ATP molecules.

Therefore, overall, one mole of glucose produces the equivalent of 38 ATP (8 through glycolysis; 6 through oxidative decarboxylation of pyruvic acid and 24 through TCA cycle).

In case of ***Glycogenesis,*** there is formation of glycogen from glucose and occurs primarily in in liver and skeletal muscles, but it can occur in every tissue to some extent. Glycogen synthase is the key enzyme which regulates the process of glycogenesis. This process can be stimulated by insulin, glucocorticoids, glucose etc and inhibited by increased concentration of glycogen, feedback inhibition, increased cyclic-AMP concentration etc.

In ***Glycogenolysis,*** there is breakdown of glycogen to glucose. It is initiated by the action of a specific enzyme present in liver and muscle i.e. phosphorylase, that brings about Phosphorolytic cleavage of α 1$\rightarrow$ 4 linkage to yield glucose-1-P. The two other pathways of Glycogenolysis those are independent of Phosphorylase enzyme include ***α-Amylolysis*** and ***γ-Amylolysis pathway.***

The regulation of glycogen metabolism is achieved by a balance in activities between Glycogen synthase and Phosphorylase enzyme such as Substrate control (through allostery); hormonal control and by end products.

The process of ***Gluconeogenesis*** involves glycolysis, the citric acid cycle and some special reactions. The main pathway is a reversal of glycolytic pathway but thermodynamic "barriers" prevent a simple reversal of glycolysis. The key enzymes involved in regulation of gluconeogenesis are Pyruvate carboxylase, Phospho-enol-Pyruvate carboxykinase (PEPCK), Fructose-1,6-biphosphatase and Glucose-6-phosphatase.

The maintenance of blood glucose within physiological limits occurs via by a balance between two sets of factors i.e. rate of glucose entrance into the blood stream and rate of its removal from the blood stream. There are two categories of endocrine influences on Carbohydrate metabolism such as those which exert a fundamental regulatory influence (e.g. hormones of pancreatic islet cells specially Insulin and hormones of adrenal cortex and anterior pituitary) and those that influence carbohydrate metabolism, but are not essential for its autoregulation under normal physiological conditions (e.g. hormones of adrenal medulla and hormones of thyroid gland).

Some ***Disorders of Carbohydrate Metabolism*** include Diabetes mellitus, Hyperinsulinism, Hypoglycemia of Baby Pigs as well as Glycogen Storage Diseases.

1. The breakdown of glycogen to blood glucose by action of a specific phosphorylase enzyme, is otherwise known as:
   a. Glycolysis b. Gluconeogenesis
   c. Glycogenolysis d. Glycogenesis
2. Glycogenesis is a process where there is storage of glucose as:
   a. Fructose b. Glycogen
   c. Maltose d. Fat
3. Which of the following involves oxidation of glucose?
   a. Glycolysis (EM Pathway) b. HMP-Shunt pathway
   c. Uronic acid pathway d. All of the above
4. Glucose is converted to fats in a process known as:
   a. Lipogenesis b. Glycogenesis
   c. Glycolysis d. Glycogenolysis
5. The process where there is formation of blood glucose by the liver from non-carbohydrate sources, such as amino acids (glucogenic), pyruvates and lactates, glycerol and propionyl-CoA is:
   a. Glycolysis b. Gluconeogenesis
   c. Both a and b d. None of the above
6. Which of the following statements are correct with respect to the process of glycolysis?
   a. Oxidation of glucose or glycogen to pyruvate and lactate is by EM pathway
   b. Glucose is degraded to pyruvate, which in presence of O_2 is completely oxidized to CO_2 and H_2O.
   c. Glycolysis occurs in all tissues and mainly in erythrocytes and nervous tissues
   d. All of the above
7. An alternative pathway for oxidation of glucose apart from glycolysis includes:
   a. HMP Shunt b. Uronic acid pathway
   c. Both a and b d. None of the above

8. Which of the following pathways can utilise O_2 if available (aerobic as well as can function in absence of O_2 (anaerobic)?
   a. Glycolysis/ Embden Meyerhof pathway
   b. Gluconeogenesis
   c. Glycogenolysis
   d. Lipogenesis
9. Which of the following statements is incorrect with respect to the aerobic phase of glycolysis?
   a. Oxidation is carried out by dehydrogenation
   b. Reducing equivalent is transferred to NAD^+
   c. Reduced NAD in presence of O_2 is oxidised in electron-transport chain producing ATP
   d. None of the above
10. Choose the correct statements related to the anaerobic phase of glycolysis.
   a. NADH cannot be oxidised in electron transport chain and hence no ATP is produced
   b. NADH is oxidised to NAD^+ by conversion of pyruvate to lactate, without producing ATP
   c. Anaerobic phase limits the amount of energy per mol. of glucose oxidise d. Therefore, more glucose must undergo glycolysis under anaerobic as compared to aerobic to provide a given amount of energy
   d. All of the above
11. Enzymes involved in glycolysis are:
   a. Extramitochondrial
   b. Mitochondrial
   c. Only b
   d. None of the above
12. Glycolysis is having biomedical importance in areas such as:
   a. Cancer therapy
   b. Haemolytic anaemias
   c. Surviving anoxic episodes by skeletal muscles
   d. All of the above
13. The mechanisms operating in liver with respect to absorption of carbohydrates that is of considerable physiological and biochemical importance include:
   a. Withdrawal of carbohydrates from blood
   b. Release of glucose by liver to the blood
   c. Both a and b
   d. None of the above
14. Which of the following statements are correct?
   a. Hepatic cells are freely permeable to glucose
   b. Intestinal mucosal and kidney tubule cells take up glucose by active transport
   c. Both a and b
   d. Only b

15. In which of the following extrahepatic tissues, insulin is associated with increasing glucose uptake?
   a. Skeletal & Heart muscle
   b. Diaphragm
   c. Adipose tissue & lactating mammary gland
   d. All of the above

16. Which of the following is provided by HMP Shunt (the pathway that operates only in certain special tissues and not all tissues)?
   a. Pentoses b. NADPH
   c. Both a and b d. D-glucuronic acid

17. Which of the following is provided by Uronic acid pathway, that is required in the formation of mucopolysaccharides (MPS) and in conjugation reaction for detoxication?
   a. D-glucuronic acid b. Ribose and deoxyribose
   c. Galactose d. Fructose

18. Which of the following constitute a part of the reactions of glycolytic pathway?
   a. Stage I: Conversion of asymmetric glucose molecule to almost symmetrical fructose 1,6-biphosphate & actual splitting of symmetrical fructose 1,6-biphosphate (Stage II)
   b. Stage III: Energy yielding reaction where an aldehyde group is oxidised to an acid
   c. Stage IV: Recovery of PO_4 group from 3-Phosphoglycerate
   d. All of the above

19. Which of the following enzymes catalyse the reaction involving conversion of glucose to glucose-6-P?
   a. Glucokinase in liver cells (specific enzyme)
   b. Hexokinase in liver and extrahepatic tissues (non-specific enzyme)
   c. Both a and b
   d. None of the above

20. An important compound at the junction of several metabolic pathways viz. glycolysis, glycogenesis, glycogenolysis, gluconeogenesis, HMP Shunt, Uronic acid pathway etc is:
   a. D-glucose b. Glucose-6-P
   c. Dihydroxyacetone-P d. D-Glyceraldehyde-3-P

21. Glucokinase differs from Hexokinase in that it:
   a. It is specific, found only in liver & can phosphorylate glucose only
   b. It is physiologically more labile & its main function is to clear glucose from blood after meals/ higher blood levels, instead of making glucose available to tissues for oxidation at lower blood glucose level
   c. It is not allosterically inhibited by Glucose-6-P and its synthesis is influenced by insulin
   d. All of the above

22. An enzyme that acts only on α-anomer of Glucose-6-P and converts it to Fructose-6-P involving an aldose-ketose isomerisation is:

    a. Phosphohexose isomerase
    b. Phosphofructokinase-1
    c. Furanose
    d. Aldolase A and B

23. Choose the incorrect statement related to conversion of fructose-6-P to fructose-1,6-bi-P.

    a. It is an irreversible reaction
    b. One ATP is utilised for phosphorylation
    c. Phosphofructokinase-1 is not the key enzyme in glycolysis that regulates glucose breakdown, is not inducible and not allosterically modified
    d. Phosphofructokinase-2 is an isoenzyme that catalyses the reaction to form fructose-2,6-bi-phosphate

24. Choose the correct statements related to steps involved in the preparatory stage of glycolytic pathway where there is conversion of asymmetric glucose to symmetrical fructose 1,6-biphosphate form.

    a. There is uptake of glucose by cells and its phosphorylation (Irreversible reaction)
    b. There is conversion of Glucose-6-P to fructose-6-P as well as conversion of fructose-6-P to fructose-1,6-bi-P
    c. There is expenditure of 2 ATP molecules for two phosphorylations and doesn't yield any energy
    d. All of the above

25. The triose phosphates obtained after splitting of fructose-1,6-bi-P by the enzyme aldolase are:

    a. Glyceraldehyde-3-P (an aldotriose)
    b. Dihydroxy acetone-P (a ketotriose)
    c. Both a and b
    d. None of the above

26. The triose phosphates such as Glyceraldehyde-3-P and Dihydroxy acetone-P are interconvertible by action of:

    a. Phosphotriose isomerase
    b. Phosphohexose isomerase
    c. Aldolase A
    d. Aldolase B

27. Which of the following statements are true for the inhibitor Bromohydroxyacetone-P?

    a. It structurally resembles dihydroxyacetone-P
    b. It binds covalently with the γ-COOH group of a glutamate residue at the active site of phosphotriose isomerase enzyme, thereby inactivating the enzyme and stopping catalysis
    c. It leads to accumulation of dihydroxyacetone-P and fructose-1,6-bi-P
    d. All of the above

28. Choose the incorrect statement with respect to the enzyme Glyceraldehyde-3-P-dehydrogenase, that is involved in oxidation of D-Glyceraldehyde-3-P to 1,3-bi-phosphoglycerate.
    a. It is NAD^+ dependent and a tetramer consisting of 4 identical polypeptides
    b. Two -SH groups are present on each polypeptide derived from cysteine residue in the chain
    c. One of the -SH group forms the 'active site' of the enzyme
    d. None of the above
29. A Substrate level phosphorylation reaction catalysed by the enzyme phosphoglycerate kinase includes:
    a. Conversion of 1,3-Biphosphoglycerate to 3-Phosphoglycerate
    b. Conversion of Glucose-6-P to fructose-6-P
    c. Oxidation of D-Glyceraldehyde-3-P to 1,3-bi-phosphoglycerate
    d. Conversion of fructose-6-P to fructose-1,6-bi-P
30. Examples of inhibitors that are involved in the stage of the Glycolytic pathway involving energy yielding reaction are:
    a. Arsenite
    b. Iodoacetate & Iodoacetamide
    c. Both a and b
    d. Only a
31. Which of the following statements are incorrect relating to the energetics of the energy yielding stage of the glycolytic pathway involving oxidation of an aldehyde group to an acid?
    a. There is net production of 6 ATPs in the reaction involving oxidation of Glyceraldehyde-3-P to 1,3-bi-phosphoglycerate (i.e., 2 NADH produced from 2 molecules of Triose-P yields=3×2=6 ATP)
    b. There is net production of 2 ATPs in the reaction involving conversion of 1,3-Biphosphoglycerate to 3-Phosphoglycerate (i.e. two ATPs produced from 2 molecules of substrate yields=1×2=2 ATP)
    c. There is a total/ net gain of 8 ATP per molecule of glucose oxidised
    d. None of the above
32. Which of the following are included in the stage of the glycolytic pathway involving recovery of PO_4 group from 3-phosphoglycerate?
    a. Conversion of 3-Phosphoglycerate to 2-Phosphoglycerate
    b. Conversion of 2-Phosphoglycerate to Phosphoenol pyruvate as well as Conversion of Phosphoenol pyruvate to Pyruvate
    c. Production of 2 ATP per molecule of glucose oxidised
    d. All of the above
33. A Substrate level phosphorylation reaction (irreversible reaction) catalysed by the enzyme pyruvate kinase includes:
    a. Conversion of 3-Phosphoglycerate to 2-Phosphoglycerate
    b. Conversion of Phosphoenol pyruvate to Pyruvate
    c. Conversion of 2-Phosphoglycerate to Phosphoenol pyruvate
    d. None of the above

34. Choose the incorrect statement related to the enzyme Enolase.
    a. It can be inhibited by Fluoride
    b. It requires either presence of Mg^{++} or Mn^{++}
    c. It catalyses the reaction i.e. conversion of 2-Phosphoglycerate to Phosphoenol pyruvate involving dehydration and redistribution of energy i.e.,
    d. None of the above
35. Choose the statements suggesting clinical significance of Fluoride.
    a. Inhibits in vitro glycolysis by inhibiting enzyme enolase
    b. Sodium fluoride is used along with K-oxalate for collection of blood for glucose estimation
    c. Acts as an anticoagulant as well as an antiseptic
    d. All of the above
36. How many ATPs are produced per molecule of glucose oxidation in Anaerobic phase of Glycolysis?
    a. 2 ATP b. 6 ATP
    c. 8 ATP d. 10 ATP
37. The aerobic phase of Glycolysis involves net gain of:
    a. 4 ATP b. 8 ATP
    c. 2 ATP d. 6 ATP
38. The regulation of glycolysis is achieved by:
    a. Changes in the rate of enzyme synthesis, Induction/repression of key enzymes
    b. Covalent modification by reversible phosphorylation
    c. Allosteric modification
    d. All of the above
39. In the anaerobic phase of glycolysis, reoxidation of NADH is achieved by conversion of pyruvate to lactate (without producing ATP) by the enzyme:
    a. Glyceraldehyde-3-P-dehydrogenase b. Lactate dehydrogenase
    c. Pyruvate kinase d. Enolase
40. An example of an inhibitor that competitively inhibits lactate dehydrogenase and prevents the reoxidation of NADH is:
    a. Oxamate b. Sodium fluoride
    c. Arsenite d. Bromohydroxyacetone-P
41. Glucose can increase the activity of key enzymes like:
    a. Glucokinase
    b. Phosphofructokinase-1 and pyruvate kinase
    c. Both a and b
    d. None of the above

42. Which of the following increase CAMP level by activating cAMP-dependant Protein kinase which can phosphorylate and inactivate the key enzyme Pyruvate kinase and, thus, inhibit glycolysis?
    a. Epinephrine
    b. Glucagon
    c. Insulin
    d. Only a and b
43. Which of the following statements are correct for Insulin?
    a. It antagonises the effects of glucocorticoids and glucagon-stimulated c-AMP in stimulating the key enzymes responsible for gluconeogenesis
    b. It enhances the synthesis of the key enzymes responsible for glycolysis
    c. Both a and b
    d. None of the above
44. Choose the correct statements related to Allosteric modification, a mechanism of glycolysis regulation.
    a. Phosphofructokinase-1 is the key regulatory enzyme subjected to 'feedback control' and is inhibited by citrate and ATP and activated by AMP
    b. When ATP is used in energy requiring processes resulting in formation of ADP, the concentration of AMP increases; thereby AMP acts as the indicator of energy status of the cell
    c. The mechanism allows the activity of the enzyme phosphofructokinase-1 to be highly sensitive to even small changes of energy status of the cell and hence it controls the amount of glucose that should undergo glycolysis prior to its entry as acetyl-CoA in TCA cycle
    d. All of the above
45. Which of the following pathway is associated with maintaining a high steady state concentration of 2,3-biphosphoglycerate (2,3-BPG), produced by a diversion in glycolytic pathway?
    a. HMP Shunt
    b. Rapoport-Luebering cycle or shunt (RLC or RLS)
    c. Citric Acid cycle
    d. All of the above
46. Choose the structural/ metabolic peculiarities of glucose oxidation by RB cells.
    a. Mature erythrocytes do not possess nucleus nor cytoplasmic subcellular structures
    b. Entirely depends on glucose for its energy; Glucose is freely permeable to erythrocytes like Liver cells
    c. The enzyme pyruvate dehydrogenase complex is absent. Hence, Pyruvic acid is not converted to "acetyl-CoA"
    d. All of the above

47. The cases where there is formation of Pyruvic Acid (PA in the body include:
   a. Oxidation of glucose (Glycolysis); Deamination of Alanine
   b. Glucogenic amino acids-pyruvate forming; Decarboxylation of oxaloacetic acid (OAA)
   c. both a and b
   d. None of the above
48. Alterations in red cell 2,3-BPG concentration occurs in:
   a. Tissue hypoxia (increase in red cell BPG level)
   b. Inherited enzyme deficiency viz. hexokinase deficiency (decrease in red cell BPG level) and pyruvate kinase deficiency (increase in red cell BPG level)
   c. Both a and b
   d. None of the above
49. In hexokinase deficient cells and pyruvate kinase deficient cells, the affinity for Oxygen, respectively
   a. Decreases, increases
   b. Increases, decreases
   c. Only a
   d. Both a and b
50. Which of the following represents the fate of pyruvic acid?
   a. Forms acetyl-CoA by oxidative decarboxylation (in presence of O_2)
   b. Forms lactic acid by reduction (in absence of O_2); direct conversion to oxaloacetic acid by CO_2-fixation reaction
   c. Forms alanine by amination and glucose by gluconeogenesis
   d. All of the above
51. Which of the following include Anaplerotic reactions?
   a. Conversion of Pyruvic acid to Oxaloacetic acid by the enzyme Pyruvate carboxylase
   b. Conversion of Pyruvic acid to Oxaloacetic acid through malic acid formation by malic enzyme
   c. Both a and b
   d. None of the above
52. Which of the following is required by the enzyme Pyruvate carboxylase for CO_2 fixation reaction?
   a. Biotin (as a prosthetic group that brings CO_2)
   b. ATP and Mg^{++}
   c. Acetyl-CoA
   d. All of the above
53. Malate dehydrogenase is associated with:
   a. Conversion of malate to oxaloacetate in presence of NAD^+
   b. Conversion of Pyruvic acid to Oxaloacetic acid
   c. Formation of malic acid in presence of CO_2 and NADPH
   d. None of the above

54. conversion of pyruvic acid to acetyl-CoA is an example of:

a. Oxidation
b. Oxidative decarboxylation
c. Reduction
d. None of the above

55. The pyruvate dehydrogenase complex that catalyses the oxidative decarboxylation reaction and exists both as inactive and active form, consists of:

a. 29 molecules of Pyruvate dehydrogenase
b. 8 molecules of flavoprotein containing dihydrolipoyl dehydrogenase
c. 1 molecule of dihydrolipoyl transacetylase
d. All of the above

56. Which of the following coenzymes/ cofactors are required for the activity of pyruvate dehydrogenase complex?

a. Thiamine pyrophosphate (TPP), NAD^+, FAD
b. Lipoic acid, CoA-SH, Mg^{++}
c. All of the above
d. None of the above

57. The energetics involved in oxidative decarboxylation of pyruvic acid include production of:

a. 6 ATP
b. 2 ATP
c. 8 ATP
d. 4 ATP

58. Pyruvate dehydrogenase complex can be inactivated by PDH kinase, which in turn is activated by:

a. Rise in ATP/ADP ratio; increased cyclic AMP in cells
b. Increase in NADH/NAD^+ ratio
c. Rise in Acetyl-CoA/CoA-SH ratio
d. All of the above

59. In which of the following conditions, the Pyruvate dehydrogenase complex and glycolysis are inhibited ?

a. High energy potential
b. Fatty acid oxidation (there is production of Acetyl-CoA and NADH that activates PDH-kinase)
c. Both a and b
d. None of the above

60. The PDH kinase can be inhibited by:

a. Increased pyruvic acid by carbohydrate diet
b. Decreased pyric acid
c. Acetyl-CoA
d. NADH

61. The biomedical importance of Citric Acid cycle involves:
    a. It is the final common pathway of breakdown /catabolism of carbohydrates, proteins and fats through formation of 2-carbon unit acetyl-CoA (Phase III of metabolism)
    b. Intermediates of the cycle plays role in the formation of heme, non-essential amino acids, fatty acid synthesis, cholesterol and steroid synthesis
    c. Both a and b
    d. None of the above
62. Which of the following vitamins play a role in the TCA Cycle?
    a. Riboflavin & Pantothenic acid
    b. Niacin & Thiamine
    c. Lipoic acid
    d. All of the above
63. The stage of the Citric acid cycle involving an irreversible, exergonic reaction and without any requirement of ATP is:
    a. Formation of Citric acid from Acetyl-CoA and OAA by action of Citrate synthase
    b. Formation of cis-aconitic acid and isocitric acid from citric acid
    c. Formation of oxalosuccinic acid and α-oxo-glutarate from isocitric acid
    d. None of the above
64. The events taking place in the formation of cis-aconitic acid and isocitric acid from citric acid are:
    a. Asymmetric dehydration, and stereospecific rehydration
    b. Catalysis by the enzyme Aconitase that requires Fe++
    c. There is no production of ATP
    d. All of the above
65. Which of the following represent types of Isocitrate dehydrogenase (ICD enzyme?
    a. NADP dependent ICD in cytosol
    b. NADP dependent ICD in mitochondria (greater activity & wide distribution)
    c. NAD^+ dependant ICD in mitochondria
    d. All of the above
66. The cofactors/ coenzymes involved in the oxidative decarboxylation of α-oxoglutarate to succinyl-CoA is:
    a. TPP, NAD^+
    b. Lipoic acid, Mg^{++}
    c. Both a and b
    d. None of the above
67. The energetics of the stage involving oxidative decarboxylation of α-oxoglutarate to succinyl-CoA includes:
    a. 6 ATP
    b. 2 ATP
    c. 4 ATP
    d. 8 ATP

68. An example of the only substrate level Phosphorylation (without participation of electron transport chain) in TCA Cycle is:
    a. Conversion of succinyl-CoA to succinic acid in presence of Succinate thiokinase
    b. Production of ATP from GTP or ITP in presence of enzyme Nucleoside diphosphate kinase
    c. Only a
    d. None of the above
69. Which of the following steps are involved in the oxidation of succinic acid to oxaloacetate?
    a. Oxidation of succinic acid to fumaric acid
    b. Formation of malic acid from fumaric acid
    c. Oxidation of malic acid to oxaloacetate
    d. All of the above
70. Choose the inhibitor that inhibits succinate dehydrogenase competitively resulting in accumulation of succinate.
    a. Arsenite b. Fluoroacetate
    c. Malonate/ Oxaloacetate d. None of the above
71. The number of ATPs produced at substrate level phosphorylation from two Succinyl-CoA as well as from the dehydrogenation reaction step (oxidation of $FADH_2$ through ETC in the TCA Cycle, respectively are:
    a. 2 ATP, 4 ATP b. 4 ATP, 2 ATP
    c. 6 ATP, 10 ATP d. 10 ATP, 6 ATP
72. The energetics of the step involving oxidation of malic acid to oxaloacetate (oxidation of $NADH_2$ through ETC includes:
    a. 2 ATP b. 6 ATP
    c. 4 ATP d. 8 ATP
73. Which of the following depict the anabolic/ synthetic role of TCA Cycle?
    a. It serves as a source of C-skeletons for the synthesis of non-essential amino acids (Transamination)
    b. Formation of glucose (gluconeogenesis); formation of acetoacetyl-CoA in extrahepatic tissues
    c. Fatty acid synthesis (Acetyl-CoA); haem synthesis (Succinyl-CoA)
    d. All of the above
74. Select the key enzymes involved in the regulation of TCA Cycle.
    a. Citrate synthase b. Isocitrate dehydrogenase
    c. α-oxoglutarate dehydrogenase d. All of the above
75. The phenomenon of inhibition of glycolysis by O_2 (anaerobic oxidative reactions) is termed as:
    a. Pasteur effect b. Crabtree effect
    c. Both a and b d. None of the above

76. Choose the pyruvate forming amino acids among the following.
    a. Glycine b. Cysteine/ cystine
    c. Both a and b d. Phenylalanine
77. Which of the following are fumarate forming amino acids?
    a. Valine/ methionine b. Arginine/ histidine
    c. Hydroxy-proline/ tryptophan d. Phenylalanine/ tyrosine
78. The α-ketoglutarate forming amino acids include:
    a. Glutamine, Arginine b. Proline, Histidine
    c. Both a and b d. None of the above
79. The overall energy production in glycolysis cum TCA Cycle under aerobic condition per molecule of glucose is:
    a. 2 ATP b. 38 ATP (30+8)
    c. 39 ATP (30+9) d. 8 ATP
80. The overall energy production in glycolysis cum TCA Cycle per molecule of glycogen is:
    a. 39 ATP (30+9) b. 38 ATP (30+8)
    c. None of the above d. Only b
81. The shuttle systems that help in the transfer of the reducing equivalents through the mitochondrial membrane via substrate pairs include:
    a. Glycerophosphate shuttle b. Malate shuttle
    c. Both a and b d. None of the above
82. When body utilises α-glycero-P-shuttle and malate shuttle, the net ATP produced by glycolysis—TCA cycle per molecule glucose oxidised, respectively will be:
    a. 36 ATP, 38 ATP b. 30 ATP, 36 ATP
    c. 2 ATP, 30 ATP d. None of the above
83. Which of the following statements is incorrect?
    a. When glycogenesis occurs, glycogenolysis does not take place and vice versa
    b. The body stores glucose as glycogen and not as glucose itself since being insoluble, it exerts no osmotic pressure, and so neither disturbs the intracellular fluid content nor diffuses from its storage sites
    c. Breakdown pathway of glycogen metabolism is a 'reversal' of synthetic pathway
    d. Liver glycogen is the only immediately available reserve store of blood glucose whereas muscle glycogen cannot directly contribute to blood glucose level
84. Which of the following enzymes are involved in the reactions of the synthetic pathway of Glycogenesis?
    a. Phosphoglucomutase b. UDP-Glc Pyrophosphorylase
    c. Glycogen synthase; Glucokinase d. All of the above
85. 'Glycogenin' is an example of:
    a. Glycogen primer b. Protein primer
    c. Both a and b d. None of the above

86. The principal key enzyme that regulates the glycogen formation and requires Glucose-6-P as an activator is:

a. Glycogen synthase
b. Nucleoside diphosphokinase
c. UDP-Glc Pyrophosphorylase
d. Glucokinase

87. A branching enzyme that establishes a branch point in the molecule when the glycogen chain has been lengthened to a minimum of 11 glucose residues:

a. Amylo-1, 4 $\rightarrow$ 1, 6-transglucosidase
b. Glucosyl transferase
c. Glucogen synthase
d. Protein phosphatase-I

88. Glycogenesis can be stimulated by

a. Insulin & Glucose (high substrate concentration)
b. Glucocorticoids
c. both a and b
d. None of the above

89. Glycogenesis can be inhibited by:

a. Increased glycogen concentration, Feedback inhibition
b. Increased concentration of cyclic-AMP
c. Both a and b
d. None of the above

90. Glycogenesis has clinical importance in

a. Treatment of hyperkalaemia
b. Treatment of diabetic ketoacidosis
c. Both a and b
d. None of the above

91. Which of the following statements is incorrect?

a. Muscle phosphorylase 'a' is inactive and a tetramer
b. Muscle phosphorylase 'b' is inactive and a dimer
c. Muscle phosphorylase 'a' is active and a tetramer
d. None of the above

92. Muscle phosphorylase differs from Liver phosphorylase by:

a. It is not affected by glucagon (no receptor on muscle)
b. There is cleavage of structure
c. Requirement of 4 molecules of pyridoxal-P (B_6-P)
d. All of the above

93. By phosphorylase activity (the rate limiting and key enzyme) in glycogenolysis, glucose is liberated as:

a. Free glucose
b. Glucose-1-P
c. None of the above
d. Only a

94. Choose the incorrect statements from the following.
   a. Muscle glycogenolysis contributes to rise in blood glucose directly by the enzyme glucose-6-phosphatase
   b. Liver glycogenolysis reflects a rise in blood glucose by removal of PO_4 group from glucose-6-P by action of glucose-6-phosphatase
   c. There is absence of glucose-6-phosphatase in muscles and the Glucose-6-P enters glycolytic cycle and forms pyruvate and lactic acid
   d. Ca^{++}-Calmodulin can bring about glycogenolysis in muscle/liver independent of cyclic-AMP

95. Choose the correct statements related to regulation of glycogenolysis by cyclic-AMP dependent protein kinase.
   a. Activation of inactive phosphorylase kinase 'b' to active phosphorylase kinase 'a' that in turn, with help of ATP, phosphorylates inactive dephosphophosphorylase 'b' to active phosphophosphorylase 'a' bringing about glycogenolysis
   b. Active protein kinase phosphorylates the protein factor 'inhibitor-1' to active inhibitor-1-p that inhibits Protein phosphatase-1
   c. Protein phosphatase-1 inhibits conversion of phosphorylase kinase a to b
   d. All of the above

96. Which of the following brings about glycogenolysis by increasing the cyclic-AMP level in cells thereby activating protein kinase?
   a. Catecholamines
   b. Glucagon and Thyroid hormones
   c. Both a and b
   d. None of the above

97. Glucagon can breakdown
   a. Liver glycogen
   b. Muscle glycogen
   c. Both a and b
   d. None of the above

98. Which subunit of Muscle phosphorylase kinase resembles calmodulin and binds 4 Ca^{++} ions?
   a. α-subunit
   b. β-subunit
   c. γ-subunit
   d. δ-subunit

99. Which of the following Ca^{++} binding, heat stable protein carries out activation of muscle contraction and glycogenolysis?
   a. Glucagon
   b. Catecholamine
   c. Calmodulin
   d. None of the above

100. Which of the following enzymes are regulated directly or indirectly by Ca^{++} through calmodulin?
   a. Adenylate cyclase
   b. Ca^{++}-dependent protein kinase; Ca^{++}/ Mg^{++} ATPase
   c. Phosphodiesterase; Myosin kinase
   d. All of the above

101. Two other pathways for breakdown of tissue glycogen other than phosphorolytic cleavage include:

a. α-Amylolysis
b. γ-Amylolysis
c. Both a and b
d. None of the above

102. Protein Phosphatase-1, a single enzyme of wide specificity, is associated with:

a. Dephosphorylation of Phosphorylase 'a'
b. Dephosphorylation of Phosphorylase kinase 'a'
c. Dephosphorylation of glycogen synthase 'b'
d. All of the above

103. Hexose Monophosphate (HMP) Shunt, an alternate pathway for oxidation of glucose, is otherwise called as:

a. Pentose phosphate pathway (PP-pathway)
b. Phosphogluconate pathway
c. Warburg-Dickens-Lipman Pathway
d. All of the above

104. HMP Pathway differs from EM Pathway in that:

a. $NADP^+$ is used as hydrogen acceptor and not NAD^+
b. CO_2 is produced and ATP is not produced
c. It is a multicyclic process and occurs in certain specialised tissues only to serve specific functions
d. All of the above

105. The similarity between HMP Pathway and EM Pathway is:

a. It operates in cytosol and the enzymes are extramitochondrial (cytosolic)
b. CO_2 is produced in both
c. both a and b
d. None of the above

106. Which of the following is included in the Oxidative phase of HMP Shunt?

a. Oxidation of glucose
b. Formation of Pentose phosphates
c. Both a and b
d. None of the above

107. Choose the steps of the non-oxidative phase of HMP Shunt.

a. Pentose-P reactions (interconversions of pentoses)
b. Conversion of pentose phosphates to hexose phosphates via transketolation and transaldolation reactions
c. Both a and b
d. None of the above

108. Choose the correct statement with respect to reactions involved in HMP Shunt.
   a. 1 Transketolation reaction and 1 transaldolation reaction
   b. 2 Transketolation reactions and 1 transaldolation reaction
   c. Both a and b
   d. None of the above
109. Regulation of HMP Shunt depends on:
   a. Cytoplasmic ratio of $[NADP^+]/[NADPH]$ i.e. a rise in the ratio enhances rate limiting reaction and HMP Pathway, whereas a decrease in the ratio inhibits both G-6-PD and 6-phosphogluconate dehydrogenase
   b. High carbohydrate diets (enhances the shunt pathway); Starvation (reduces the shunt pathway)
   c. Increase in Fatty acid and Steroid synthesis (enhances the shunt pathway)
   d. All of the above
110. The major function of Uronic acid pathway is:
   a. Production of D-Glucuronic acid
   b. Transketolation reaction
   c. Transaldolation reaction
   d. None of the above
111. Which of the following enzymes are involved in the metabolic pathway of formation of Uridine-diphosphate glucose (UDP-G) from glucose?
   a. Phosphoglucomutase
   b. UDP-G Pyrophosphorylase
   c. Both a and b
   d. None of the above
112. In Uronic acid pathway, the oxidation of UDP-G by the enzyme UDP-G dehydrogenase (requiring NAD^+) results in formation of active form of:
   a. L-Gulonic acid
   b. UDP-Glucuronic acid
   c. D-Glucuronic acid
   d. None of the above
113. Which of the following is not synthesised in humans, guinea-pigs, other primates?
   a. Ascorbic acid
   b. 3-keto-L-Gulonic acid
   c. L-Xylulose
   d. All of the above
114. The direct precursor of Ascorbic acid, in those animals that are capable of synthesising this vitamin, is:
   a. L-Gulonic acid
   b. D-Glucuronic acid
   c. Both a and b
   d. None of the above
115. Which of the following drug administration in rats results in a significant increase in the conversion of glucose to glucuronic acid, L-Gulonic acid and ascorbic acid?
   a. Barbital or chlorobutanol
   b. Aminopyrine
   c. Antipyrine
   d. All of the above
116. Important substances that undergo conjugation with D-glucuronic acid include:
   a. Aromatic acids (e.g. Benzoic acid)
   b. Bile pigments (e.g. Bilirubin)
   c. Certain antibiotics and hormones (e.g. chloramphenicol; thyroid hormones, steroid hormone derivatives etc)
   d. All of the above

117. D-glucuronic acid is associated with synthesis of mucopolysaccharides (MPS) such as:
   a. Hyaluronic acid & Heparin
   b. Chondroitin & Chondroitin SO_4
   c. Both a and b
   d. None of the above

118. In mammals, the principal organs involved in gluconeogenesis (i.e. the process of formation of glucose or glycogen from non-carbohydrate sources) are:
   a. Liver & Kidneys
   b. Heart & Lungs
   c. Both a and b
   d. None of the above

119. Which of the following are the Substrates for Gluconeogenesis?
   a. Glucogenic amino acids
   b. Lactates and pyruvates
   c. Glycerol and Propionic acid (in ruminants)
   d. All of the above

120. Which of the following are involved in gluconeogenesis?
   a. Glycolysis
   b. Citric acid cycle and some special reactions
   c. Both a and b
   d. None of the above

121. The main pathway of gluconeogenesis is a reversal of glycolytic pathway and the energy barriers which are irreversible and prevent such reversal occur:
   a. Between pyruvate and phosphoenol pyruvate
   b. Between fructose-1, 6-bi-phosphate and fructose-6-P
   c. Between glucose-6-P and glucose as well as between glucose-1-P and glycogen
   d. All of the above

122. The energy barrier between pyruvate and phosphoenol pyruvate can be circumvented by special adaptations such as action of important enzymes that include:
   a. Pyruvate carboxylase (a mitochondrial enzyme)
   b. Phosphoenol pyruvate carboxykinase (an enzyme present mainly in cytosol and in small amounts in mitochondrion)
   b. Both a and b
   d. None of the above

123. A key enzyme in gluconeogenic pathway, whose presence determines whether or not a tissue is capable of forming glucose and/or glycogen not only from pyruvate/lactate but also from triosephosphates, is:
   a. Pyruvate carboxylase
   b. Fructose-1,6-biphosphatase
   c. Malate dehydrogenase
   d. None of the above

124. The enzymes involved in circumventing the energy barrier between glucose-6-P and glucose include:
   a. Glucose-6-phosphatase
   b. Glycogen synthase
   c. Phosphorylase
   d. None of the above

125. Which of the following constitutes the principal and major gluconeogenic pathway?
    a. Net conversion of both glucogenic amino acids via Pyruvate for formation of glucose/glycogen (i.e. after transamination or deamination, glucogenic amino acids form either Pyruvic acid or intermediates of TCA cycle)
    b. Net conversion of lactates via Pyruvate for formation of glucose/glycogen
    c. both a and b
    d. None of the above

126. Some special pathways for Gluconeogenesis other than the major pathway include:
    a. Conversion of Glycerol to Glucose
    b. Conversion of Propionic Acid to Glucose
    c. Both a and b
    d. None of the above

127. Vitamin B_{12} deficiency in animals and humans results in excretion of large amounts of:
    a. Methylmalonic acid
    b. Propionic acid
    c. D-glucuronic acid
    d. None of the above

128. The hormones that increase gluconeogenesis include:
    a. Glucagon
    b. Glucocorticoids
    c. Both a and b
    d. None of the above

129. An example of Oxaloacetate forming amino acids is:
    a. Glycine
    b. Aspartic acid
    c. Proline
    d. Glutamate

130. Which of the following enzymes are involved in propionic acid metabolism?
    a. Acyl-CoA synthase
    b. Propionyl-CoA carboxylase
    c. Methylmalonyl-CoA racemase & Methylmalonyl-CoA isomerase
    d. All of the above

131. Choose the incorrect statement with respect to "Cori Cycle".
    a. Once formed Lactic acid can be further metabolised only by its reconversion to pyruvate
    b. Lactates and pyruvates can readily diffuse out from the cells in which they are produced and pass into the circulation
    c. Muscles can convert Glucose-6-P to glucose due to lack of the enzyme Glucose-6-Phosphatase
    d. All of the above

132. The Steps of the reactions involved in the Lactate-Propanediol Pathway include:
   a. Lactic acid is first reduced to form Lactaldehyde
   b. Conversion of lactaldehyde to Acetol
   c. Acetol in turn is reduced, in presence of NADH, to form 1,2-propanediol either "free" form or "Phosphorylated" form
   d. All of the above

133. In the metabolic pathway of Galactose, the reaction where Galactose is phosphorylated to Galactose-1-P using Galactokinase (an adaptive enzyme), is a:
   a. Irreversible
   b. Reversible
   c. Both a and b
   d. None of the above

134. Galactose-1-P reacts with UDP-Glucose to form UDP-Galactose and glucose-1-P, in presence of the enzyme:
   a. Galactokinase
   b. Galactose-1-P-uridyl transferase
   c. Epimerase
   d. None of the above

135. What brings about the transfer of galactosyl moiety to D-glucose to form Lactose in the lactating mammary gland?
   a. Binding of α-lactalbumin modifier to the catalytic subunit of Lactose synthetase enzyme
   b. Involvement of Galactosyl transferase
   c. Both a and b
   d. None of the above

136. Which of the following include the disorders of carbohydrate metabolism in animals?
   a. Diabetes Mellitus and Glycogen Storage Diseases
   b. Hyperinsulinism
   c. Hypoglycaemia of Baby Pigs
   d. All of the above

137. The main Glucose transporter in the liver cell plasma membrane is:
   a. GLUT-5
   b. GLUT-3
   c. GLUT-2
   d. None of the above

138. The most widely used methods for blood glucose levels that are used in manual, automated and in point-of-care testing modules are:
   a. Hexokinase (HK)
   b. Glucose Dehydrogenase (GD)
   c. Glucose Oxidase (GO)
   d. All of the above

139. The Normal fasting plasma glucose concentration in monogastrics and ruminants, respectively is approximately around:
   a. 4-6 mmol/l and 3-5mmol/l
   b. 1-2 mmol/l and 1-2 mmol/l
   c. 2 mmol/l and 3 mmol/l
   d. 1-3 mmol/l and 2-3 mmol/l

140. The respective renal thresholds for glucose in cows and dogs are:

a. 70-130 mg/dl; 180-200 mg/dl   b. 98-102 mg/dl; 180-220 mg/dl

c. 160-200 mg/dl; 70-100 mg/dl   d. None of the above

141. The approximate Serum Insulin concentrations in Canine Diabetes of Type II Obese and Type III Obese approximately are:

a. 5-20 μU/ml; 0-5 μU/ml   b. 20-130μU/ml; 8-60 μU/ml

c. 0-5 μU/ml; 20-30 μU/ml   d. None of the above

142. A consistent finding in bovine ketosis and in ovine pregnancy toxemia is:

a. Hypoglycemia   b. Hyperglycemia

c. Both a and b   d. None of the above

143. Which of the following constitute the two major pathways of glucose catabolism?

a. Glycolysis   b. TCA Cycle

c. Both a and b   d. None of the above

144. Pyruvate, generated through glycolysis, has different fates, depending on the conditions of the animal and the cell type such as:

a. Lactic acid production   b. Acetyl CoA production

c. Both a and b   d. None of the above

145. The enzyme that links glycolysis with the TCA cycle by converting pyruvate into acetyl CoA is:

a. Pyruvate dehydrogenase   b. Lactate dehydrogenase

c. Hexokinase   d. All of the above

146. The main precursor for the TCA cycle, lipogenesis, and ketogenesis (during negative balance) whose production occurs in the aerobic state is:

a. Thiamine   b. Acetyl CoA

c. Lactic acid   d. None of the above

147. Choose the correct statements related to the role of TCA Cycle intermediates.

a. Citrate for fatty acid synthesis

b. α-ketoglutarate for glutamic acid (amino acid synthesis

c. Oxaloacetate for non-essential amino acid synthesis

d. All of the above

148. Choose the correct statement with respect to the fate of volatile fatty acids in ruminant carbohydrate metabolism.

a. Acetate—precursor to Acetyl CoA (TCA cycle; fat synthesis)

b. Propionate—precursor to glucose (glycolysis, milk lactose)

c. Butyrate—precursor to Acetyl CoA (TCA cycle)

d. All of the above

149. A high fiber and a high concentrate diet favours the respective production of:

a. Acetate; Propionic acid   b. Butyric acid; Acetate

c. Both a and b   d. None of the above

150. For every glucose molecule fully metabolized to CO_2 and H_2O, the efficiency of converting glucose bond energy into ATP high-energy P bond is:

a. 10% b. 45%

c. 20% d. 80%

Answer Key

1	c	2	b	3	d	4	a	5	b	6	d	7	c
8	a	9	d	10	d	11	a	12	d	13	c	14	c
15	d	16	c	17	a	18	d	19	c	20	b	21	d
22	a	23	c	24	d	25	c	26	a	27	d	28	b
29	a	30	c	31	d	32	d	33	b	34	d	35	d
36	a	37	b	38	d	39	b	40	a	41	c	42	d
43	c	44	d	45	b	46	d	47	c	48	d	49	b
50	d	51	c	52	d	53	a	54	b	55	d	56	c
57	a	58	d	59	c	60	a	61	c	62	d	63	a
64	d	65	d	66	c	67	a	68	b	69	d	70	c
71	a	72	b	73	d	74	d	75	a	76	c	77	d
78	c	79	b	80	a	81	c	82	a	83	c	84	d
85	b	86	a	87	a	88	c	89	c	90	c	91	a
92	d	93	b	94	a	95	d	96	c	97	a	98	b
99	c	100	d	101	c	102	d	103	d	104	d	105	a
106	c	107	c	108	b	109	d	110	a	111	c	112	b
113	a	114	a	115	d	116	d	117	c	118	a	119	d
120	c	121	d	122	c	123	b	124	a	125	c	126	c
127	a	128	c	129	b	130	d	131	c	131	d	132	d
133	a	134	b	135	a	136	d	137	c	138	d	139	a
140	b	141	b	142	a	143	c	144	c	145	a	146	b
147	d	148	d	149	a	150	b						

11

Biochemistry of Protein Metabolism

Suraksha Subedi Deka[1], Manoj Kumar Kalita[1] and Prerona Patowary[2]

[1]Lakhimpur College of Veterinary Science, Assam Agricultural University Joyhing North Lakhimpur, Assam

[2]Assam Agricultural University-Goat Research Station, Burnihat, Assam

Introduction

Protein metabolism is a complex and multifaceted process that plays a crucial role in the overall health and function of living organisms. At the most fundamental level, protein metabolism involves the synthesis, breakdown, and utilization of proteins, which are essential macromolecules that serve a wide range of structural, functional, and regulatory roles within the body.

The process of protein synthesis, or translation, begins with the transcription of genetic information stored in DNA into messenger RNA (mRNA) molecules. These mRNA molecules then serve as templates for the assembly of specific sequences of amino acids into polypeptide chains, which ultimately fold into the three-dimensional structures of functional proteins. This highly regulated process is essential for the production of the diverse array of proteins required for cellular processes, tissue repair, immune function, and numerous other physiological activities. In contrast, protein degradation, or catabolism, refers to the breakdown of proteins into their constituent amino acids. This process is mediated by various proteolytic enzymes, such as endopeptidases, exopeptidases, and dipeptidases, which cleave the peptide bonds that hold the amino acid residues together Protein degradation serves important functions, such as the recycling of amino acids for energy production or the synthesis of new proteins, the removal of damaged or misfolded proteins, and the regulation of cellular signaling pathways.

The balance between protein synthesis and degradation, known as protein turnover, is crucial for maintaining homeostasis and ensuring the proper functioning of cells and tissues. Factors that can influence protein turnover include the availability of amino acids, the activity of proteolytic enzymes, the presence of hormones and growth factors, and the overall energy status of the cell. Disruptions in protein metabolism can have significant implications for human health, as evidenced by the numerous diseases and disorders associated with aberrant protein synthesis, folding, or degradation. For example, neurodegenerative diseases such as Alzheimer's and Parkinson's have been linked to the accumulation of misfolded proteins and the failure of cellular protein quality control mechanisms. Conversely, the upregulation of protein degradation pathways, such as the ubiquitin-proteasome system and autophagy, has been observed in certain cancers, where it may contribute to the rapid turnover of cellular proteins required for tumour growth and metastasis the study of protein metabolism also provides valuable insights into the fundamental biological processes and the evolution of living organisms. By understanding the mechanisms that govern protein synthesis, folding, and degradation, researchers can gain a deeper appreciation for the complexity and adaptability of life at the molecular level.

Understanding protein metabolism has significant implications for disease prevention and therapeutic interventions. Targeting protein synthesis, degradation pathways, or protein quality control mechanisms represents potential strategies for treating diseases characterized by protein misfolding, aggregation, or deficiency. Emerging therapies aim to modulate protein metabolism to enhance muscle growth and repair, mitigate neurodegeneration, and improve metabolic health in diverse patient populations. Protein metabolism encompasses a series of interconnected processes that maintain cellular function and adaptability. The following chapter covers multiple-choice questions on protein metabolism, reflecting their significance in biological sciences and medical research.

1. Sakaguchi test is done for the detection of which of the following amino acids?
   a. Methionine   b. Lysine
   c. Arginine   d. Leucine
2. all naturally occurring proteins are made of
   a. D amino acids   b. L amino acids
   c. Either D or L amino acids   d. Neither D nor L amino acids
3. Which structure of the protein is unaffected by the denaturation process?
   a. Primary structure   b. Secondary structure
   c. Tertiary structure   d. None of the above
4. Which of the following amino acids is a lipotropic factor?
   a. Serine   b. Leucine
   c. Lycine   d. Methionine
5. Number of ATP(s) required for synthesis of molecule of urea in the Kreb's Hansleit cycle is
   a. 1   b. 2
   c. 3   d. 4
6. α helix of protein is stabilized by
   a. Peptide bonds   b. Disulphide bonds
   c. Polar bonds   d. Hydrogen bonds
7. The largest subunit in in prokaryotic RNA polymerase is
   a. α b. β
   c. σ d. β'
8. Hartnup's diseases is associated withlow serum levels of
   a. Tryptophan   b. Threonine
   c. Tyrosine   d. Phenylalanine

9. Which of the following amino acids does not participate in transamination?
   a. Threonine
   b. Lysine
   c. All of the above
   d. None of the above
10. Which of the following statements is not true for Shine Dalgarno sequence?
   a. It is recognition sequence of initiation codonin prokaryotes and eukaryotes.
   b. It binds with 16S RNA
   c. It is located 6-10 bases upstream of the AUG codon in mRNA
   d. All of the above
11. Which of the following is responsible for ribosomal translocation in protein synthesis?
   a. EF- T
   b. EF- Tu
   c. EF- Ts
   d. EF- G
12. Puromycin enters the A site of ribosomes and inhibit translation in
   a. Prokaryotes only
   b. Eukaryotes only
   c. Both prokaryotes and Eukaryotes
   d. None of the above
13. Wobble synthesis of degeneracy of genetic code was proposed by
   a. R.W Hollcy
   b. Francis Crick
   c. M. Nirenberg
   d. H. Khorana
14. D- Amino acid oxidase needs which of the following coenzymes?
   a. NAD
   b. NADP
   c. FMN
   d. FAD
15. The enzyme trypsin specifically hydrolyses peptide bonds of
   a. Basic amino acid
   b. Acidic amino acid
   c. Aromatic amino acids
   d. Neutral amino acids
16. which of the following is not a chaperone?
   a. HsP 70
   b. HsP 40
   c. PPI
   d. BiP
17. Which of the following conditionsis related to prions?
   a. Mad cow disease
   b. Creutzfeldt-Jacob disease
   c. Alzheimer's Disease
   d. All of the above
18. Proteins can be separated according to size by
   a. Ion exchange chromatography
   b. Affinity chromatography
   c. Molecular Exclusion Chromatography
   d. All of the above
19. The technique used to determine the 3D structure of protein is
   a. X ray crystallography
   b. Mass Spectrometry
   c. Protein Microarrays
   d. Zeta potential
20. Antibiotics contain which of the following?
   a. Protein amino acids
   b. Non protein amino acids
   c. None of the above
   d. Both of the above

21. The molecular basis for sickle cell anemia is substitution of
    a. Glutamic acid by valine
    b. Valine by glutamic acid
    c. Glycine by valine
    d. Valine by glycine
22. Which of the following is Sanger's reagent?
    a. 1-fluoro- 2,3 dinitrobenzene
    b. 1-fluoro- 2,4 dinitrobenzene
    c. 2-fluoro- 2,3 dinitrobenzene
    d. 2-fluoro- 2,4 dinitrobenzene
23. Edman degradation is used for identification o
    a. C terminal amino acids
    b. N terminal amino acids
    c. 5′ end of nucleic acids
    d. 3′ end of nucleic acids
24. The average molecular weight of an amino acid residue in a protein is
    a. 210
    b. 140
    c. 130
    d. 110
25. In SDS PAGE separationof proteins is based on which of the following properties?
    a. Molecular weight, shape and charge
    b. Molecular weight and charge
    c. Molecular weight and shape
    d. Molecular weight only
26. Which of the following is reducing agent in SDS PAGE?
    a. SDS
    b. SLS
    c. 2- mercaptoethanol
    d. Bisacrylamide
27. The immediate precursor of heme in its biosynthesis is
    a. Protoporphyrin IX
    b. Uroporphyrinogen
    c. Porphobilinogen
    d. Coproporphyrinogen
28. Tyrosine is associated with which of the following inborn errors of metabolism?
    a. Tyrosinemia and phenylketonuria
    b. Tyrosinemia and cystinuria
    c. Tyrosinemia and alkaptonuria
    d. Tyrosinosis and citrullinemia
29. An amino acid not found in protein is
    a. Histidine
    b. Threonine
    c. Cysteine
    d. β alanine
30. Trypsinogen is converted to its active form trypsin by
    a. Gastric HCl
    b. Bile salts
    c. Enterokinase
    d. Calcium
31. The enzymes of urea cycle are located in
    a. Mitochondria
    b. Cytosol
    c. Both a and b
    d. Ribosomes
32. Which of the following amino acids is (are) exclusively ketogenic?
    a. Leucine
    b. Isoleucine
    c. Histidine
    d. All of the above
33. Histamine is formed from histidine by which of the following process?
    a. Decarboxylation
    b. Deamination
    c. Dehydrogenation
    d. Hydration

34. The most abundant immunoglobin found in plasma is
  a. Ig E b. Ig M
  c. Ig G d. Ig D
35. Which of the following is an imino acid?
  a. Serine b. Threonine
  c. Leucine d. Proline
36. Which of the following statement is not true for Bence Jones proteins?
  a. It is a dimer of light chains
  b. It is made of Kappa and Lamba chains
  c. It is found in urine of patients with multiple myeloma
  d. It is a type of immunoglobulin
37. The major metabolism for removal of ammonia in brain is the formation of
  a. Glutamate b. Glutamine
  c. Aspartate d. Urea
38. Which of the following is used for separation of plasma proteins?
  a. Ultracentrifugation
  b. Salting out with ammonium sulfate
  c. Salting in
  d. All of the above
39. The coenzyme required by all transaminase is
  a. Pyridoxal phosphate b. Thiamine Pyrophosphate
  c. Biotin d. Coenzyme A
40. Which amino acid (s) undergoesoxidative deamination at a significant rate to release ammonia?
  a. Aspartate b. Glutamate
  c. Both of the above d. None of the above
41. The coenzyme utilized by glutamate dehydrogenase is
  a. NAD^+ b. $NADP^+$
  c. Either NAD^+ or $NADP^+$ d. None of the above
42. The end product of protein/ amino acid metabolism is
  a. Urea b. Uric acid
  c. Ammonia d. Purine
43. Which of the following has peptidyl transferase activity?
  a. 16S rRNA b. 5S rRNA
  c. 23SrRNA d. 21S rRNA
44. The compound that serves as link between TCA and Urea cycle is
  a. Malate b. Fumarate
  c. Citrate d. Succinate

45. Which of the following causes misreading of the mRNA
    a. Chloramphenicol b. Cyclohexamine
    c. Erythromycin d. Streptomycin
46. Urea has two amino groups; one is derived from ammonia and the other from _______.
    a. Aspartate b. Arginosuccinate
    c. Fumarate d. None of the above
47. Carbamoyl PhosphateSynthetase I is located in
    a. Cytosol b. Mitochondria
    c. Both a and b d. Nucleus
48. Ribozyme is
    a. RNA having immunological properties b. RNA with catalytic activity
    c. RNA without sugar d. RNA without phosphate
49. An example of negative acute phase protein
    a. Albumin b. Globulin
    c. Ceruloplasmin d. C reactive protein
50. Which among the following is fibrous protein?
    a. Histones b. Prolamines
    c. Protamine d. Elastin
51. Which of the following bonds is not responsible for protein structure?
    a. Phosphodiester bond b. Disulfide bond
    c. Hydrogen bond d. Electrostatic bond
52. Glycine is not required for the synthesis of
    a. Hemoglobin b. Creatinine
    c. Taurocholic acid d. Glutathione
53. Name the lipoprotein with the fastest electrophoretic mobility and the lowest triglyceride content is
    a. HDL b. LDL
    c. Chylomicrons d. IDL
54. Pepsinogen is converted to its active form pepsin by
    a. Bile salts b. Trypsin
    c. Pancreatic amylase d. HCl
55. Cofactor for the enzyme carbamoyl phosphate synthetase is
    a. Magnesium b. Sodium
    c. Zinc d. Calcium
56. Which amino acid is not optically active?
    a. Glycine b. Alanine
    c. Valine d. Serine

57. The main purpose of glucose alanine cycle is
   a. To convert glucose to alanine
   b. To increase protein catabolism
   c. Transport enzymes of gluconeogenesis
   d. To deliver amino groups from muscle to liver
58. Biuret reaction is specific for
   a. -(NH)NH_2 b. –CO-NH-linkages
   c. Both of the above d. None of the above
59. Which of the following is simple protein found in nucleoproteins of sperm?
   a. Protamine b. Prolamine
   c. Globulin d. Albumin
60. Which among the following disrupts the non-covalent bonds between peptide linkages of protein molecules?
   a. Perfomic acid b. Guanidine hydrochloride
   c. Uric acid d. Trypsin
61. Which of the statements is not true for peptide bond
   a. It is rigid and planar
   b. It is partial double bond
   c. It generally exists in trans form
   d. It is written from C- terminal residue to N- terminal residue.
62. The alpha-helix and beta-pleated sheet conformation of proteins were proposed by
   a. Watson and Crick b. Carl Neuberg
   c. Pauling and Corey d. M Nirenberg
63. Which amino acid has an indole group?
   a. Proline b. Tryptophan
   c. Histidine d. Cystine
64. In birds, ammonia is removed in the form of
   a. Uric acid b. Urea
   c. Both of the above d. None of the above
65. Which condition is characterized by deficiency ofprotein ?
   a. Kwashiorkor b. Marasmus
   c. Rye's syndrome d. Gaucher's disease
66. All following are conjugated proteins except
   a. Gycoproteins b. Chromoproteins
   c. Casein d. Proteans
67. Systematic name of alanine is
   a. 2,6 diaminohexanoic acid b. 2-Aminopropanoic acid
   c. 2- Aminobutanedioic acid d. 2- Amino 3- propanoic acid

68. Which of the following bonds is not broken by denaturation?
    a. Disulfide bond b. Ionic bond
    c. H bond d. Peptide bond
69. Protoporphyria (erythrohepatic is caused by the deficiency of
    a. ALA hydratase b. Protoporphyrin oxidase
    c. ALA Synthase d. Ferrochelatase
70. Which is the largest Immunoglobulin?
    a. Ig A b. Ig M
    c. Ig D d. Ig G
71. Creatine is made up of
    a. Glycine, cysteine and glutamate b. Glutamine, serine and cystine
    c. Glycine, threonine and methionine d. Glycine, arginine and methionine
72. Glutathione is composed of
    a. Glycine, cysteine and glutamate b. Glutamine, serine and cystine
    c. Glycine, threonine and methionine d. Glycine, arginine and threonine
73. Which of the following amino acid is not polar?
    a. Methionine b. Alanine
    c. Proline d. All of the above
74. Hydroxylation of proline requires the following except
    a. Succinate b. Vitamin C
    c. Proline hydroxylase d. Iron
75. Which is the most abundant protein in the human body?
    a. Albumin b. Globulin
    c. Collagen d. Myosin
76. Aspartic acid is
    a. Aromatic amino acid b. Dicarboxylic mono amino acid
    c. Monocarboxylic di amino acid d. Non polar amino acid
77. Parkinson's diseases is associated with reduced levels of
    a. Epinephrine b. GABA
    c. dopamine d. Serotonin
78. Tryptophan is a precursor for synthesis of
    a. Coenzymes of niacin b. Serotonin
    c. Melatonin d. All of the above
79. Ubiquitin is a highly conserved protein containing ____________ number of amino acids.
    a. 75 b. 76
    c. 78 d. 79

80. A signal sequence is
   a. A peptide located at the N terminal of nascent protein which facilitates is transport to the correct location
   b. Short peptide sequences attached to a protein that initiates its degradation
   c. Sequence for glycosylation
   d. Peptide sequence that identifies the origin of translation
81. Which of the following is not a type of typical post translational modification?
   a. Protein folding b. Glycosylation
   c. Intein splicing d. Phosphorylation
82. In N - glycosylation, the carbohydrate moiety is attached to which amino acid?
   a. Serine b. Threonine
   c. Asparagine d. Valine
83. Which of the following is not required for activation of amino acids for translation?
   a. Amino acyl transferase b. ATP
   c. GTP d. Mg^{2+}
84. Diphtheria toxin inhibits the process of protein synthesis by
   a. Inhibiting the peptide bond formation
   b. Inhibiting binding of amino acyl tRNA
   c. ADP ribosylation of eEF2
   d. Inactivation of 60 S subunit of ribosomes
85. Translocation during protein synthesis is the movement of
   a. DeacetylatedtRNA from A site to P site
   b. DeacetylatedtRNA from P site to A site
   c. Dipeptidyl -tRNA from P site to E site
   d. Dipeptidyl -tRNA from A site to P site
86. Which of the following is not a characteristic of genetic code?
   a. Overlapping b. Degeneracy
   c. Universality d. Specificity
87. Which one is not a stop codon?
   a. UGA b. AUG
   c. UAA d. UAG
88. Carbamoyl phosphate synthase I is allosterically inhibited by
   a. ATP b. Acetyl Co- A
   c. Glutamate d. N acetyl glutamate
89. What is the source of carbon atom for synthesis of urea in the Urea cycle?
   a. CO_2 b. Citrulline
   c. Aspartate d. Glutamate

90. Trypsin is the activator of which of the following pancreatic enzymes?
    a. Chymotrypsinogen
    b. Proelastase
    c. Procarboxypeptidase A and B
    d. All of the above

91. Which statement is not true for aminotransferase?
    a. They catalyse ping pong reactions
    b. They catalyse irreversible reactions
    c. Pyridoxal phosphate is covalently bond to the active site of the enzyme
    d. Most of the aminotransferases are specific for α ketoglutarate as acceptor of amino group

92. α ketoglutarate is the precursor for the synthesis of following amino acids except
    a. Glutamine
    b. Leucine
    c. Asparagine
    d. Proline

93. One carbon transfer during synthesis of glycine from serine is mediated by
    a. Tetrahydrofolate
    b. PLP
    c. Biotin
    d. TPP

94. 2,3 Biphosphoglyceratebinds with oxygen in the RBCs and cause
    a. Shift of oxyhemoglobin dissociation curve to the right
    b. Shift of oxyhemoglobin dissociation curve to the left
    c. No effect in oxyhemoglobin dissociation curve
    d. Increases affinity of Hb for oxygen

95. Maple syrup urine disease is a genetic disease caused by deficiency of enzyme
    a. Homogentisatedioxidase
    b. Branched chain amino transferase
    c. Branched chain α-keto acid dehydrogenase complex
    d. Pyruvate dehydrogenase complex

96. Pepsinogen is secreted by ______________ cells of gastric glands
    a. Chief cells
    b. Parietal cells
    c. Both (a and b)
    d. Neither (a nor b)

97. Which of the following proteolytic enzymes are zymogens?
    a. Trypsinogen
    b. Pepsinogen
    c. Procarboxypeptidase
    d. All of the above

98. Thalassemias are haemolytic disorders caused by impairment in synthesis of
    a. Heme
    b. Globin
    c. Haemoglobin
    d. Protoporpyrin

99. Primary hyperoxaluria or deposition of oxalates in different tissues is associated with metabolic disorder of ________
    a. Serine
    b. Arginine
    c. Glutathione
    d. Glycine

100. At neutral pH, a mixture of amino acids in solution will exists mainly
a. Non polar b. Dipolar ions
c. Hydrophobic d. None of the above

101. Histamine is synthesised in which part of the body?
a. basophils b. Mast cells
c. brain d. All of the above

102. GABA receptors increases the permeability of cell membrane to
a. Na^+ b. K^+
c. Cl^+ d. Mg^{++}

103. An amino acid containing disulphide bond is
a. Cysteine b. Cystine
c. Homocysteine d. Methionine

104. Which of the following histone pairs form tetramers in solution?
a. H3, H4 b. H2A, H2B
c. H2A, H3 d. H1, H2A

105. After completion of protein synthesis, in which sequence the following leave the ribosome?
a. Polypeptide chain, mRNA, tRNA
b. Polypeptide chain, tRNA, mRNA
c. mRNA, Polypeptide chain, tRNA
d. tRNA, mRNA, Polypeptide chain,

106. Holozyme binds to
a. Single stranded DNA b. Doubled stranded DNA
c. Single stranded RNA d. Double stranded RNA

107. Which step of translation does not consume high energy phosphate bond?
a. Initiation b. Amino acid activation
c. Translocation d. Peptidyl transferase reaction

108. The binding site of tRNA with amino acids is
a. -CCA 3'arm b. Anticodon arm
c. DHU loop d. Variable loop

109. The binding site of tRNA with mRNA is
a. -CCA 3'arm b. Anticodon arm
c. DHU loop d. Variable loop

110. In protein synthesis, the tRNA carrying initiating amino acids enter which site of ribosome?
a. A site b. E site
c. P site d. Initiation site

111. A complete protein is one which contains
a. All essential amino acids b. All 20 amino acids
c. All non-essential amino acids d. All D amino acids

112. One amino acid differs from another based on
    a. Amino group b. COOH group
    c. Peptide bond d. R group
113. The turnover number of enzymes is related to
    a. Protein nature b. Non protein group
    c. Efficiency d. Catalytic activity
114. Ninhydrin test is positive for
    a. Alpha amino acids b. Beta amino acids
    c. Acidic amino acids d. Basic amino acids
115. What percentage of mammalian DNA codes for protein ?
    a. 1-2% b. 2-4%
    c. 80-90% d. 90-100%
116. The carbon skeleton of which of the following is not converted to acetyl coA
    a. Glycine b. Lysine
    c. Leucine d. Tryptophan
117. The first protein sequenced by Federick Sanger was
    a. Haemoglobin b. Keratin
    c. Albumin d. Insulin
118. Trypsinogen is converted to trypsin by
    a. HCl b. Bicarbonate
    c. Enterokinase d. Pepsin
119. An example of essential sulphur containing amino acid
    a. Cystine b. Cysteine
    c. Methionine d. All of the above
120. Name the intermediate of TCA cycle that participates in heme synthesis
    a. Citrulline b. Succinyl CoA
    c. α Ketoglutaric acid d. Fumarate
121. Cryoelectronmicroscopy is used to determine the 3D structure of protein in which the samples are frozen in ____________ to preserve its structure.
    a. Liquid Nitrogenb. Liquid Helium
    c. Iced. Liquid CO_2
122. Which enzymes do not require co-enzymes for their activity?
    a. Proenzymes b. Intracellular enzymes
    c. Extracellular enzymes d. All of the above
123. Ribosomes are made of
    a. RNA b. DNA
    c. RNA and protein d. RNA, DNA and protein

124. Hypoproteinaemia leads to oedema because of
   a. Increased hydrostatic pressure at the capillaries
   b. Decreased hydrostatic pressure at the capillaries
   c. Increased colloidal osmotic pressure across capillary wall
   d. Decreased colloidal osmotic pressure across capillary wall
125. Which of the following proteins promotes rouleaux formation?
   a. Prothrombin b. Fibrinogen
   c. Thrombin d. Albumin
126. Which of the following techniques uses antibodies to visualise specific protein?
   a. Southern blotting b. Western Blotting
   c. SDS PAGE d. Chromatography
127. The function of protein microarray in proteomics is
   a. To study protein- protein interactions b. To study protein structure
   c. To study protein synthesis d. All of the above
128. In two dimensional gel electrophoresis:
   a. Two types of protein with same molecular weight tend to migrate at same position
   b. Proteins with similar migration tend to locate near each other
   c. A large number of proteins can be determined
   d. None of the above
129. The most abundant protein in bone is
   a. Collagen Type I b. Collagen Type II
   c. Collagen Type III d. Collagen Type IV
130. Highest concentration of cystine can be found in
   a. Myosin b. Keratin
   c. Collagen d. Melanin
131. Low density lipoproteins are rich in
   a. Cholesterol b. Proteins
   c. Phospholipids d. Apoproteins
132. Urea synthesis takes place in
   a. Kidney b. Liver
   c. Kidney and Liver d. Blood
133. Deficiency of tryptophan and nicotinate in diet leads to
   a. Beri beri b. Pernicious anaemia
   c. Megaloblastic anaemia d. Pellagra
134. Which of the following amino acids produces a vasodilator on decarboxylation?
   a. Glutamate b. Aspartate
   c. Histidine d. Threonine

135. The spliceosome activity is at
  a. 5' splice site b. 3' splice site
  c. Branch point sequence d. All of the above

136. Which of the following statement is true for codon anticodon reaction?
  a. Inosine in the 5' position of anticodon can base pair with A, U or C in 3' codon position
  b. Inosine in the 3' position of anticodon can base pair with A, U or C in 5' codon position
  c. Inosine in the 5' position of anticodon can base pair with A, U or G in 3' codon position
  d. Inosine in the 3' position of anticodon can base pair with A, U or G in 5' codon position

137. Transmethylation of guanido acetic acid leads to biosynthesis of
  a. Choline b. Creatinine
  c. Nicotine d. Purine

138. The amino acid which not optically active is
  a. Valine b. Leucine
  c. Lysine d. Glycine

139. An example of scleroprotein is
  a. Keratin b. Collagen
  c. Elastin d. All of the above

140. The H- bonds in the secondary and tertiary structure of proteins are directly attacked by
  a. Acid b. Salts
  c. Alkalis d. Detergents

141. Which of the following amino acids doesnot exist as α helix?
  a. Phenylalanine b. Cysteine
  c. Proline d. Tryptophan

142. Collagen molecule contains _____________ number of helices.
  a. 2 b. 3
  c. 4 d. 5

143. Ribosomes bound to endoplasmic reticulum synthesise almost all integral membrane proteins except the proteins of
  a. Mitochondria b. Chloroplast
  c. Chloroplast and nucleus d. Chloroplast and mitochondria

144. ppGpp stands for
  a. Guanosine tetraphosphate b. Biphospho guanyl diphosphate
  c. Unusual guanine phosphate d. Guanine phospho hydrate

145. Wilson's disease is associated with which of the following proteins?
  a. Albumin b. Ceruloplasmin
  c. Transferrind.c- reactive protein

146. Ribosomes were discovered by
   a. George A Palade
   b. Leibig
   c. Robert Hook
   d. Watson and Crick
147. Nuclear localization signal is rich in
   a. Glutamate and aspartate
   b. Glutamine and asparagine
   c. Lysine and arginine
   d. Threonine and serine
148. Secretory proteins are synthesised by
   a. Ribosomes on ER
   b. Mitochondria
   c. Free ribosomes
   d. Ribosomes on cell membrane
149. SDS PAGE was discovered by
   a. Karry Mullis
   b. Federick Sanger
   c. Arne Tiselius
   d. U.K Laemili
150. L amino acids are absorbed from intestine by
   a. Active transport
   b. Passive transport
   c. Facilitated diffusion
   d. Free diffusion
151. Which of the following is not tertiary structure of protein?
   a. Fibrous
   b. Beta sheet
   c. 3-D arrangement
   d. Domains
152. The destruction of the tertiary structure of a protein and loss in its biological activity is called
   a. Deproteination
   b. Deamination
   c. Denaturation
   d. None of the above
153. Which compound is accumulated in the defective Ornithine trans-carboxylase enzyme?
   a. Ammonia
   b. Citrulline
   c. Ornithine
   d. All of the above
154. What is the isoelectric pH of alanine?
   a. 7.0
   b. 6.09
   c. 6.02
   d. 6.90
155. Thymol turbidity test is done for non-specific measurement of
   a. Globulins
   b. Albumin
   c. Threonine
   d. Total Protein
156. Gamma heavy chains is present in
   a. IgA
   b. Ig D
   c. Ig E
   d. Ig G
157. Serum amylase is increased in
   a. Jaundice
   b. Acute pancreatitis
   c. Pancreatic cancer
   d. All of the above

158. Anion exchange resin linked to cellulosebackbone is
   a. DEAE cellulose b. Cholestyramine
   c. Sodium polystyrene sulphonate USP d. Sephadex
159. Which of the following is the slowest process
   a. Transcription b. Translation
   c. DNA replication d. Splicing
160. Which of the following is the most energetically expensive process?
   a. Transcription b. Translation
   c. Post translational modification d. Splicing
161. Which of the following is not a property of open reading frame?
   a. Specifies a single protein
   b. Non-overlapping
   c. Segments between start and stop codon
   d. It is the part of the genome translating into protein
162. Shine – Dalgarno sequence is also known as the ________
   a. Ribosome binding site b. ORF
   c. TATA box d. Start codon
163. How many unsual bases are present in tRNA?
   a. 2 b. 3
   c. 5 d. 6
164. Charging of tRNA molecules requires acyl linkage between the carboxyl group of the amino acid to the ___________
   a. 3' OH group of C b. 3' OH group of A
   c. 5' OH group of T d. None of the above
165. How many types of tRNA synthetases are found in cell?
   a. 64 b. 20
   c. 30 d. 21
166. Which of the following is a decapeptide?
   a. Vasopressin b. Oxytocin
   c. Angiotensin I d. All of the above
167. When $V_0 = V_{max}/2$, what is the substrate concentration?
   a. K_m b. 0
   c. S/2 d. ½ K_m
168. What are the advantages of immobilised enzymes?
   a. Reusability and Stability b. For maximum reaction
   c. To minimise substrate use d. None of the above
169. Which of these methods is not a type of continuous enzyme assay?
   a. Colorimetric method b. Fluorometric method
   c. Chemilumiscent method d. Radiometric assay

170. Which of the following statements is true for glucokinase?
   a. It is inhibited by glucose 6 phosphate   b. It is present in all the cells
   c. It has higher Km for glucose   d. It has higher affinity for glucose

171. Which of the following statements about uncompetitive inhibition of an enzymeare true?
   A. Uncompetitive inhibitor binds to both free enzyme as well as an enzyme substrate complex.
   B. Addition of uncompetitive inhibitor lowers the Vmax of the reaction.
   C. Apparent KM of the enzyme is lowered
   D. Uncompetitive inhibitor binds to Enzyme substrate complex
   a. A, B and C are correct   b. B, C and D are correct
   c. A, C and D are correct   d. A, B, C and D are correct

172. Fe-S are prosthetic group that carry electrons in the following except
   a. Cytochrome C oxidase   b. NADH dehydrogenase
   c. Succinate dehydrogenase   d. Cytochrome C reductase

173. Hexokinase belongs to which class of enzymes?
   a. Oxidoreductase   b. Lyase
   c. Ligase   d. Transferase

174. Puromycin inhibits protein synthesis by
   a. Premature termination of translation   b. Inhibit peptidyl transferase
   c. Inhibition of ADP ribosylation of EF 1   d. Block DNA polymerase

175. During eukaryotic Translation, guanine nucleotide exchange factor is
   a. eIF 2 A   b. eIF 2 B
   c. eIF 4 F   d. eIF 4 B

176. Which of the following is not involved in regulation of enzyme activity?
   a. Allosteric interaction   b. Feedback inhibition
   c. Competitive inhibition   d. Suicide inhibition

177. Which of the following is not a serine protease?
   a. Acetylcholine esterase   b. Fibrinolysin
   c. Aspartate transaminase   d. Thrombin

178. Initiation of protein synthesis in most of the eukaryotes requires
   a. Poly A tail   b. 5' cap
   c. Both of the above   d. None of the above

179. Kozak sequence is associated with
   a. Transcription in prokaryotes   b. Transcription in eukaryotes
   c. Translation in prokaryotes   d. Translation in eukaryotes

180. Which of the following is used in detoxification of benzoic acid to form hippuric acid?
   a. Glutamine   b. Glutamic acid
   c. Glycine   d. Glutathione

Answer Key

1	c	2	b	3	a	4	d	5	c	6	d	7	d
8	a	9	c	10	a	11	d	12	c	13	b	14	d
15	a	16	c	17	d	18	c	19	a	20	b	21	a
22	b	23	b	24	d	25	d	26	c	27	a	28	c
29	d	30	c	31	c	32	a	33	a	34	c	35	d
36	d	37	b	38	d	39	a	40	b	41	c	42	a
43	c	44	b	45	d	46	a	47	b	48	b	49	a
50	d	51	a	52	c	53	a	54	d	55	a	56	a
57	d	58	b	59	a	60	b	61	d	62	c	63	b
64	a	65	a	66	d	67	b	68	d	69	d	70	b
71	d	72	a	73	d	74	a	75	c	76	b	77	c
78	d	79	b	80	a	81	a	82	c	83	c	84	c
85	d	86	a	87	b	88	d	89	a	90	d	91	b
92	c	93	a	94	a	95	c	96	a	97	d	98	b
99	d	100	b	101	d	102	c	103	b	104	a	105	b
106	b	107	d	108	a	109	b	110	c	111	a	112	d
113	c	114	a	115	a	116	a	117	d	118	c	119	c
120	b	121	b	122	a	123	c	124	d	125	b	126	b
127	a	128	d	129	a	130	b	131	a	132	b	133	d
134	c	135	d	136	a	137	a	138	d	139	d	140	c
141	c	142	b	143	d	144	a	145	b	146	a	147	c
148	a	149	d	150	a	151	b	152	c	153	a	154	c
155	a	156	d	157	b	158	a	159	b	160	b	161	d
162	a	163	c	164	b	165	b	166	c	167	a	168	a
169	d	170	c	171	b	172	a	173	d	174	a	175	b
176	d	177	c	178	c	179	d	180	c				

12

Biochemistry of Lipid Metabolism

***Sasmita Barik*[1] *and Shiv Kumar Yadav*[2]**

[1]*Department of Veterinary Physiology and Biochemistry, College of Veterinary Sciences and Animal Husbandry, Guru Angad Dev Veterinary and Animal Scienes Univeristy, Ludhiana, Punjab*

[2]*KVK, Shahjahanpur, Uttar Pradesh*

Introduction

Lipids (dietary or body reserve) serves as the major source of energy for the body at the time of carbohydrate depletion. Triacyl glycerol (TG) forms the major part of lipids alongwith phospholipids, cholesterol and fat-soluble vitamins. The different forms of lipids are utilised by the body for generation of energy in the form of ATP. In addition, it serves as the source of essential fattyacids and vitamins for different metabolic purpose.

Dietary triacylglycerols (TG) are digested by lipase group of enzymes (lingual, gastric, pancreatic and intestinal) secreted by the digestive tract into free fatty acids and 2-monoacylglycerols. The 2-monoacylglycerols are either absorbed as such or hydrolysed into glycerol and fatty acids which are then absorbed independently. The glycerol and fatty acids are distributed to different tissues through circulation and utilised in the following ways-

i. Storage in fat cells of adipose tissue in the form of triacylglycerols.
ii. Oxidised in peripheral tissues for production of energy.
iii. converted to glucose in hepatic cells in the process of gluconeogenesis.
iv. Synthesis of other derived compounds like steroids and eicosanoids in gonadal and other tissues
v. Synthesis of phospholipids and cholesteryl esters.

Lipogenesis is the biochemical process of synthesis of triacyclglycerols from free fatty acids and glycerol. The process commonly occurs in cytosol of adipose tissue. In the process the fatty acids and glycerol are activated to fatty acyl CoA and glycerol phosphate by the enzyme fattyacyl coA synthetase and glycerol kinase followed by formation of triacyl glycerol by acyl transferase. The process of lipogenesis is stimulated by the hormone insulin in full fed state whereas it is inhibited by the hormone glucagon during fasting state. Lipolysis is the hydrolysis of triacylglycerols into glycerol and free fatty acids that occurs in the cytosol of adipose tissue cells by the enzyme lipase. The hormone sensitive triacylglycerol lipase controls the process of lipolysis by active phosphorylation and dephosphorylation. The hormones epinephrine, norepinephrine and glucagon stimulate whereas insulin inhibits the process of lipolysis.

The free fatty acids released by the process of lipolysis undergoes oxidation with sequential removal of a two-carbon fragment in the form of acetyl CoA with production of energy in the form of ATP. The glycerol produced in the adipose tissue is transported to liver to be utilised in the process of gluconeogenesis. The free fatty acids released in the cytosol is transported into the mitochondrial matrix in the form of acyl CoA through a carrier protein carnitine. Inside the mitochondrial matrix the Acyl co A undergoes cyclic process of oxidation, dehydration, oxidation and cleavage to release a two-carbon fragment in the form of acetyl CoA that further enters into the TCA cycle to produce energy. The 16 carbons containing palmitic acid undergoes 7 of beta oxidation (each cycle producing 5 ATPS) generating 8 acetyl CoASo total 131 ATPs are produced with utilization of 2 ATPs in the activation step. Net 129 ATPs are produced in the beta oxidation of palmitic acid.

There are 2 mechanisms for fatty acids synthesis: cytoplasmic and microsomal. Cytoplasmic system for fatty acid synthesis aka extramitochondrial system or de novo synthesis of fatty acids occurs in cutosol in liver, adipose tissue, mammary gland, lung and kidney producing mainly palmitate (16 C). Acetyl CoA, $NADPH^{+}H^{+}$ and fatty acid synthase complex are collectively required this. Acetyl CoA provided by glucose through pyruvate in glycolysis condenses with oxaloacetate in the mitochondria in the presence of citrate synthase to form citrate. Then citrate diffuses out of mitochondria to cytosol where it is splitted again by citrate lyase into acetyl CoA and oxalaoacetate. $NADPH^{+}H^{+}$ is synthesized in pentose phosphate pathway. Fatty acid synthase complex is a dimer, with each unit containing 7 enzymes and a acyl carrier protein (ACP). ACP is the part of pantothenic acid in the form of phosphopantotheine and it carries the acyl group. Each monomer contains 2 -SH groups, one provided by phosphopantotheine and attached to ACP. The other is provided by cysteine attached to the enzyme 3- ketoacyl synthase. The 2 monomers are arranged head to tail, so the -SH group of ACP of one monomer is very close to the -SH group provided by 3- ketoacyl synthase of the other monomer. A molecule of acetyl CoA combines with a pantotheine -SH group of the first monomer by acetyl (acyl) transacylase enzyme. Then acetyl group is transferred to the cysteine -SH group of the other monomer of fatty acid synthase. A molecule of malonyl CoA then combines with a pantetheine -SH group of the first monomer catalyzed by malonyl transacylase enzyme. This leads to the formation of acetyl (acyl)-malonyl-enzyme. Then acetyl group attacks the malonyl group to liberate C02 and to form 3 ketoacyl enzyme (acetoacetyl enzyme) that attached to pantotheine -SH group and to let the cysteine-SH group. The 3-ketoacyl group is reduced, dehydrated and reduced again to form the corresponding acyl-enzyme (4 carbon saturated fatty acyl enzyme). The 4 carbons saturated fatty acyl group is then transferred to cysteine -SH group of the other monomer of fatty acid synthase leaving the pantetheine -SH group of the first monomer for the second molecule of malonyl CoA. The sequence of reactions is then repeated 6 more times to produce fatty acids of 6,8,10,12,14 and finally 16 carbons (palmitic acid). Free palmitate is formed by the action of thioesterase enzyme of the multi-enzyme complex, which adds H20 and hydrolyzes the palmitoyl enzyme.

The key enzyme of cytoplasmic pathway is acetyl CoA carboxylase enzyme. Insulin stimulates fatty acid synthesis through both acetyl CoA carboxylase and pyruvate dehydrogenase and inhibits lipolysis Glucagon and epinephrine inhibits fatty acid synthesis through cyclic AMP and also stimulates lipolysis of long chain fatty acids. Long chain acyl CoA inhibits Fatty acid synthesis inhibiting allosterically acetyl CoA carboxylase and transport of citrate from mitochondria to cytosol.

Acetone, acetoacetate and beta hydroxybutyrate are the major ketone bodies are produced in the body and used as a source of energy in skeletal muscles, cardiac muscles, kidneys in prolonged fasting and starvation. Brain tissue can also oxidize ketone bodies within 5 to 6 days of starvation whereas, liver does not contain enzymes for ketone bodies oxidation (ketolysis). These are produced in mitochondria in liver from acetyl CoA derived from fatty acids oxidation and ketogenic amino acids. Acetoacetate is the first ketone body produced Then both beta-hydroxy butyrate and acetone are derived from It., Insulin secreted, following a meal inhibits lipolysis and ketogenesis whereas anti-insulin hormones glucagon secreted fasting stimulates lipolysis and ketogenesis. Excessive lipolysis in adipose tissue leads to very high level of plasma free fatty acids (FFA) which in liver is activated to acyl CoA that undergoes beta oxidation to give acetyl CoA that enters into the citric acid cycle. But if the amount of acetyl CoA molecules is more than the capacity of TCA cycle in liver, they are used to form ketone bodies. Oxidation of ketone bodies (ketolysis) occurs intracellularly in mitochondria in extra hepatic tissues like muscles. Ketolysis do not occur in liver. Acetone is volatile and removed in the expired air. Beta-hydroxybutyrate is converted in to acetoacetate by hydroxybutyrate dehydrogenase enzyme. Acetoacetate is then activated in to acetoacetyl CoA by thiophorase enzyme in the presence of succinyl CoA and acetoacetyl CoA synthetase enzyme. In the presence of ATP acetoacetyl CoA is split into two molecules or acetyl CoA which are oxidized in citric acid cycle each producing12 ATP. Ketonemia is the increase of blood ketone bodies above normal concentration. It occurs when the rate of formation of ketone bodies (ketogenesis) is greater than the rat e of their oxidation (ketolysis). ketonemia may lead to acidosis (ketosis). Ketonuria is the increase of urine ketone bodies concen tration above normal concentration. It usually occurs with ketonemia Starvation, severe diabetes mellitus and hypercatabolic states e.g. diarrhea and fever are the main causes of ketonemia.

Cholesterol is an animal sterol having -OH group at C3. It is formed in the body almost in all nucleated cells from Acetyl-CoA Liver is the major site of cholesterol synthesis along with other tissues e.g. intestine, adrenal cortex, gonads and skin. Condensation of two molecules of acetyl CoA gives acetoacetyl CoA that gives rise to cholesterol in a series of reactions. HMG CoA reductase is the key enzyme for cholesterol synthesis. It is present in two forms active dephosphorylated and Inactive phosphorylated. It Is Regulated through Feedback Inhibition. Glucagon inhibits HMG CoA reductase through stimulation of cAMP and protein kinase. Insulin stimulates HMG CoA reductase through stimulation of phosphodiesterase and phosphatase enzymes. Lovastatin and mevastatin are drugs, which Inhibit HMG CoA reductase by reversible competitive Inhibition. They are used to decrease plasma cholesterol levels in patients with hypercholesterolemi A Cholesterol is transported in plasma in the more soluble lipoprotein forms like LDL, VLDL and HDL. Free cholesterol is removed from tissues by HDL and transported to be excreted by the liver. Cholesterol ester Is the storage form of cholesterol in both tissues and plasma. In tissues like liver, cholesterol is esterified by ACAT enzyme (acyl CoA cholesterol acyl transferase) whereas in plasma, cholesterol is esterified by LCAT enzyme (lecithin cholesterol acyl transferase). LCAT is associated with HDL.VLDL contains triacylglycerols, TG, Cholesterol esters, phospholipids and protein content apo B100, apo E and apo C (CII) and it carries lipids from liver to the blood to the peripheral tissues. The particles released from the liver are called nascent VLDL and contain B1oo. When it reaches the plasma, it receives- from circulating HDL- two apollpoproteins; E and C and converted into VLDL. The triacylglycerols component of VLDL will be hydrolyzed into glycerol and fatty acids. by lipoprotein lipase enzyme, which is activated by apo Cll. The remaining particles are called Intermediate density lipoproteins (IDL). IDL is converted I to LDL by transferring phospholipids, apo Cll, and apo E to HDL. LDL are removed from circulation by tissues as muscles and VLDL particles also transfer phospholipids (PL) and TG to HDL. At the same time HDL transfer cholesterol esters (CE) to VLDL. These reactions are catalyzed by cholesterol ester transfer protein. Low density lipoproteins (LDL) contains cholesterol, cholesteryl esters, phospholipids and apoproteins like apo B1oo· The primary function of LDL particles is to provide cholesterol to the peripheral tissues by deposition of free cholesterol on cell membranes or by binding to receptors on cell membranes that recognize apo B100· The LDL receptors are negatively charged glycoprotein molecules grouped in pits in cell membranes. The intracellular side of the pits is coated with a protein called clathrin. After binding with receptors, the LDL are internalized as intact particles by endocytosis. The vesicle containing the LDL rapidly loses its clathrin coat and fuses with other similar vesicles, forming large vesicle called endosomes. The pH of the contents of endosomes falls, allowing separation of the LDL from its receptors. The receptors then migrate to one side of the endosome while the LDL stays free within the lumen of the vesicle. The receptors can be returned to the cell membrane. The lipoprotein remnants are hydrolyzed by lysosomal enzymes releasing cholesterol, amino acids, fatty acids and phospholipids.High density lipoproteins (HDL) synthesized in liver is the reservoir of apoC-II that is transferred to chylomicrons and VLDL to activate lipoprotein lipase enzyme and remove free cholesterol from extrahepatic tissue esterifying with lecithin cholesterol acyl transferase (LCAT). The apo A-1 of HDL activates LCAT. HDL particles carry cholesterol esters to VLDL and LDL in liver where the HDL is hydrolyzed and cholesterol released Free fatty acids (FFA are transported in conjugation with albumin. Plasma FFA are produced by lipolysis in adipose tissue by lipoprotein lipase in chylomicron & and VLDL. Their level increases in all conditions associated with excessive lipolysis e.g. fastingproduce ketone bodies.

Eicosanolds are cyclic compounds that derived from arachidonic acid (20 C after cyclization of its carbons chain to form a ring. It includes prostanolds that comprise prostaglandins, prostacyclins and thromboxanes. And leukotrlens that are present In leucocytes, platelets and mast cells. The immediate precursor of prostanoids is arachidonic acid Arachidonic acid Is derived from Phospholipids present In all cell membranes by the action of phospholipase A2 enzyme. The first step In the synthesis of prostanoids is the oxidation and cyclization of arachidonic acid to give PGG2 and PGH2. These reactions are catalyzed by two microsomal enzymes, Fatty acid cyclo-oxygenase, which requires 2 oxygen molecules and peroxidase, which Is dependent on reduced glutathione (G-SH). PGH2 is the precursor all prostanoids. Cortisol inhibits the phospholipase A2 activity. Aspirin, indomethacin and phenylbutazone -which are antiinflamatory agents- Inhibit cyclooxygenas. These agents do not affect synthesis of the leukotrienes. In neutrophils, arachidonic acid Is converted to 5-hyroperoxy 6, 8, 11, 14 eicosatetraenoic acid (5-HPETE). This reaction is. catalyzed by 5- llpooxygenase enzyme. 5-HPETE is converted to a series of leukotrienes like LTA4, LTB4 , L TC4 , LTD4 and LTE4. C In contrast to prostanoids synthesis, no drugs are known specifically to inhibit the lipoxygenase pathway. Thromboxane is produced by platelets and it stimulates platelets aggregations. Prostacyclin produced by endothelial cells of the blood vessels inhibits platelets aggregationcauses vasodilatation. Prostaglandin F2a (PGF2A) produced by most tissues causes vasoconstriction and contraction of smooth muscles. Leukotrlenes B4 (LTB4) cause movement and aggregation of white blood cells at the site of lnflammation and release of lysosomal enzymes.

1. Fats get deposited in adipose tissues in the form of
   a. Steroids
   b. Ketone
   c. Triacylglycerol
   d. Lipoproteins
2. The molecular weight of free fatty acids are determined by
   a. Iodine value
   b. Acid number
   c. RM value
   d. Saponification value
3. Ketone bodies are produced as a result of excessc oxidation of
   a. Glucose
   b. Glycerol
   c. Protein
   d. Fatty acids
4. Acetyl CoA can be converted into all of the following except
   a. Protein
   b. Cholesterol
   c. Fatty acid
   d. Ketone body
5. Fatty acid synthase complex does not include
   a. Enoyl reductase
   b. Acetyl CoA carboxylase
   c. Acyl transacetylase
   d. Ketoacyl synthase
6. Which of the following is used for Fatty acid synthesis
   a. Enoyl reductase
   b. Acetyl CoA carboxylase
   c. Acyl transacetylase
   d. All of the above
7. The major lipid of mitochondrial membrane is
   a. Cardiolipin
   b. Phosphitidyl inosital
   c. Plasmalogen
   d. Cholesterol
8. The triacyl glycerol found in plasma lipoproteins are hydrolysed by
   a. Lingual lipase
   b. Pancreatic lipase
   c. Lipoprotein lipase
   d. Adipokinetic lipase
9. Bile serves as an important excretory route for
   a. Lipids
   b. Proteins
   c. Cholesterol
   d. Fatty acids
10. The calorific value of lipid is
    a. 4.0 Kcal/gm
    b. 9.0 Kcal/gm
    c. 6.0Kcal/gm
    d. 12 Kcal/gm
11. Inherited deficiency of enzyme cerebrosidase produces
    a. Gaucher's disease
    b. Neimann-Pick disease
    c. Krabbe's disease
    d. Tay-Sach's disease
12. Phospholipase is activated for Prostaglandin synthesis by
    a. Insulin
    b. Glucagon
    c. Angiotensin II
    d. All of the above

13. Cholesterol scavengeing lipoprotein is
    a. VLDL b. LDL
    c. HDL d. None of the above
14. PG-E is catabolised by oxidation of secondary hydroxyl group at
    a. C7 b. C9
    c. C15 d. None of the above
15. An alcoholic amine residue is present in which of the following lipids?
    a. Phosphatidic acid b. Sphingomyelin
    c. Ganglioside d. cholesterol
16. Brain cannot utilize free fatty acid because they usually complexed to
    a. Albumin b. Globuline
    c. cholesterol d. Glucuronic acid
17. PG-Es lowers cyclic adenosine monophosphate level in
    a. Adipose tissue b. Spleen
    c. Lungs d. Thyroids
18. PG-E2 when infused intravenously has the following action on the kidneys
    a. Decrease the renal plasma flow
    b. Decrease in glomerular filtration rate
    c. Increase the excretion of sodium
    d. Decrease rennin secretion from juxtra glomerular cells
19. The leucotrienes are characterized by all of the following except
    a. Are formed from arachidonate
    b. One of the leucotrienes chemotaxis and chemokinesis of neutrophils
    c. All of them contain cyclopentane ring
    d. Lipooxigenase system is responsible for conversion of arachidonate to leucotrienes
20 PG-synthesis is aerobic process and requires two molecules of reduced
    a. Glutathione b. NAD+
    c. NADP+ d. FAD
21. All the PGs have in common in addition to cyclopentane ring one double bond between
    a. C5 and C6 b. C9 and C10
    c. C7 and C8 d. C13 and C14
22. Pancreatic α-lipase when an act on triacylglycerols produces
    a. 2- acylglycerol and free fatty acids b. Glycerol and free fatty acids
    c. 1-acylglycerol and free fatty acids d. 3-acylglycerol and free fattyacids
23. The lipoprotein synthesized from absorbed lipids in the intestinal mucosa are
    a. HDL b. VDL
    c. VLDL d. Chylomicrons

24. The acid number of an oil indicate
    a. Volatile fatty acid
    b. Free fatty acids
    c. Molecular weight of fatty acids
    d. Unsaturated fatty acids
25. Which of the following is a ketogenic substance?
    a. Leucine
    b. Lysine
    c. Fatty acids
    d. All of the above
26. Hypercholesterolemia is observed in the disorder of
    a. Diabetes
    b. Nephrotic syndrome
    c. Hypothyroidism
    d. all of the above
27. The nitrogenous base present in lecithin is
    a. Choline
    b. Ethanolamine
    c. Phosphatadic acid
    d. Plasmalogen
28. Which of the organelle is absent in Zellweger's syndrome?
    a. Lysosome
    b. Mitochondria
    c. Ribosome
    d. Peroxisome
29. The two final products in the β-oxidation of odd chain fatty acids are
    a. Acctyl CoA and malonyl CoA
    b. Acetyl CoA and propionyl CoA
    c. Acetyl CoA and acetyl CoA
    d. Succinyl CoA and acetyl CoA
30. Regarding arachidonic acid which statement is not true
    a. It is a twenty-carbon fatty acid with five double bonds
    b. It can form cyclic endopeoxydase PG-H2
    c. It is a precursor of Tx-A2
    d. It is precursor of PG-I2
31. Acetyl CoA is necessary for
    a. Fatty acid synthesis
    b. Glucose storage
    c. amino acid
    d. all of the above
32. The release of arachidonic acid from membrane phospholipids is inhibited by
    a. By administration of aspirin
    b. A specific protein inducedby glucocorticoids
    c. Catacholamines
    d. All of the above
33. Transport of fatty acids through mitochondrial membrane is by
    a. Diffusion
    b. Active transport
    c. Facilitated transport
    d. Osmosis
34. All PGs have a structure based on prostanoic acid which contains a cyclopentane ring and having carbon atom
    a. 10
    b. 15
    c. 20
    d. 18

35. Which one of the following is the most important essential fatty acid in the diet?
    a. Arachidonic acid   b. Oleic acid
    c. Linoleic acid   d. Palmitic acid
36. The product of oxidation of odd chain fatty acids will be
    a. Propionyl CoA   b. Acetyl CoA
    c. both a and b   d. None of the above
37. Fatty acid synthesis occurs in
    a. Peroxisome   b. Mitochondria
    c. Cytoplasm   d. Ribosome
38. Which of the following is not a method of fatty acid oxidation?
    a. α oxidation   b. β oxidation
    c. gamma oxidation   d. Omega oxidation
39. Cholesterol is required for biosynthesis of
    a. Gonadotropins   b. Plasma membrane
    c. Adrenal medullary hormones   d. All of the above
40. Prostaglandins are derived from
    a. Linolenic acid   b. Arachidonic acid l
    c. Cholestero   d. None of the above
41. Coconut oil is rich in
    a. Polyunsaturated fatty acid
    b. Medium chain unsaturated fatty acids
    c. Medium chain saturated fatty acids
    d. All of the above
42. The sugar component of cerebrosides is
    a. Fructose   b. Glucose
    c. Sucrose   d. Galactose
43. The level of which enzyme is decreased during starvation
    a. Fatty acid synthase   b. Citrate lyase
    c. CoA carnitine transferase   d. Lipoprotein lipase
44. Prostaglandins are derived from
    a. Cholesterol   b. Arachidonic acid
    c. Linolenic acid   d. None of the above
45. Which of the following organs do not utilize ketone bodies as fuel?
    a. Heart   b. Brain
    c. Liver   d. Kidney
46. One of the following is not a ketone body
    a. Acetone   b. Acetyl CoA
    c. Acetoacetate   d. Isopropanol

47. Ketone bodies are produced in Lactating cow from
    a. Mammary tissue
    b. Rumen
    c. Liver
    d. All of the above
48. FAD is act as a coenzyme in a reaction catalysed by following enzymes
    a. Acyl CoA synthatase
    b. Acyl CoA Dehydrogenase
    c. Hydroxy acyl CoA dehydrogenase
    d. β-ketothiolase
49. Micelles formed in the intestine have which of the following properties?
    a. They can mostly triaceylglycerol
    b. They are absorbed intact in the duodenum
    c. They are mainly absorbed from stomach wall
    d. They facilitate transfer of hydrolytic product of triacylglycerol to intestinal mucosa
50. Aginomotto is chemically
    a. Monoaminoglycolate
    b. Monosodium glutamate
    c. N acetyl glutamate
    d. N acetyl glycine
51. Which one is a phospholipid that does not contain glycerol
    a. Cephalin
    b. Lecithin
    c. Cardiolipin
    d. Sphingomyelins
52. The basic ring skeleton seen in all the steroids is
    a. Cyclopentane
    b. Tetraapyrrole
    c. Porphyrin
    d. Cyclopentanoperhydrophenanthrene
53. The ketogenic effect on liver is shown by following
    a. GH
    b. Insulin
    c. Androgen
    d. Glucose
54. Hexadecanoic acid is also known as
    a. Myristic acid
    b. Stearic acid
    c. Palmitic acid
    d. Oleic acid
55. Dietary triacylglycerols are absorbed from the intestinal lumen after hydrolysis mainly as
    a. Acyl CoA and glycerol
    b. Glycerol phosphate and fatty acids
    c. Fatty acids and two monoacylglycerol
    d. Fatty acids and glycerol
56. The process of conversion of vegetable oils to vanaspati is called
    a. Hydrogenation
    b. Hydration
    c. Oxygenation
    d. Halogenation

57. The gastric lipase is inactive because of following reason except
    a. The enzyme is secreted in small quantity
    b. The gastric juice is highly acidic
    c. The concentration of bile salt is high in gastric juice
    d. Emulsification of fat does not occur in stomach
58. Peroxysomes are absent in the following diseaase
    a. Sickle cell disease b. Zellweger's syndrome
    c. Cystic fibrosis d. None of the above
59. Ketone bodies are byproduct of the metabolism of
    a. Fat b. Carbohydrate
    c. Protein d. All of the above
60. Which of the following compound is not a ketone body?
    a. Acetic acid b. Acetoacetate
    c. Acetone d. β-OH butyrate
61. Which of the following compound is not a phospholipid?
    a. Cerebroside b. Lecithin
    c. Cephalin d. Sphingomyelin
62. A pathway that requires NADPH as a cofactor is
    a. Glycogenesis
    b. Gluconeogensis
    c. Ketogenesis
    d. Extramitochondrial de novo fatty acid synthesis
63. β-oxidation of odd carbon fatty acid chain produces
    a. Acetoacetyl CoA b. Acetyl CoA
    c. Propionyl CoA d. Succinyl CoA
64. LCAT activity is associated with which of the lipoprotein complex
    a. HDL b. LDL
    c. VLDL d. Chylomicrons
65. The energy yield from complete oxidation of products generated by second reaction cycle of β-oxidation of palmitoyl CoA will be
    a. 34 ATP b. 42 ATP
    c. 17ATP d. 12 ATP
66. Which of the following are used as coenzymes in β-oxidation of fatty acids?
    a. FAD and FMN b. NAD+ and NADP+
    c. FAD and NAD+ d. FAD and NADP+
67. beta oxidation occurs in which of the following organells
    a. Cytoplasm b. Mitochondria
    c. Ribosome d. Endoplasmic reticulum

68. The committed step in the biosynthesis of cholesterol from acetyl CoA is
    a. Formation of acetoacetyl CoA from acetyl CoA
    b. Formation of lanosterol from squalene by cyclisation
    c. Formation of mevalonate from HMG-CoA
    d. Formation of squalene-by-squalene synthetase

69. The most important source of reducing equivalents for fatty acid synthesis in liver is
    a. HMP-shunt b. Kreb's cycle
    c. Glycolysis d. Gluconeogenesis

70. All of the following compounds are produced during each cycle of β-oxidation of fatty acid except
    a. FADH2 b. Acety CoA
    c. acyl CoA d. H2O

71. The lipoproteins having fastest electrophoretic mobility and the lowest TG content are
    a. VLDL b. LDL
    c. HDL d. chylomicrons

72. In synthesis of TG from α-glycero-PandacylcoA, the first intermediate formed is
    a. Phosphatidic acid b. Lysophosphatide
    c. Acyl carnitine d. α,β-diacyl glycerol

73. The major source of cholesterol in arterial smooth muscle cells is from
    a. LDL b. HDL
    c. VLDL d. Chylomicrons

74. If ethanolamine replaces the choline moity the resultant compound produced is
    a. Cerebroside b. Cephalin
    c. Sphingomyelin d. Plasmalogen

75. Triglycerides in serum are transported
    a. HDL b. Chylomicrons
    c. VLDL d. LDL

76. The lipotropic factors are
    a. Betanin b. Cholin
    c. Methionine d. All of the above

77. Ketosis is caused partly due to
    a. Under production of acetyl CoA b. Over production of acetyl CoA
    c. Over utilization of Glucose d. A reduction in lipid metabolism

78. NADPH is required for
    a. Gluconeogenesis b. Lipogenesis
    c. Glycogenolysis d. HMP shunt

79. Ketone bodies are synthesized from fatty acid oxidation products by which qaof the following organs
    a. Kidney
    b. Liver
    c. RBC
    d. Brain
80. All the statements regarding ketone bodies are true except
    a. They are formed in kidney
    b. They may result from starvation
    c. They may be excreted in urine
    d. It includes acetoacetic acid and acetone
81. Chain elongation of fatty acids occurring in mammalian liver takes place in which of the following subcellular fraction of the cell
    a. Microsomes
    b. Lysosome
    c. Ribosomes
    d. Golgi body
82. Which of the following cofactors of their derivatives must be present for the conversion of acetyl CoA to malonyl CoA in fatty acid synthesis?
    a. ACP
    b. FMN
    c. FAD
    d. Biotin
83. All the statements regarding 3-OH-3-methyl glutaryl CoA are true except
    a. Involved in the synthesis of fatty acid
    b. Required in ketogenesis
    c. It is formed in cytoplasm
    d. Enzyme involved in HMG CoA synthase
84. The rate limiting step in cholesterol biosynthesis is
    a. Thiolase
    b. HMG-CoA synthetase
    c. HMG-CoA reductase
    d. Squalene synthetase
85. Brown adipose tissue is characterized by the following s
    a. Absent in hibernating animals
    b. Oxdation and phosphorylation are tightly coupled
    c. Present in large quantities in adult humans
    d. Mitochondrial content higher than white adipose tissue
86. Correct statement regarding to β-oxidation is
    a. Requires GTP for its activity
    b. Produces acetyl CoA as a product
    c. Forms CoA thioesters
    d. Requires β-ketoacyl CoA as a substrate
87. Ketosis is partily ascribed to
    a. Increased fat utilization
    b. Increased carbohydrate utilization
    c. Increased pyruvate in liver
    d. Over production of glucose

88. Biosynthesis of triglycerides and lecithin both requires an intermediate
   a. Phosphatidyl adenylate
   b. Phosphatidyl ethanolamine
   c. Phosphatidyl cytidylate
   d. Phosphatidic acid
89. Which of the following lipoproteins would contribute to a measurement of plasma cholesterol in a normal individual following a 12 hours fast?
   a. LDL
   b. Chylomicrons
   c. VLDL
   d. Both LDL and VLDL
90. Which of the following statement is false regarding to ketone bodies?
   a. May be excreted in urine
   b. They include acetone and β-OH butyrate
   c. They are produced in kidney
   d. Its concentration is increased in uncontrolled diabetes mellitus
91. The free fatty acid found in blood are
   a. Mainly bound to serum albumin
   b. Stored in fat depots
   c. Metabolically inactive
   d. Mainly bound to β-lipo-proteins
92. Acetyl CoA required for extramitochondrial fatty acid synthesis is produced by
   a. Acetyl CoA synthease
   b. Thiolase
   c. Carnitine-acyltransferase
   d. Citrate lyase
93. Triacyl glycerol found in VLDL is hydrolysed by
   a. Lipoprotein lipase
   b. Pancreatic lipase
   c. Intestinal lipase
   d. Hormone sensitive TGlipase
94. Propionyl CoA is produced by beta oxidation of
   a. Odd chain fatty acids
   b. Even chain fatty acids
   c. Unsaturated fatty acids
   d. All of the above
95. Which of the following is involved in the synthesis of carnitine?
   a. Serine
   b. Choline
   c. Lysine
   d. Threonine
96. A metabolite which is common to pathways cholesterol biosynthesis from acetyl CoA and cholecalciferol formation from cholesterol is
   a. Pregnenolone
   b. Zymosterol
   c. Ergosterol
   d. 7-dehydrocholesterol
97. Net yield of ATP from beta oxidation of one molecule of palmitic acid is
   a. 88
   b. 96
   c. 112
   d. 129
98. Which of the following aids in prevention of fatty liver condition?
   a. Thiamine
   b. dietary choline
   c. Guanidocetate
   d. dimethyl propiothenate
99. Hypolipidemic agent act on
   a. HMG CoA synthetase
   b. HMG CoA mutase
   c. HMG CoA oxygenase
   d. HMG CoA reductase

100. Phospholipids include all the following except

a. Ceramide b. Plasmalogens

c. Cardiolipin d. Lecithin

101. Fatty acid synthesis takes place in which of the following organells

a. Cytoplasm b. Mitochondria

c. Peroxisome d. Endoplasmic reticulum

102. desaturation of fatty acid takes place in the

a. Cytoplasm b. Endoplasmic reticulum

c. Peroxisome d. Mitochondria

103. The compound which stimulates the transfer of acetate from cytosol into mitochondria is

a. TPP b. Citrate

c. Carnitine d. Acetyl CoA

104. β-oxidation in peroxisome is differentiated from that occurring in mitochondria by

a. Acetyl CoA b. NADH is required

c. HMG CoA d. H2O2

105 Ketone bodies are not utilized by which organ

a. Liver b. Spleen

c. Brain d. Kidney

106. The lipoprotein which contains highest concentration of lipid and lowest concentration of protein is

a. VLDL b. LDL

c. Chylomicrons d. HDL

107. Ligand for low density lipoprotein is

a. Apo 48 b. Apo A 11

c. Apo E d. Apo B 100

108 Which of the following organ can utilize fatty acid, ketone bodies and glucose?

a. Brain b. RBC

c. Liver d. Skeletal muscle

109. Cholesterol is an/a

a. Ester b. Lipoprotein

c. Sterol d. Phospholipid

110. The important intermediate product in biosynthesis of fatty acid is

a. Malonyl CoA b. Thioesterase

c. Acetyl CoA d. Cholesterol

111. Which of the following enzyme activity is not decreased during starvation?

a. Acetyl CoA carboxylase b. Fatty acid synthetase

c. Lipoprotein lipase d. Carnitine palmitoyl transferase-I

112. The main type of lipids present in tissues in starving individual are in end of first week of fasting

a. Cholesterol
b. Glycolipids
c. Triacylglycerol
d. Phospholipids

113. Glucogenic VFA is

a. Propionic acid
b. Acetic acid
c. Butyric acid
d. All of the above

114. RQ of oxidation of fat

a. 7.0
b. 0.7
c. 1.0
d. 1.1

115. The RQ of a mixed diet is

a. 0.85
b. 0.75
c. 0.80
d. 1.00

116. In which type of hypertriglyceridemia increase in chylomicron and VLDL remnants occurs?

a. Type I
b. Type III
c. Type II A
d. Type IV

117. Which of the following reaction is catalysed by HMG-CoA reductase ?

a. Acetyl CoA + CO2 + ATP→ Malonyl CoA + ADP + Pi
b. β-OH β-methyl glutaryl CoA→ Mevalonic acid
c. L- methyl malonyl CoA→ Succinyl CoA
d. Lactose + H2 O→ Glucose+ Galactose

118. Rothera's test is used for detection of

a. Lipid
b. Ketones
c. Cholesterol
d. All of the above

119 Ketonemia occurs due to increased catabolism of

a. Protein
b. Glycerol
c. Fatty acid oxidation
d. Glucose catabolism

120 Which enzyme is required for conversion of cholesterol to preganalone

a. 3β- hydroxylase
b. 11β- hydroxylase
c. 17β-hydroxylase
d. Cytochrome P450

121. Tay-sachsdisease isdue todeficiency of

a. β- glucosidase
b. β- galactosidase
c. β - galactosidase
d. Hexosaminidase- A

122. Fabry'sdisease isdue todeficiency of

a. α- galactosidase
b. β- glucosidase
c. Hexosaminidase- A
d. β- galactosidase

123. Which one of the following is not a Ketone body

a. Acetone
b. Acetyl CoA
c. D-Hydroxy Butyrate
d. Aceto acetic acid

124. High rate of B-oxidation of fatty acids causes increased production of
    a. Oxalo acetate   b. Ethyl acetate
    c. Butane acetate   d. Aceto acetate
125. In high yielding cows Ketone bodies are majorly produced in
    a. Liver   b. Mammary gland
    c. Both of the above   d. None of the above
126. Transport of Endogenous TG are transported mainly through
    a. Chylomicrons   b. LDL
    c. VLDL   d. HDL
127. How many acetyl co A are produced from β oxidation of one molecule of palmitic acid
    a. 7   b. 8
    c. 9   d. 10
128. Total ATP molecules produced from complete oxidation of one molecule of palmitic acid?
    a. 129   b. 96
    c. 131   d. 119
129. Net ATP molecules produced from complete oxidation of one molecule of palmitic acid?
    a. 129   b. 96
    c. 131   d. 119
130. Which of the following enzyme controls cholesterol biosynthesis?
    a. HMG-CoA reductase   b. HMG-CoA oxidase
    c. HMG-CoA hydratase   d. HMG-CoA peroxidase
131. The phospholipids is hydrolysed by phospholipase C to form
    a. Phosphatidyl choline   b. Inositol
    c. Phosphatidyl inositol bisphosphate   d. Diacyl glycerol
132. Protoglandine are synthesized from
    a. Oleicacid   b. Linoleic acid
    c. Linolenic acid   d. Arachidonic acid
133. Which of the following component of cell do not contains lipids
    a. GM2 gangliosides   b. Sphingomyelin
    c. Cholesterol   d. Triglycerol
134. The function of Lipotropic factor is to
    a. Fat removal from liver   b. Cholesterol removal from gall
    c. Cholesterol removal from liver   d. Fat removal from kidney
135. Fatty acid biosynthesis is controlled by
    a. Acetyl CoA   b. Palmitoyl CoA
    c. Malonyl CoA   d. NADH

136. Which of the following enzyme is not used in ketogenesis?
   a. HAMG CoA lyase
   b. HMG CoA synthase
   c. HMG CoA reductase
   d. beta hydroxyl butyrate De- hydrogenase

137. Which of the following compound is precursor of steroid hormones?
   a. Sterol
   b. Free Fatty acid
   c. Stearic acid
   d. Palmitic acid

138. Cholesterols are the precursor of
   a. Vitamin C
   b. Vitamin D
   c. Vitamin B
   d. Vitamin A

139. Myocardium normally utilizes
   a. Lipids
   c. Glucose
   b. Ketone body
   d. Amino acids

140. Amphipathic lipid include
   a. Bile salt
   b. Phospholipids
   c. Sphingolipids
   d. All of the above

141. Steatorrhea is a condition characterized by the loss of
   a. Proteins in feces
   c. Sugars in feces
   b. Lipids in feces
   d. All of the above

142. The true statement regarding to the absorption of lipids from the intestine is
   a. The TAG carried by chylomicrons is degraded to free fatty acids and glycerol by lipoprotein lipase on the endothelial surface of capillaries in muscle and adipose primarily
   b. Fatty acids that contain ten carbon or less are absorbed and enter the circulation primarily via lymphatic system
   c. Deficiencies in the ability to absorb fat result in excessive amounts of chylomicrons in the blood
   d. Dietary triacylglycerol must be completely hydrolysed to free fatty acids and glycerol before absorption

143. Steatorrhea is commonly seen in disorders associated with
   a. Pancreas
   b. Severe liver dysfunction
   c. Biliary obstrction
   d. All of the above

144. Orlistat is a
   a. Analog of triacylglycerol
   b. Analog of cholesterol
   c. Both a and b
   d. None of the above

145. Which of the following events occurs during fasting
   a. Hormone sensitive lipase is phosphorylated and activated by cAMP- activated protein kinase
   b. Stored fatty acids are released from adipose tissue into the plasma as components of the serum lipoprotein particle, VLDL
   c. Free fatty acids are produced at a high rate in plasma by action of lipoprotein lipase on chylomicrons
   d. Glycerol obtained from the breakdown of triacylglycerol is an important source source of energy for the fibroblast and adipocytes
146. Olestra is a synthetic lipid, produced by esterification of natural fattyacids with
   a. Sucrose b. Glycerol
   c. Both a and b d. None of the above
147. Which of the following is a synthetic lipid
   a. Orlistat b. Olestra
   c. Both a and b d. None of the above
148. Ketone bodies are mainly produced during starvation due to
   a. Decreased activity of hormone-sensitive lipase in the adipose tissue
   b. Inhibition of β-oxidation of fatty acids in liver
   c. Reduced synthesis of acetyl CoA in the liver
   d. Increased levels of free fatty acids in the blood
149. The basic ring skeleton seen in all the steroids is
   a. cyclopentane
   b. Tetraapyrrole
   c. Porphyrin
   d. cyclopentanoperhydrophenanthrene
150. The ketogenic effect on liver is shown by following
   a. GH b. Insulin
   c. Androgen d. Glucose

Answer Key

1	c	2	d	3	d	4	a	5	b	6	d	7	a
8	c	9	c	10	b	11	a	12	c	13	c	14	c
15	b	16	a	17	a	18	c	19	c	20	a	21	d
22	a	23	d	24	b	25	d	26	d	27	a	28	d
29	b	30	a	31	a	32	b	33	c	34	c	35	c
36	c	37	c	38	c	39	b	40	b	41	c	42	b
43	a	44	b	45	c	46	b	47	d	48	b	49	d
50	b	51	d	52	d	53	d	54	c	55	c	56	a
57	c	58	b	59	a	60	a	61	a	62	d	63	c
64	a	65	a	66	c	67	b	68	c	69	a	70	d
71	c	72	a	73	a	74	b	75	c	76	d	77	b
78	b	79	b	80	a	81	a	82	d	83	a	84	c
85	d	86	c	87	a	88	d	89	a	90	c	91	a
92	d	93	a	94	a	95	c	96	d	97	d	98	b
99	d	100	a	101	a	102	b	103	c	104	d	105	a
106	c	107	d	108	d	109	c	110	a	111	d	112	d
113	a	114	b	115	a	116	b	117	b	118	b	119	c
120	d	121	d	122	a	123	b	124	d	125	c	126	c
127	b	128	c	129	a	130	a	131	c	132	d	133	a
134	a	135	b	136	c	137	a	138	b	139	a	140	d
141	b	142	a	143	d	144	a	145	a	146	a	147	c
148	d	149	d	150	d								

13

Biochemistry of Vitamins

Sasmita Barik[1] and Shiv Kumar Yadav[2]

[1]Department of Veterinary Physiology and Biochemistry, College of Veterinary Sciences and Animal Husbandry, Guru Angad Dev Veterinary and Animal Scienes Univeristy, Ludhiana, Punjab

[2]KVK, Shahjahanpur, Uttar Pradesh

Introduction

Vitamins are the organic derived accessory food factors apart from carbohydrate, lipid and proteins meant for specific biological functions, optimum growth and health of an organism. These factors are are required in minute amount in the diet for proper functioning of biological enzymes. The term accessory factors were given by Hopkins to the essential nutrients present in the natural foods. Funk (1913) coined the term vitamine to the active principal present in rice polishings. Vitamins are classified into two categories like fat soluble A and water-soluble b Vitamins A, D, E, K are fat soluble whereas Vitamins B and C are water soluble. The B group of vitamins include vitamin B1, B2, B6, biotin folic acid, B12 etcall the fat-soluble vitamins are isoprenoid in nature consisting of repeating isoprenoid units. And meant for diversified functions. The water-soluble vitamins are heterogenous group of compounds generally not stored in the body and readily excreted in urine. These are mostly act as coenzymes for the vital biological enzymes deficiency of which reflects in the form of various deceases.

Vitamin A, include retinoid group of compounds like retinol, retinal and retinoic acid Retinol is a primary alcohol containing β-ionone ring with isoprenoid units, double bonds and hydroxyl group. Naturally it exists as ester of long chain fatty acids. Retinal is the aldehyde form whereas Retinoic acid is the acid form. Carotene is provitamin A normally found in plant origin foods that in the intestine gives rise to two moles of retinal by enzyme carotene 15-15-dioxygenase. Diet contains retinol esters and p carotene. Retinol esters are hydrolyzed into fatty acids and retinol that absorbed into intestinal mucosal cells. p-carotene Is absorbed and converted into retinal by p-carotene dioxygenase. Retinal then converted into retinol. In the intestinal mucosal cells, retinol re-esterifies with fatty acid to form retinol ester. Retinol esters are absorbed through lymph vessels into general circulation and transported to the liver, where 90% of the body's vitamin A is stored. When the body cells need vitamin A, stored retinol esters are hydrolysed and free retinol combines with a protein formed by the liver called retinol binding protein (RBP). RBP carries retinol to the retina and target cells. In retina, retinol is converted into retinal that essential for visions. In other target cells retinol is oxidized into retinoic acid which binds to nuclear receptors. Retinoic acid receptor complexes stimulate genes. This mode of action is similar to that of hormones. Retinal is essential for night vision. Retinol is essential for reproduction as it supports sperm formation (spermatogenesis) in males and maintains fetal life in females. Retinol is essential for normal growth and bone & teeth formation. Retinol and retinoic acid are essential for normal differentiation of epithelial cells. This is important for smoothness of skin and mucus membranes. Retinol is also essential for intact cornea Retinoic acid is important for a glycoprotein synthesis, phospholipids synthesis in the lungs and cell differentiation. Retinoids and carotenoids (carotenes) act as antioxidants and protect tissues from toxic effect of some oxidants leading to epithelial tissue cancer. Deficiency of vitamin A causes night blindness, impaired dark adaptation, Xerophthalmia, dryness/roughness of cornea, Growth retardation, roughness of skin and mucus membranes of different body systems leading to infection.

Ultraviolet rays of sun generate the vitamin D from the provitamin ergosterol (in plants) and 7-dehydrocholesterol (in human and animals). Apart from this liver, egg, yeast and fish liver oils are rich in vitamin dactive vitamin D is a steroid hormone. 1,25 dihydroxycholecalciferol (calcitriol) acts as a hormone. It normalization the serum calcium. Calcitriol maintains serum calcium level through its effects on intestine, bones and kidneys. On Intestine, it stimulates synthesis of calcium binding protein (calbindin) that responsible for calcium absorption. On bones, it stimulates calcium reabsorption from bones. On kidneys, it increases renal tubular reabsorption of calcium. In small doses, calcitriol helps bone mineralization by providing calcium and phosphate. In large doses calcium and phosphate move from bone to blood. Osteocalcin is calcium binding protein present in bones and is important for proper mineralization of bones. 1,25(OH)2D3 stimulates its synthesis in the form of proosteocalcin. 24, 25 dihydroxycholecalciferol is biologically inactive. Hypocalcemia releases parathyroid hormone that activation of renal1 hydroxylase enzyme that converts 25(OH)D3 into 1,25 (OH)2D3. Hypophosphatemia causes direct activation of renal 1hydroxylase enzyme that converts 25 D3 into 1,25 (OH)2 D3. In the Intestinal mucosal cells, 1,25 (OH)2 D3 is bound to specific cytoplasmic receptors forming a complex. This complex enters the nucleus, stimulating DNA to produce specific mRNA. This mRNA is responsible for synthesis of calcium binding protein (calbindin), which helps the absorption of calcium. Absorption of phosphate is similar to the previous mechanism but it occurs secondary to calcium absorption.

Deficiency of vitamin D causes demineralization of bones that leads to rickets in children and osteomalacia in adults. In chronic renal failure there is a deficient formation of active form of the vitamin D3. Hypervitaminosis D3 leads to abnormal calcification of tissues and deposition of calcium and phosphate in different systems e.g. renal stones.

There are three forms (vitamers) of vitamin K ie. K1, K2 and K3. The difference between K1 and K2 lies in side chain R. K3 is synthetic vitamin with no R side chain. The main source of vitamin K1 is the Intestinal bacteria Vitamin K2 Is present in plants. Vitamin K3 is synthetic It is water soluble and more potent than vitamin K1 & K2. Vit K helps in synthesis of some blood clotting factors (prothrombin (factor II), factors VII, IX and X) in liver and osteocalcin (calcium binding protein) in bones. Prothrombin is a protein formed in the liver as inactive form called prothrombin precursor. It contains 10 glutamic acid residues. Carboxylation of these glutamic acid residues into y-carboxy glutamate converts the molecule into active thrombin. The same carboxylation reactions occur to factors VII, IX and X. Deficiency of vitamin K causes impairment of blood clotting. Long use of dicumarol and warfarin (anticoagulants) causes deficiency as they act as competitive inhibitors with vitamin K for its site of action. Osteocalcin is a calcium binding protein present in bones. 1,25 (OH) 2D3 stimulates its synthesis in the form of proosteocalcin. Vitamin K converts pro-osteocalcin into active osteocalcin by mechanism similar to that of prothrombin i.e. carboxylation of glutamic acid residues.

Vitamin E includes tocopherols (α, β, γ, €) that contain tocol ring. The most active member is a tocopherol. The α, β, γ tocopherols differ from a tocopherol in number and position of - CH3 groups attached to the tocol ring. Vegetables, seed oils and fish liver oil are the major source of Vitamine E. It majorly serves as an antioxidant that prevent non-enzymatic oxidation of cell components (e.g. polyunsaturated fatty acids, DNA and cell membranes) by molecular oxygen or free radicals. Vitamin E removes peroxide formation in polyunsaturated fatty acids. It prevents oxidation of LDL preventing atherosclerosis and heart disease. Deficiency of the vitamin E causes haemolysis of RBCs, anemia and muscle breakdown.

Vitamin C is the L-ascorbic acid mostly present in citrus fruits (lemon, orange), melon and strawberry, green leafy vegetables as lettuce, tomatoes, potatoes, raw cabbage and green peppers. Guava is very rich in vitamin canimal tissues contains both Land D ascorbic acid in active form that upon oxidation gives oxalic acidascorbic acid is acidic because it contains two enol groups (C-OH). Ascorbic acid is essential for the conversion of the procollagen into collagen. Procollagen is a protein containing proline and lysine. Hydroxylation of both amino acids is catalyzed by hydroxylase enzymes and by vitamin C as a coenzyme. This converts procollagen into collagen. Collagen is essential for the synthesis of connective tissue, bone, cartilage and teeth. Ascorbic acid is a potent reducing agent, keeping iron in ferrous state. Ascorbic acid acts as a coenzyme for many hydroxylase enzymes required for bile acids synthesis, osteocalcin synthesis, carnitine synthesis. Vitamin C acts as antioxidant and protect tissues from toxic effect of some oxidants that may lead to cancer. Deficiency of vitamin C causes scurvy which is manifestated by decreased collagen formation, bleeding into gum, muscles, joints, kidneys, gastrointestinal tract and pericardium, defective formation of bone and teeth, defective healing of wounds. While excess of vitamin C intake causes hyperoxaluria leading to stone formation.

Thiamin (vitamin B1) consists of a substituted pyrimidine ring connected to a substituted thiazole ring through a methylene bridge (CH3). The active form of B1 is thiamine diphosphate (TPP)/thiamine pyrophosphate formed by thiamine kinase enzyme. TPP acts as coenzyme in two separate reactions in carbohydrate metabolism. First one in oxidative decarboxylation of ketoacids by pyruvate dehydrogenase and a-ketoglutarate dehydrogenase. Second one is in transketolation reactions by transketolase, in pentose phosphate pathway. Thiamin is also essential for the process of nerve conduction and structure of nerve membrane. Thiamin triphosphate acts as phosphate donor for phosphorylation of sodium transport channel of the nerve membrane. Deficiency of vitamin B1 causes Beriberi with impaired carbohydrate carbohydrate metabolism with impaired cellular functions reflecting neuronal disorders.

Vitamin B2 is known as riboflavin with flavin ring attached to ribitol. The sources include milk, milk products, eggs, liver and green leafy vegetables. Riboflavin functions in the form of flavin mononucleotide (FMN) and flavin adenine dinucleotide (FAD). FMN is formed by phosphorylation of riboflavin by intestinal flavokinase enzyme whereas, FAD is formed by the transfer of AMP moiety from ATP to FMN. Both FMN and FAD are coenzyme for flavoenzymes like L -Amino acid oxidase and Succinate dehydrogenase and act as hydrogen or electron carriers. Deficiency causes photophobia cheilosis, glossitis and dermatitis.

Niscin is nicotinic acid (B3) is synthesized endogenously from the amino acid tryptophan. Each 60 mg tryptophan can be converted to 1 mg niacin with the help of B6 as coenzyme. The sources are whole grain cereals, milk, meat, liver, and yeast. Meat is rich in tryptophan, wheareas corn is poor in both niacin and tryptophan. Niacin is a pyridine derivative that is converted to active form nicotinamide with amide group in the liver cells. The NAD^+ and $NADP^+$ are present in two forms oxidized and reduced Reduction of pyridine ring occurs by accepting a hydride ion. Niacin lowers plasma cholesterol inhibiting of free fatty acids (FFa from adipose tissue blocking the supply of aetyl Coadeficiency of niacin causes pellagra, a disease affects the skin, GIT and central nervous system. It is manifested by diarrhoea, dermatistis, dementia Genetically deficiency in tryptophan absorption from intestine and reabsorption from renal tubules causes Hartnup's disease.

Pantothenic acid is formed of pantoic acid (α and γ dihydroxy beta dimethyl butyric acidconnected to β alanlne. Pantothenic acid forms the structure of coenzyme A (Coaand acyl carrier protein. Coenzyme A acts in the transfer of acyl groups e.g. acetyl CoA, succinyl CoA, malonyl CoA and other carboxylic acids in the metabolism process, heme synthesis and fatty acid synthesis. ACP is a component of fatty acid synthase enzyme required for fatty acid synthesis. Deficiency of pantothenic acid causes no effect in human.

Biotin consists of thiophene ring connected to urea with valeric acid as side chain. Biotin acts as CO2 carrier. It attaches to carboxylase enzyme to form biocytin a reaction catalysed by holocarboxylase synthetase enzyme. CO2 is attached to biotin to form. CO2 biotin enzyme complex. The CO2 group is then transferred to the substrate for carboxylation. It acts as coenzyme for carboxylase enzymes in carboxylation reactions like carboxylation of acetyl CoA to malonyl CoA in fatty acid synthesis, carboxylation of pyruvate to oxaloacetate in gluconeogenesis, carboxylation of propionyl CoA to give succinyl Coa The biotin deficiency is manifested by muscle pain, dermatitis, glossitis, loss of appetite and nausea Vitamin B12 or cobalamine consists of corin ring formed of 4 pyrrole rings connected by methenyl groups (=CH-)]. Cobalt ion is present at the center of corin ring that gives red color. Cyano group (CN) attached to cobalt ion forming cyanocobalamin that is the most stable form.

Meat, egg, milk, milk products and intestinal microorganisms are the major sources whereas it is absent in plants. Vitamin B12 is required for synthesis of methionine, tetrahydrofolate and myelin sheath. Deficiency causes megaloblastic anemia and neuronal symptoms.

Folic acid is formed of pteroic acid conjugated to glutamic acid residues. Pteroic acid consists of pteridine ring (2 amino, 4 hydroxy, 6 methyl pteridine) connected to para-aminobenzoic acid (PABA). It is absorbed in jejunum in the form of pteroylmonoglutamate. Then folate enters the liver through the portal circulation where it is converted to dihydrofolate (H2 folate) and tetrahydrofolate (H4folate). The liver converts some of tetrahydrofolate monoglutamate to tetrahydrofolate polyglutamate which is then stored Some are excreted in the bile as N5-methyltetrahydrofolate (MeH4 folate). The active form is tetrahydrofolic acid (H4 folate) which functions as a carrier for one-carbon groups which is utilized for the synthesis of DNA and RNA through synthesis of purines, synthesis of nonessential amino acids e.g. serine and glycine and conversion of homocysteine to methionine. The deficiency is manifested by pancytopenia, megaloblastic anemia, leucopenia, thrombocytopenia, impaired growth and neural tube defects in fetus.

1. Vitamins are
   a. Accessory food factors
   b. Generally synthesized in the body
   c. Produced in endocrine glands
   d. Proteins in nature
2. Which of the following statement is true about the vitamin B12?
   a. It is found in plant products
   b. The cofactor form is vitamin B12 itself
   c. Involves in transfer of amino groups
   d. It requires a specific glycoprotein for its absorption
3. Fat soluble vitamins are
   a. Soluble in alcohol
   b. One or more Propene units
   c. Stored in liver
   d. all of the above
4. Regarding to the vitamin D, the correct statement is
   a. Chronic renal failure requires the oral administration of 1, 25-dihydroxycholecalciferol
   b. 25-hydroxycholecalciferol is the active form of the vitamin
   c. It is required in the diet of the individuals exposed to sun light
   d. Deficiency of vitamin D leads to an hyper secretion of calcitonin
5. Retinal is reduced to retinol in intestinal mucosa by a
   a. Retinal reductase
   b. Retinal dehyde
   c. Retinal oxygenase
   d. Retinal dioxygenase
6. The true statement regarding to retinol
   a. Mediates actions of retinoids
   b. Is dephosphorylated and phosphorylated during the visual cycle
   c. In its ester form is transported from intestine to liver in chylomicrons
   d. None of the above
7. Retinol is transported in blood bound to
   a. Retinol binding protein
   b. α2-Globulin
   c. β-Globulin
   d. Albumin
8. Vitamin K
   a. Is a water soluble vitamin
   b. Is synthesized by intestinal bacteria
   c. Plays a key role in the prevention of thrombosis
   d. Increases the coagulation time in new born infants suffering with hemorrhagic disease
9. Richest source of Vitamin D is
   a. Fish liver oils
   b. Egg yolk
   c. Margarine
   d. Butter

10. Which of the following enzymes have impaired activity in thiamine deficiency?
    a. Isocitrate dehydrogenase and enolase
    b. Aconitase and aldolase
    c. Transketolase and pyruvate dehydrogenase
    d. Hexokinase and glucokinase
11. Calcitriol synthesis involves
    a. Both liver and kidney b. Intestine
    c. Adipose tissue d. Muscle
12. All are antioxidant except
    a. Vitamin A b. Vitamin D
    c. Vitamin C d. Vitamin E
13. The proteins present in maize are deficient in
    a. Lysine b. Threonine
    c. Tryptophan d. Tyrosine
14. Correct statement regarding to vitamin B12
    a. Intrinsic factor of castle b. Cyanocobalamine
    c. Extrinsic factor of castle d. Both b and c
15. Niacin is present in maize in the form of
    a. Niacin b. Nicotin
    c. Niacytin d. Nicyne
16. Vitamin A or retinal is a
    a. Steroid b. Polyisoprenoid compound
    c. Isoprenoid derivative d. Pentathione
17. β-Carotene, precursor of vitamin A, is oxidatively cleaved by
    a. β-Carotene dioxygenase b. Oxygenase
    c. Hydroxylase d. Transferase
18. Preformed Vitamin A is supplied by
    a. Milk, fat and liver b. Fat
    c. Liver d. All of the above
19. The dehydrogenase that converts Retinol to retinal require
    a. NAD or NADP b. NADH + H+
    c. NADPH d. FAD
20. One international unit of vitamin A is equivalent to the activity caused by
    a. 0.3 μg of retinol b. 0.344 μg of retinol
    c. 0.6 μg of retinol d. 1.0 μg of retinol
21. Riboflavin is a coenzyme in the reaction catalysed by the enzyme
    a. Acyl CoA synthetase b. Acyl CoA dehydrogenase
    c. β-Hydroxy acyl CoA d. Enoyl CoA dehydrogenase

22. One manifestation of vitamin A deficiency is
    a. Arthritis
    b. Night blindness
    c. Loss of hair
    d. Thickening of long bones
23. Deficiency of Vitamin A causes
    a. Xeropthalmia
    b. Thrombinemia
    c. Anemia
    d. Cancer
24. An important function of vitamin A is
    a. Coenzyme
    b. Protein synthesis
    c. Prevent hemorrhages
    d. Integrity of epithelial tissue
25. Retinal is a component of
    a. Iodopsin
    b. Cardiolipin
    c. Rhodopsin
    d. Glycoproteins
26. Retinoic acid participates in the synthesis of
    a. Iodopsin
    b. Glycoprotein
    c. Rhodopsin
    d. Cardiolipin
27. On exposure to light rhodopsin forms
    a. All trans-retinal
    b. Retinol
    c. Cis-retinal
    d. Retinoic acid
28. Post translational modification of clotting factor requires
    a. Vitamin K
    b. Vitamin C
    c. Vitamin A
    d. Vitamin E
29. When eggs are cooked
    a. Biotin is destroyed but avidin remains unaffected
    b. Avidin is inactivated but biotin remains unaffected
    c. Both avidin and biotin are inactivated
    d. Both avidin and biotin remain unaffected
30. Which of the following vitamins also act as hormone ?
    a. Vitamin A
    b. Vitamin E
    c. Vitamin D
    d. Vitamin K
31. Biotin is required as a coenzyme by
    a. Anaerobic dehydrogenases
    b. decarboxylases
    c. aerobic dehydrogenases
    d. carboxylases
32. Vitamin K
    a. Is a water soluble vitamin
    b. Is synthesized by intestinal bacteria
    c. Tissue damage
    d. All of the above
33. Which of the following compounds inhibit blood clotting?
    a. Heparin
    b. citrate
    c. Fluoride
    d. all of the above

34. Biotin is a coenzyme for
    a. Pyruvate carboxylase
    b. Acetyl CoA carboxylase
    c. Propionyl CoA carboxylase
    d. All of these
35. Regarding to the vitamin D, the correct statement is
    a. Chronic renal failure requires the oral administration of 1, 25-dihydroxy-cholecalciferol
    b. 25-hydroxycholecalciferol is the active form of the vitamin
    c. It is required in the diet of the individuals exposed to sun light
    d. Deficiency of vitamin D leads to an hyper secretion of calcitonin
36. Lipoic acid is a conenzyme for
    a. Pyruvate dehydrogenase
    b. α-Ketoglutarate dehydrogenae
    c. both a and b
    d. None of these
37. Bioflavonoidsare commonly knownas
    a. Vitamin B7
    b. Vitamin P
    c. Vitamin B9
    d. None of the above
38. Chemically, lipoic acid is
    a. Saturated fatty acid
    b. Unsaturated fatty acid
    c. Amino acid
    d. Sulphur containing fatty acid
39. Which of the following compound is/are act as antioxidant?
    a. β-carotene
    b. Ascorbic acid
    c. Tocopherol
    d. All of the above
40. When eggs are cooked
    a. Biotin is destroyed but avidin remains unaffected
    b. Avidin is inactivated but biotin remains unaffected
    c. Both avidin and biotin are inactivated
    d. Both avidin and biotin remain unaffected
41. Which of the following vitamin is essential for purine synthesis?
    a. Thiamine
    b. Ascorbic acid
    c. Folic acid
    d. Biotin
42. Biotin is required as a coenzyme by
    a. Anaerobic dehydrogenases
    b. Decarboxylases
    c. Aerobic dehydrogenases
    d. Carboxylases
43. Which vitamin is necessary for CoA synthesis?
    a. Vitamin C
    b. Vitamin B2
    c. Biotin
    d. Pantothenic acid
44. Cyanocobalamin is absorbed in the
    a. Stomach
    b. Proximal ileum
    c. Duodenum
    d. Terminal ileum

45. Which of the following vitamins also act as hormone ?
   a. Vitamin A   b. Vitamin E
   c. Vitamin D   d. Vitamin K
46. Pantothenic acid act as coenzyme for the reaction
   a. Reduction   b. Decarboxylation
   c. Oxidation   d. Acetylation
47. The structure shown below is of
   a. Cholecalciferol   b. 25-Hydroxycholecalciferol
   c. Ergocalciferol   d. 7-Dehydrocholesterol
48. Vitamin D absorption is increased in
   a. Acid pH of intestine   b. Alkaline pH of intestine
   c. Impaired fat absorption   d. Contents of diet
49. Cyanocobalamin is absorbed in the
   a. Stomach   b. Proximal ileum
   c. Duodenum   d. Terminal ileum
50. Increased carbohydrate consumption increases the dietary requirement for
   a. Thiamine   b. Pyridoxine
   c. Riboflavine   d. Folic acid
51. The most potent Vitamin D metabolite is
   a. 25-Hydroxycholecalciferol   b. 1,25-Dihydroxycholecalciferol
   c. 24, 25-Dihydroxycholecalciferol   d. 7-Dehydrocholesterol
52. Post translational modification of clotting factor requires
   a. Vitamin K   b. Vitamin C
   c. Vitamin A   d. Vitamin E
53. Deficiency of vitamin D causes
   a. Ricket and osteomalacia   b. Tuberculosis of bone
   c. Hypthyroidism   d. Skin cancer
54. The disease in which pyruvate utilization decreases in tissue
   a. Beriberi   b. Pellagra
   c. Scurvy   d. Pernicious anemia
55. Vitamin required for the conversion of p hydroxyphenylpyruvate to homo gentisate is
   a. Folacin   b. Cobalamin
   c. Ascorbic acid   d. Niacin
56. A hypochromic microcytic anaemia with increased Fe stores in the bone marrow may be
   a. Folic acid responsive   b. Pyridoxine responsive
   c. Vitamin B12 responsive   d. Iron responsive

57. Transketolase activity is affected in
    a. Bitoin deficiency
    b. Pyridoxine deficiency
    c. PABA deficiency
    d. Thiamine deficiency
58. The activity of following enzymes is affected by biotin deficiency
    a. Carboxylase
    b. Dehydrogenase
    c. Oxidase
    d. Reductase
59. The deficiency of which one of the following vitamin causes creatinuria?
    a. Vitamin E
    b. Vitamin A
    c. Vitamin K
    d. Vitamin B6
60. The β-ring of 7-dehydrocholesterol is cleaved to form cholecalciferol by
    a. Infrared light
    b. Dim light
    c. Ultraviolet irridation with sunlight
    d. Light of the tube lights
61. The hydrolysis of glucose-6-PO4 is catalyzed by a phosphatase that is not found in which of the following?
    a. Liver
    b. Kidney
    c. Muscle
    d. Small intestine
62. Insignificant amount of Vitamin E is present in
    a. Wheat germ oil
    b. Sunflower seed oil
    c. Safflower seed oil
    d. Fish liver oil
63. The activity of tocopherols is destroyed by
    a. Commercial cooking
    b. Reduction
    c. Conjugation
    d. all of the above
64. The requirement of vitamin E is increased with greater intake of
    a. Carbohydrates
    b. Proteins
    c. Polyunsaturated fat
    d. Saturated fat
65. Vitamin E reduces the requirement of
    a. Iron
    b. Selenium
    c. Zinc
    d. Magnesium
66. The most important natural antioxidant is
    a. Vitamin D
    b. Vitamin B12
    c. Vitamin E
    d. Vitamin K
67. Tocopherols prevent the oxidation of
    a. Vitamin A
    b. Vitamin K
    c. Vitamin D
    d. Vitamin C
68. Creatinuria is caused due to the deficiency of vitamin
    a. A
    b. E
    c. K
    d. D

69. All the following conditions produce a real or functional deficiency of vitamin K except
    a. Prolonged oral, broad-spectrum antibiotic therapy
    b. Total lack of red meat in the diet
    c. The total lack of green leafy vegetables in the diet
    d. Being a new born infant
70. Vitamin K is found in
    a. Green leafy plants   b. Meat
    c. Fish   d. Milk
71. Function of Vitamin A
    a. Maintaining epithelial   b. Gene regulation
    c. Protein synthesis   d. All of the above
72. Which of the following compound is/are act as antioxidant?
    a. β-carotene   b. Ascorbic acid
    c. Tocopherol   d. All of the above
73. The colour of cyanomethmoglobin is
    a. Pale yellow   b. Pink
    c. Brown   d. Bright red
74. Tocopherols prevent the oxidation of
    a. Vitamin A   b. Vitamin D
    c. Vitamin K   d. Vitamin C
75. Which of the following is regarded as "Vitamin in another vitamin"?
    a. Riboflavin   b. PABA
    c. Thiamin   d. Ascorbic acid
76. Bioflavonoids are commonly known as
    a. Vitamin B7   b. Vitamin P
    c. Vitamin B9   d. None of the above
77. Lipoic acid is therapeutically useful as an antioxidant to prevent
    a. Myocardial infraction   b. Stroke
    c. both a and b   d. None of the above
78. Vitamin K2 was originally isolated from
    a. Soyabean   b. butter
    c. liver   d. Putrid fish meal
79. Vitamin synthesized by bacterial in the intestine is
    a. A   b. D
    c. C   d. K
80. Vitamin K is involved in posttranslational modification of the blood clotting factors by acting as cofactor for the enzyme:
    a. Carboxylase   b. Hydroxylase
    c. Decarboxylase   d. Oxidase

81. Vitamin K is a cofactor for
   a. Gamma carboxylation of glutamic acid residue
   b. β-Oxidation of fatty acid
   c. Formation of γ-amino butyrate
   d. Synthesis of tryptophan

82. Hypervitaminosis K in neonates may cause
   a. Porphyria b. Pellagra
   c. Jaundice d. Prolonged bleeding

83. Dicoumarol is antagonist to
   a. Riboflavin b. Menadione
   c. Retinol d. Tocopherol

84. The Vitamin B1 deficiency causes
   a. Ricket b. Nyctalopia
   c. Beriberi d. Pellagra

85. The vitamin which would most likely become deficient in an individual who develop a completely carnivorous life style is
   a. Thiamin b. Niacin
   c. Vitamin C d. Cobalamin

86. In human body highest concentration of ascorbic acid is found in
   a. Liver b. Adrenal cortex
   c. Adrenal medulla d. Spleen

87. The vitamin required for the formation of hydroxyproline (in collagen) is
   a. Vitamin C b. Vitamin A
   c. Vitamin D d. Vitamin E

88. Vitamin required for the conversion of p hydroxyphenylpyruvate to homo gentisate is
   a. Folacin b. Cobalamin
   c. ascorbic acid d. Niacin

89. Vitamin required in conversion of folic acid to folinic acid is
   a. Biotin b. Cobalamin
   c. Ascorbic acid d. Niacin

90. Ascorbic acid can reduce
   a. 2, 6-Dibromobenzene b. 2, 6-Diiodoxypyridine
   c. 2, 6-Dichlorophenol indophenol d. 2, 4-Dinitrobenzene

91. Sterilised milk lacks in
   a. Vitamin A b. Vitamin D
   c. Vitamin C d. Thiamin

92. Scurvy is caused due to the deficiency of
   a. Vitamin A b. Vitamin D
   c. Vitamin K d. Vitamin C

93. Both Wernicke's disease and beriberi can be reversed by administrating
   a. Retinol b. Thiamin
   c. Pyridoxine d. Vitamin B12
94. The Vitamin B1 deficiency causes
   a. Ricket b. Nyctalopia
   c. Beriberi d. Pellagra
95. Concentration of pyruvic acid and lacticacid in blood is increased due to deficiency of the vitamin
   a. Thiamin b. Riboflavin
   c. Niacin d. Pantothenic acid
96. Vitamin B1 coenzyme (TPP) is involved in
   a. Oxidative decarboxylation b. Hydroxylation
   c. Transamination d. Carboxylation
97. Increased glucose consumption increases the dietary requirement for
   a. Pyridoxine b. Niacin
   c. Biotin d. Thiamin
98. Thiamin is oxidized to thiochrome in alkaline solution by
   a. Potassium permanganate b. Potassium ferricyanide
   c. Potassium chlorate d. Potassium dichromate
99. Riboflavin is a coenzyme in the reaction catalysed by the enzyme
   a. Acyl CoA synthetase b. Acyl CoA dehydrogenase
   c. β-Hydroxy acyl CoA d. Enoyl CoA dehydrogenase
100. In pernicious anemia, urine contains high amounts of
   a. Methyl malonic acid b. FIGLU
   c. VMA d. 5 HIAA
101. Anti sterility Vitamin is
   a. Vitamin B1 b. Vitamin B2
   c. Vitamin E d. Vitamin K
102. Riboflavin deficiency causes
   a. Cheilosis b. Loss of weight
   c. Mental deterioration d. Dermatitis
103. Niacin can be synthesised in human beings from
   a. Histidine b. Tyrosine
   c. Phenylalanine d. Tryptophan
104. Cholesterol is a precursor in the biogenesis of
   a. Vitamin A b. Vitamin D
   c. Vitamin E d. None of these
105. The pellagra preventive factor is
   a. Riboflavin b. Pantothenic acid
   c. Niacin d. Pyridoxine

106. Symptoms of pellagra are
    a. Dermatitis and diarrhea only
    b. Dermatitis and Dermentia only
    c. Diarrhea and dermentia only
    d. Diarrhea, Dermatitis and dementia
107. Niacin or nicotinic acid is a monocarboxylic acid derivative of
    a. Pyridine b. Pyrimidine
    c. Flavin d. Adenine
108. Niacin is synthesized in the body from
    a. Tryptophan b. Tyrosine
    c. Glutamate d. Aspartate
109. Biotin deficiency is characterized by the following except
    a. Muscular pain b. Anaemia
    c. Nausea d. Dermatitis
110. Deficiency of thiamine causes
    a. Beri beri b. Scurvy
    c. Night blindness d. Rickets
111. Vitamin C enhances the intestinal absorption of
    a. Potassium b. Iodine
    c. Iron d. None of these
112. Provitamin D3 is
    a. Cholecalciferol b. Ergosterol
    c. 7-Dehydrocholesterol d. Ergocaliferol
113. The enzymes with which nicotinamide act as coenzyme are
    a. Dehydrogenases b. Transaminases
    c. Decarboxylases d. Carboxylases
114. The Vitamin which does not contain a ring in the structure is
    a. Pantothenic acid b. Vitamin D
    c. Riboflavin d. Thiamin
115. Pantothenic acid is a constituent of the coenzyme involved in
    a. Decarboxylation b. Dehydrogenation
    c. Acetylation d. Oxidation
116. A water soluble form of vitamin K is
    a. Phylloquinone b. Farnoquinone
    c. Menadione d. None of these
117. The precursor of CoA is
    a. Riboflavin b. Pyridoxamine
    c. Thiamin d. Pantothenate

118. Burning foot syndrome' has been ascribed to the deficiency of
   a. Pantothenic acid
   b. Thiamin
   c. Cobalamin
   d. Pyridoxine

119. Prothrombin time is prolonged in
   a. Vitamin K deficiency
   b. Liver damage
   c. Both a and b
   d. None of these

120. Pyridoxal phosphate is central to
   a. Deamination
   b. Amidation
   c. Carboxylation
   d. Transamination

121. A synthetic form of vitamin K is
   a. Menadione
   b. Farnoquinone
   c. Phylloquinone
   d. None of these

122. The vitamin required as coenzyme for the action of transaminases is
   a. Niacin
   b. Pantothenic acid
   c. Pyridoxal phosphate
   d. Riboflavin

123. Retinal is reduced to retinol by retinene reductase in presence of the coenzyme
   a. NAD+
   b. NADP+
   c. NADH + H+
   d. NADPH + H+

124. Vitamin B6 deficiency may occur during therapy with
   a. Isoniazid
   b. Terramycin
   c. Sulpha drugs
   d. Aspirin

125. Carotenes are transported with the
   a. Minerals
   b. Proteins
   c. Lipids
   d. Lipoproteins

126. Deficiency of vitamin B6 may occur in
   a. Obese person
   b. Alcoholics
   c. Thin person
   d. Diabetics

127. The drugs that form complexes with pyridoxal are
   a. Isoniazid
   b. Penicillamine
   c. Rifampicin
   d. Both a and b

128. Vitamin B12 is
   a. Not stored in the body
   b. Stored in bone marrow
   c. Stored in liver
   d. Stored in RE cells

129. Biotin is a coenzyme of the enzyme
   a. Carboxylase
   b. Decarboxylase
   c. Hydroxylase
   d. Deaminase

130. The coenzyme required for conversion of pyruvate to oxaloacetate is
   a. FAD
   b. TPP
   c. NAD
   d. Biotin

131. Vitamin B12 is synthesized by
  a. Bacteria only b. Animals only
  c. Plants only d. Both a and c
132. Extrinsic Factor of Castle is a
  a. Mucoprotein b. Glycoprotein
  c. Mucopolysaccharide d. Cyanocobalaminm
133. In biotin-containing enzymes, the biotin is bound to the enzyme by
  a. An amide linkage to carboxyl group of glutamines
  b. A covalent bond with CO_2
  c. An amide linkage to an amino group of lysine
  d. An amide linkage to α-carboxyl group of protein
134. Intrinsic factor is chemically a
  a. Protein b. Glycoprotein
  c. Mucopolysaccaride d. Peptide
135. A molecule of CO_2 is captured by biotin when it acts as coenzyme for carboxylation reaction. The carboxyl group is co valently attached to
  a. A nitrogen (N1) of the biotin molecule b. Sulphur of thiophene ring
  c. α-Amino group of lysine d. α-Amino group of protein
136. Vitamin B12 is transported in blood by
  a. Albumin b. Transcortin
  c. Transcobalamin I d. Transcobalamin II
137. Consumption of raw eggs can cause deficiency of
  a. Biotin b. Riboflavin
  c. Pantothenic acid d. Thiamin
138. Absorption of Vitamin B12 requires the presence of
  a. Pepsin b. Intrinsic factor
  c. Hydrochloric acid d. Both b and c
139. The cofactor or its derivative required for the conversion of acetyl CoA to malonylCoA is
  a. FAD b. NAD+
  c. ACP d. Biotin
140. Vitamin B12 forms coenzymes known as
  a. Cobamide b. Transcobalamin I
  c. Transcobalamin II d. Both b and c
141. Niacin can be synthesised in human beings from
  a. Histidine b. Tyrosine
  c. Phenylalanine d. Tryptophan
142. Methylcobalamin is required for formation of
  a. Serin from glycine b. Glycine from serine
  c. Methionine from homocysteine d. All of the above

143. Riboflavin deficiency symptoms are
   a. Glossitis b. Vomitting
   c. Stomatis d. both a and b
144. Conversion of folate into tetrahydrofolate requires
   a. NADH b. FMNH2
   c. NADPH d. FADH2
145. A cofactor required in oxidative decarboxylation of pyruvate is
   a. Lipoate b. Pantothenic acid
   c. Biotin d. Para aminobenzoic acid
146. The central structure of B12 referred to as corrin ring system consists of
   a. Cobalt b. Magnesium
   c. Manganese d. Iron
147. The central heavy metal cobalt of vitamin B12 is coordinately bound to
   a. Cyanide group b. Amino group
   c. Carboxyl group d. Sulphide group
148. Vitamin B12 has a complex ring structure (corrin ring) consisting of four
   a. Purine rings b. Pyrrole rings
   c. Pyrimidine rings d. Pteridine rings
149. Lipoic acid is a conenzyme for
   a. Pyruvate dehydrogenase b. α-Ketoglutarate dehydrogenae
   c. both a and b d. None of these
150. Chemically, lipoic acid is
   a. Saturated fatty acid b. Unsaturated fatty acid
   c. Amino acid d. Sulphur containing fatty acid

Answer Key

1	a	2	d	3	d	4	a	5	c	6	c	7	a
8	b	9	a	10	c	11	a	12	b	13	c	14	d
15	c	16	a	17	a	18	d	19	a	20	a	21	b
22	b	23	a	24	d	25	c	26	b	27	a	28	a
29	b	30	a	31	d	32	c	33	d	34	d	35	c
36	c	37	a	38	d	39	d	40	b	41	d	42	d
43	d	44	b	45	a	46	d	47	a	48	a	49	b
50	a	51	b	52	a	53	a	54	a	55	d	56	c
57	d	58	a	59	b	60	c	61	c	62	d	63	a
64	c	65	b	66	c	67	a	68	b	69	b	70	a
71	d	72	d	73	d	74	d	75	b	76	b	77	c
78	d	79	d	80	a	81	a	82	b	83	c	84	c
85	d	86	d	87	a	88	d	89	c	90	c	91	c
92	d	93	b	94	c	95	a	96	a	97	d	98	b
99	b	100	a	101	c	102	a	103	d	104	b	105	b
106	d	107	a	108	a	109	b	110	a	111	c	112	c
113	a	114	a	115	c	116	c	117	d	118	a	119	c
120	d	121	a	122	c	123	c	124	a	125	b	126	b
127	d	128	c	129	a	130	a	141	d	142	c	143	d
144	b	145	c	146	a	147	a	148	c	149	c	150	d

14

Biochemistry of Minerals

Sasmita Barik[1] and Shiv Kumar Yadav[2]

[1]Department of Veterinary Physiology and Biochemistry, College of Veterinary Sciences and Animal Husbandry, Guru Angad Dev Veterinary and Animal Scienes Univeristy, Ludhiana, Punjab

[2]KVK, Shahjahanpur, Uttar Pradesh

Introduction

According to the body needs, minerals may be divided into 2 groups like macrominerals and microminerals. Macrominerals are required in amounts greater than 100 mg/day. They include 6 elements like calcium, phosphorus, magnesium, sodium, potassium and chloride. Whereas microminerals are also known as trace elements and are required in amounts less than 100 mg/day. They include 10 elements like chromium, cobalt, copper, fluoride, iodine, iron, manganese, molybdenum, selenium, zinc and silicon. Some minerals are always required since small amounts of inorganic salts are always excreted Fruits, vegetables and cereals are the chief sources of the mineral elements in the diet. Milk products supply the majority of the calcium and phosphorus in the diet.

Milk and milk products are the richest source of calcium along with beans, leafy vegetables and egg yolk. It is absorbed from upper small intestine. Absorption of calcium is active process and requires calcium binding protein present in the intestinal mucosal cells. The absorption is regulated by vitamin D, parathyroid hormone, high protein diet, pH, high dietary lactate and citrate are the factors that promotes calcium absorption. Whereas high dietary phosphate, alkalinity and impaired fat absorption are the factors that inhibits calcium absorption. Of the total body calcium, 99 % present in bones and teeth in the form of hydroxyapatite and 1 % is present in body fluids and other tissues. Calcium in bones acts as a reservoir, which helps to stabilize calcium ions in plasma and extracellular fluid Parathyroid hormone and active vitamin D stimulate osteoblasts while estrogen hormone inhibits osteoclasts. Plasma calcium is present in two forms; ionized and non-ionized Ionized /diffusible form is the active fraction and its deficiency causes tetany. Non ionized/diffusible form complexes with organic ions (citrate), protein (albumin) and its deficiency occur with conditions of hypoproteinemia and causes no tetany.The hormones like parathyroid hormone, active vitamin D (calcitriol) and calcitonin are the factors tp maintain calcium homeostasis.The function include: calcification of bones and teeth, regulation of transmission of nerve impulses, regulation of contraction of muscles, decrease of neuromuscular excitability, cardiac conduction, second messenger for hormonal action, blood and milk clotting, maintenance of cell membrane permeability, activation of certain enzymes e.g. pyruvate kinase. Hypercalcemia is caused by primary hyperparathyroidism, malignancy, malignancy, Milk-alkali syndrome whereas, hypocalcemia is caused by hypoparathyroidism, alkalosis, kidney diseases.

Phosphorus is absorbed in the mid jejunum in the form of phosphate and enters blood stream via portal circulation. Absorption is regulated by active vitamin D (calcitriol). Most of phosphorus (Bo%) is present in the skeleton (bones and teeth) in the form of hydroxyapatite (Ca3(P04)2, Ca (OH)2). The other 20 % is present in other tissues (mostly intracellular) and body fluids. In plasma it is present as phospholipids and in RBCs it is present as organic phosphate e.g. ATP, glucose-6-phosphate. PTH decreases blood phosphorus by stimulating its excretion through inhibiting its renal tubular reabsorption. Calcitriol increases blood phosphorus through absorption of phosphorus from the intestine, bone resorption i.e. mobilization of phosphorus from bones. It forms the major form of bones and teeth (in the form of hydroxyapatite), plasma buffers (phosphate buffers), cellular components of DNA, RNA, Phospholipids, phosphoproteins, coenzymes (NAD, NADP) and high energy phosphate compounds (ATP, GTP, creatine). Hpyoparathyroidism, acidosis, hypervitaminosis D and RBCs Hemolysis increases serum phosphate. Hyperparathyroidism, Vitamin D deficiency, Renal tubular disease, chronic alcoholism decreases serum phosphate. 70% of body phosphorous is in the skeleton (bones and teeth) and the remaining 30% is present in the other tissues and body fluids mostly intracellular. It activates many enzymes like kinases. It is required for the active transport of other cations (Ca^{++}, Na^{+}, K^{+}) across the cell membrane. Also, it is important for muscle contraction, nerve impulse transmission and it decreases neuromuscular excitability.

The main source of sodium is table salt. Its absorption occurs in small intestine.Aldosterone, the rennin angiotensin system, atrial natriuretic peptide are the factors affecting plasma sodium level. It is responsible for maintenance of osmotic pressure and volume of plasma andextracellular fluid It causes transmission of nerve impulses, contraction of muscle, regulation of acid base balance. Sodium acts as substrate for Na+fK+ ATPase enzyme (sodium potassium pump). Hypernatremia is caused by cushing syndrome, glucocorticoids, conn's disease, diabetes insipidus, and drugs like ACTH or cortisone. Hyponatremia is caused by Addison's disease, aldosterone, renal failure, and diuretics like thiazides.

Vegetables, fruits and nuts are the rich source of potassium. Its absorption occurs in the small intestine which is regulated by aldosterone. The 2/3 of potassium is present in tissues and body fluids. Potassium is the main intracellular cation (3.5-5 mmol/L.). About 1/3 is present in skeleton. It is responsible for maintenance of osmotic pressure and volume of intracellular fluid It causes transmission of nerve impulses, contraction of muscle, acid base balance, substrate for Na+ /K+ ATPase. excess plasma potassium is known as hyperkalemia it is caused by addison's disease, acidosis, tissue necrosis, acute renal failure, advanced chronic renal failure, uncontrolled diabetes mellitus. Acute hyperkalemia occurs when plasma level gets more than 6.5 mmol/L that cause cardiac arrhythmias and even cardiac arrest. Decreased plasma potassium is known as hypokalemia it is caused by alkalosis, hyperglycemia, excessive vomiting, diarrhea, cushing syndrome, hyper-aldosteronism and diuretic.

Chloride is the main extracellular anion. Together with sodium, it maintains the osmotic pressure and volume of plasma and extracellular fluidchloride ions are essential for formation of HCl in the stomach and activation of enzymes like salivary and pancreatic amylase enzymes. The absorption occurs in small intestine. Plasma chloride level is 96-106 mmol/L. Hyperchloremia occurs in hyperchloremic acidosis, renal tubular acidosis, hyperventilation, glomerulonephritis and eclampsia Hypochloremia occurs in hypochloremic alkalosis, addison's disease, diabetes insipidus.

Absorption of iron occurs in the duodenum and the proximal part of the jejunum. The total body iron is distributed in RBCs as hemoglobin (66%), tissue (33%) and plasma (1%). Ferritin is the main storage form of iron. ii- It is formed of a protein called apoferritin, which can carry 3500-4000 atoms of iron to form ferritin. It is present in iron stores: liver, spleen, bone. Iron eforms the major component of hemoglobin, myoglobin, cytochrome P 45o, catalase, peroxidase and tryptophan oxygenase. Absorbed iron enters in the portal blood in ferrous state (Fe++). In the plasma, it is rapidly oxidized to ferric state (Fe+++). A protein containing copper called ceruloplasmin catalyzes this oxidation. Then ferric ions are carried by a transferrin, which is taken mostly by bone marrow to synthesize hemoglobin. Iron, from iron stores (ferritin) can be released into plasma and carried by transferrin to be utilized by bone marrow and other tissues. Iron excreted in the feces is mainly exogenous i.e. dietary iron that has not been absorbed.

Iron deficiency occurs in insufficient intake, impaired absorption: e.g. steatorrhea, abdominal Surgery and excessive loss e.g. menstrual loss, gastrointestinal bleeding due to some parasites (anchylostoma). Deficiency causes decreased plasma iron, increased plasma TIBC, decreased plasma ferritin and hypochromic/microcytic anaemia. Iron overload caused by repeated blood transfusion and intravenous administration of iron. Hemochromatosis (hemosiderosis, bronze diabetes) is a rare hereditary disease characterized by abnormal increase of iron absorption. Iron is deposited in the form of hemosiderin in liver causing liver cirrhosis. It is associated with increased plasma iron, decreased plasma TIBC, increased plasma ferritin.

50% of copper in body are found in muscles and the remaining present in other tissues including liver and bones.Copper is essential for hemoglobin synthesis, bone formation, maintenance of myelin of the nerves. It forms component of several metaloenzymes like ceruloplasmin, superoxide dismutase, cytochrome oxidase. It also activates many enzymes like tyrosinase, uricase and dopamine hydroxylase. Ceruloplasmin is considered as acute phase protein i.e. its plasma level is increased in infections and malignancy. Decreased plasma level causes anemia mostly hypochromic and microcytic, alongwith impaired bone mineralization and wilson's disease manifested by hepatolenticular degeneration.

The micromineral zinc absorption occurs mainly in small intestine. About 20 % of total body zinc is present in the skin. The remaining is present in skeleton (bones and teeth), spermatozoa, prostate, epididymis and pancreas. Zinc is essential for growth and reproduction. It plays a role in tissue repair and wound healing. It forms a complex with insulin in islet cells of thepancreas. This helps crystallization, storage and release of insulin. Zinc is required for mobilization of vitamin A from the liver and subsequently maintains the normal concentration of vitamin A in plasma It forms component of a number of enzymes like alkaline phosphatase, carbonic anhydrase, superoxide dismutase and carboxypeptidase. Zinc deficiency causes hypogonadism, poor healing of wounds, poor appetite, liver cirrhosis, diarrhea and dermatitis.

Manganese is essential for, normal bone structure, reproduction (spermatogenesis and ovulation) and normal function of the central nervous system. It is a component of Pyruvate carboxylase, superoxide dismutase and arginase enzyme.

Chromium is the micromineral that acts only together with insulin to promote glucose utilization. Its deficiency leads to impairment of glucose utilization by tissues. It is involved in lipoprotein metabolism by decreasing serum low density lipoproteins, increases high density lipoproteins decreases total serum cholesterol level. Chromium deficiency causes disturbances in carbohydrate, lipid and protein metabolisms whereas its toxicity causes to liver and kidney damage.

Selenium is the mineral that act as antioxidantsa as it forms major component of the enzyme glutathioneperoxidase. It prevents the development of hepatic necrosis and muscular dystrophy. It forms component of enzyme deiodinase that converts thyroxine (T4) to triiodothyronine and thioredoxin reductase that is involved in purine nucleotide metabolism. Its deficiency is associated with increased risk of cardiovascular disease, and various cancers.

Cobalt forms a component of vitamin B12, which is necessary for normal blood cell formation. It forms a component of vitamin B12 dependant enzymes like methylmalonyl CoA mutase, methyl tetrahydro folate, oxidoreductase, homocysteine methyltransferase and ribonucleotide reductase. Deficiency of cobalt causes pernicious anaemia whereas prolonged administration becomes toxic resulting in polycythemia.

Molybedenum forms a component of oxidase enzymes e.g. xanthine oxidase, aldehyde oxidase, sulfite oxidase and nitrite reductase. excessive consumption causes molybdenosis manifestations by impairment in growth, diarrhea and anemia.

Flourine forms major component of bones and teeth. Its deficiency causes dental carries and osteoporosis. It inhibits the activities of certain enzymes enolase in glycolysis. Similarly fluoroacetate inhibits aconitase of citric acid cycle.Excess flouride leads to fluorosis with mottling and discoloration of the enamel of teeth and changes in bones.

Iodine in the form of iodinized table salt is absorbed from small intestine. In the body iodine is present in thyroid gland as thyroglobulin and in other tissues as T3 and T4. The only known function of iodine is the formation of thyroid hormones (T3 - T4). Deficiency causes ypothyroidism reflected as myxodema in adults and cretinism in children.

1. All following are essential trace elements except
   a. Iron b. Iodine
   c. Zinc d. Cadmium
2. All following are macro minerals except
   a. Sodium b. Potassium
   c. Selenium d. Iron
3. The general functions of minerals are
   a. The structural components of body tissues
   b. In the regulation of body fluids
   c. In acid-base balance
   d. All of the above
4. Cobalt is essential component of
   a. Vitamin B1 b. Vitamin B12
   c. Vitamin B6 d. All of the above

5. Iodine is required in human body for
   a. Formation of thyroxine
   b. Formation of Glutathione
   c. Formation of potassium iodide
   d. Adrenalin
6. Calcium is excreted by
   a. Kidney
   b. Intestine
   c. Both
   d. None
7. All the following statements regarding calcium are correct except
   a. It diffuses as a divalent cation
   b. It freely diffuses across the endoplasmic reticulum of muscle cells
   c. It can exist in the blood as ionic form and also protein bound
   d. It is found in high concentration in bones
8. A deficiency of ionized fraction of serum calcium causes
   a. Tetany
   b. Rickets
   c. Goitre
   d. Osteoporosis
9. In kidneys the active transport of Ca is regulated by
   a. Cholecalciferol
   b. 25-OH cholecalciferol
   c. 1, 25-di-OH-cholecalciferol
   d. All of the above
10. Menke kinky syndrome is characterized by congenital deficiency of
    a. Copper binding ATPase
    b. Serum copper
    c. Serum ceruloplasmin
    d. None of these
11. Iron transport oxygen in which state
    a. Fe+2
    b. Fe+3
    c. Fe
    d. None of these
12. In haemochromatosis, the liver is infiltrated with
    a. Lipids
    b. Chromium
    c. Manganese
    d. Iron
13. In which of the following conditions iron therapy is ineffective:
    a. Thalassaemia minor (α-chain thalassaemia)
    b. Hypochromic anaemia of pregnancy
    c. Impaired absorption of Fe
    d. Chronic blood loss
14. An increased serum iron and decreased Fe-binding capacity are found in
    a. Anaemia of chronic disorders
    b. Fe-deficiency anaemia
    c. Thalassaemia
    d. Sideroblastic anaemia
15. Zinc is a constituent of
    a. Carbonic anhydrase
    b. Aldolase
    c. Amylase
    d. All of the above
16. A rise in blood calcium may indicate
    a. Paget's disease
    b. Rickets
    c. Osteomalacia
    d. Hypervitaminosis D

17. An increase in carbohydrate metabolism is accompanied by temporary decrease in serum:
    a. Calcium
    b. Phosphate
    c. Iron
    d. Sodium
18. An inherited or acquired renal tubular defect in the reabsorption of phosphate is characterize with
    a. Normal serum Phosphate
    b. High serum phosphate
    c. A low blood phosphorous with elevated alkaline Phosphate
    d. A high blood phosphorous with decreased alkaline phosphatase
19. Iron is a component of
    a. Hemoglobin
    b. Ceruloplasmin
    c. Transferase
    d. Transaminase
20. In iron deficiency anemia
    a. The plasma bound iron is low
    b. The plasma bound iron is high
    c. Total iron binding capacity is low
    d. Both the plasma bound iron and total iron binding capacity are low
21. In hepatic diseases
    a. Both the bound iron and total iron binding capacity of the plasma may be low
    b. Both the bound iron and total iron binding capacity of the plasma may be high
    c. Only bound iron may be high
    d. Only the total iron binding capacity may be high
22. The percent of total iron in body in hemoglobin is
    a. 10–20
    b. 30–40
    c. 20–30
    d. 60–70
23. Which of the following is the active form of calcium?
    a. Ionized calcium
    b. Protein bound calcium
    c. Albumin bound calcium
    d. Phosphate bound calcium
24. Minute to minute regulation of calcium ions is carried out by
    a. Parathyroid
    b. Calcitonin
    c. Calcitriol
    d. Thyroxin
25. The iron containing nonporphyrin is
    a. Hemosiderin
    b. Cytochrome C
    c. Catalase
    d. Peroxidase
26. A rise in blood Ca may indicate
    a. Cushing disease
    b. Hypervitaminosis D
    c. Vitamin D deficiency
    d. All of the above

27. The absorption of iron is increases in
   a. Iron deficiency anemia
   b. Pregnancy
   c. Spherocytosis
   d. Sickle cell anemia
28. All of the following are true of hypochromic anaemias not due to iron deficiency, except
   a. Iron therepy is effective
   b. Vitamin B6 deficiency
   c. Stainable iron in bone marrow
   d. Serum Fe is high
29. An increased serum iron and decreased iron binding capacity is found in
   a. Fe deficiency anemia
   b. Sideroblastic anemia
   c. Folate deficiency anemia
   d. Sickle cell anemia
30. Which of the following essential trace element catalyses the formation of Hb in the body
   a. Cu
   b. Fe
   c. Se
   d. Mn
31. The normal route of calcium excretion is
   a. Kidney and intestine
   b. Pancreas, liver and kidney.
   c. Kidney, intestine and pancreas
   d. Kidney and liver
32. A hypochromic microcytic anemia with increased iron stores in the bone marrow may be
   a. Iron responsive
   b. Pyridoxine responsive
   c. Vitamin B12 responsive
   d. Folate responsive
33. Best indicator of iron deficiency is
   a. Serum iron
   b. Serum ferritin
   c. Transferrin
   d. None of these
34. Iron is mainly absorbed from
   a. Stomach and duodenum
   b. Ileum
   c. Caecum
   d. Colon
35. In vitamin D poisoning
   a. Both serum and urinary Ca are low
   b. The serum Ca is increased and urinary Ca is normal
   c. The serum Ca is low and urinary calcium high
   d. Both serum and urinary Ca are high
36. Molecular iron is
   a. Stored primarily in the spleen
   b. Exreted in the urine as Fe2+
   c. Stored in the body in combination with ferritin
   d. Absorbed in the ferric form
37. In hemochromatosis, the liver is infiltrated with
   a. Iron
   b. Molybdenum
   c. Copper
   d. Fats

38. Hypocalcaemia affects
    a. Skeletal muscles + smooth muscles
    b. Skeletal muscles + smooth muscles + cardiac muscles
    c. Smooth muscles
    d. Cardiac muscles
39. Wilson's disease is a condition of toxicosis of
    a. Iron b. Copper
    c. Chromium d. Molybdenum
40. The cytosolic superoxide dismutase enzyme contains
    a. $Cu2+$ b. $Cu2+$ and $Zn2+$
    c. $Zn2+$ d. $Mn2+$
41. The deficiency of copper decreases the activity of the enzyme:
    a. Lysine oxidase b. Lysine hydroxylase
    c. Tyrosine oxidase d. Proline hydroxylase
42. Glutathione peroxidase contains
    a. Se b. Zn
    c. Ca d. Cu
43. In Wilson's disease
    a. Copper fails to be excreted in the bile
    b. Copper level in plasma is decreased
    c. Ceruloplasmin level is increased
    d. Intestinal absorption of copper is decreased
44. Menke's disease is due to an abnormality in the metabolism of
    a. Iron b. Manganese
    c. Magnesium d. Copper
45. The activity of following enzymes is affected by biotin deficiency
    a. Carboxylase b. Dehydrogenase
    c. Oxidase d. Reductase
46. The trace element catalyzing hemoglobin synthesis is
    a. Manganese b. Magnesium
    c. Copper d. Selenium
47. The disease in which pyruvate utilization decreases in tissue
    a. Beriberi b. Pellagra
    c. Scurvy d. Pernicious anemia
48. Mitochondrial superoxide dismutase contains
    a. Zinc b. Copper
    c. Magnesium d. Manganese
49. Glutathione peroxidase contains
    a. Se b. Zn
    c. Ca d. Cu

50. Mitochondrial pyruvate carboxylase contains

a. Zinc b. Zinc

c. Manganese d. Magnesium

51. A hypochromic microcytic anaemia with increased Fe stores in the bone marrow may be

a. Folic acid responsive b. Pyridoxine responsive

c. Vitamin B12 responsive d. Iron responsive

52. In human beings' molybdenum is mainly absorbed from

a. Liver b. Kidney

c. Intestine d. Pancreas

53. In human beings' molybdenum is mainly excreted in

a. Faeces b. Sweat

c. Urine d. Tears

54. Molybdenum is a constituent of

a. Hydroxylases b. Oxidases

c. Transaminases d. Transferases

55. A deficiency of copper affects the formation of normal collagen by reducing the activity of which of the following enzyme?

a. Lysyl oxidase b. Galactosyl transferase

c. Lysyl hydroxylase d. Glucosyl transferase

56. A nonspecific intracellular antioxidant is

a. Chromium b. Magnesium

c. Selenium d. Nickel

57. Molecular iron (Fe), is

a. Stored in the body in combination with feritin

b. Absorbed in the Ferric, Fe+++ form

c. Excreted in the urine as Fe++

d. Absorbed in the intestine by transferring

58. Cobalt forms an integral part of the vitamin

a. B1 b. B6

c. B12 d. Folate

59. Which of the following statement regarding calcium is incorrect?

a. It freely diffuses across the endoplasmic reticulum of muscle cells

b. Required as a cofactor in some of reactions

c. It diffuses as a divalent cation

d. It can exist in the blood as ionic form and also protein bound

60. Selenium is a constituent of the enzyme:

a. Glutathione peroxidase b. Homogentisate oxidase

c. Tyrosine hydroxylase d. Phenylalanin hydroxylase

61. A hypochromic microcytic anaemia with increased Fe stores in the bonemarrow may be
    a. Folic acid responsive
    b. Pyridoxine responsive
    c. Vitamin B12 responsive
    d. Iron responsive
62. Metallic constituent of "Glucose tolerance factor" is
    a. Sulphur
    b. Cobalt
    c. Chromium
    d. Selenium
63. Iron is absorbed from
    a. Ileum
    b. Stomach
    c. Caecum
    d. Duodenum and jejunum
64. Intestinal absorption of chromium is shared with
    a. Mn
    b. Mg
    c. Ca
    d. Zn
65. Which of the following vitamin is essential for purine synthesis?
    a. Thiamine
    b. Ascorbic acid
    c. Folic acid
    d. Biotin
66. Chromium is potentiator of
    a. Insulin
    b. Glucagon
    c. Thyroxine
    d. Parathromone
67. The essential trace element which catalyzes the formation of Hb in the body is
    a. Mn
    b. Mg
    c. Se
    d. Cu
68. Which of the following is true? Hypochromic anaemia is not due to iron deficiency except
    a. Serum 'Fe' is high
    b. Normal/low transferrin
    c. Stainable iron in bone marrow
    d. Iron therapy is affective
69. Cytosolic superoxide dismutase contains
    a. Zn only
    b. Zn and Cu
    c. Cu only
    d. Mn
70. Iron therapy is ineffective in which of the following conditions:
    a. Chronic blood loss
    b. Inadequate Fe intake
    c. Hypochromic anaemia of pregnancy
    d. Thalassaemia minor
71. A rise in blood 'Ca' may indicate
    a. Paget's disease
    b. Vitamin D deficiency
    c. Cushing's disease
    d. Hypervitaminosis D
72. In hoemochromatosis, the liver is infiltrated with
    a. Copper
    b. Manganese
    c. Iron
    d. Chromium

73. An increased serum 'Iron' and decreased 'Fe' binding capacity are found in
   a. Fe-deficiency anaemia   b. Sideroblastic anaemia
   c. Thalassaemia   d. Anaemia of chromic disorders
74. Cobalt may act as cofactor for the enzyme:
   a. Glycl-glycine dipeptidase   b. Elastase
   c. Polynucleotidases   d. Phosphatase
75. Zinc is a constituent of the enzyme:
   a. Succinate dehydrogenase   b. Carbonic anhydrase
   c. Mitochondrial superoxide dismutase   d. Aldolase
76. Excess intake of cobalt for longer periods leads to
   a. Polycythemia   b. Megaloblastic anemia
   c. Pernicious anemia   d. Microcytic anemia
77. The Fe containing pigments is
   a. Haematoidin   b. Hemasiderin
   c. Bilirubin   d. Urobilinogen
78. Serum inorganic phosphorous decreases in all the following conditions except
   a. Hyperparathyroidism   b. Intestinal malabsorption
   c. Osteomalacia   d. Chronic renal failure
79. Sulphur is made available to the body by the amino acids:
   a. Cystine and methionine   b. Taurine and alanine
   c. Proline and hydroxyproline   d. Arginine and lysine
80. Magnesium ions are required in the reactions involving
   a. NAD   b. ATP
   c. FAD   d. CoA
81. All of the following are true of Wilson's disease except
   a. Low total plasma Cu   b. Elevated urinary copper
   c. Arthritis   d. Aminoaciduria
82. Sodium is involved in the active uptake of
   a. D-Glucose   b. L-Amino acids
   c. D-Galactose   d. All of the above
83. Sulphur containing coenzyme is
   a. NAD   b. FAD
   c. Pyridoxal phosphate   d. Biotin
84. Hyponatraemia occurs in the following condition
   a. Addison's disease   b. Chronic renal failure
   c. Severe diarrhoea   d. All of the above
85. Iodine is stored in
   a. Thyroid gland as thyroglobulin   b. Liver
   c. Intestine   d. Skin

86. Concentration of the following is higher in intracellular fluid than in extracellular fluid:
   a. Sodium b. Chloride
   c. Potassium d. Bicarbonate

87. Normal range of serum potassium is
   a. 2.1-3.4 mEq/L b. 3.5-5.3 mEq/L
   c. 5.4–7.4 mEq/L d. 7.5–9.5 mEq/L

88. Normal range of serum chloride is
   a. 24–27 mEq/L b. 70–80 mEq/L
   c. 100–106 mEq/L d. 120–140 mEq/L

89. An extracellular fluid having a higher concentration of chloride than serum is
   a. Bile b. CSF
   c. Sweat d. Pancreatic juice

90. Iodine is the constituent of
   a. T3 and T4 b. Glucagon
   c. Insulin d. Serotonin

91. Fluorosis occurs due to
   a. Drinking water containing less than 0.2 ppm of fluorine
   b. Drinking water containing high calcium
   c. Drinking water containing greater than 1.2 ppm of fluroine
   d. Drinking water containing heavy metals

92. Hypocalcaemia can occur in all the following except
   a. Rickets b. Osteomalacia
   c. Hyperparathyroidism d. Intestinal malabsorption

93. Metal required for polymerization of insulin is
   a. Copper b. Chromium
   c. Cobalt d. Zinc

94. Metalloenzyme-retinene for polymerization of insulin is
   a. Copper b. Zinc
   c. Cobalt d. Manganese

95. Normal range of serum sodium is
   a. 30–70 mEq/L b. 70–110 mEq/L
   c. 117–135 mEq/L d. 136–145 mEq/L

96. An important zinc containing enzyme is
   a. Carboxypeptidasea b. Isocitrate dehydrogenase
   c. Cholinesterate d. Lipoprotein lipase

97. Each haemoglobin molecule contains
   a. One iron atom b. Four iron atoms
   c. Two iron atoms d. Six iron atoms

98. Each myoglobin molecule contains
   a. One iron atom
   b. Four iron atoms
   c. Two iron atoms
   d. Six iron atoms
99. Iron is stored in the form of
   a. Ferritin and transferrin
   b. Transferrin and haemosiderin
   c. Haemoglobin and myoglobin
   d. Ferritin and haemosiderin
100. Acrodermatitis enteropathica is due to defective absorption of
   a. Manganese
   b. Molybdenum
   c. Iodine
   d. Zinc
101. Hypogonadism develops due to deficiency of
   a. Sulphur
   b. Cobalt
   c. Zinc
   d. Manganese
102. Tetany can occur in
   a. Hypocalcaemia
   b. Hypercalcaemia
   c. Alkalosis
   d. Hypocalcaemia and alkalosis
103. Intestinal absorption of calcium occurs by
   a. Active takeup
   b. Simple diffusion
   c. Facilitated diffusion
   d. Endocytosis
104. Intestinal absorption of calcium is hampered by
   a. Glucose
   b. Proteins
   c. Phytate
   d. Lactose
105. Calcitriol facilitates calcium absorption by increasing the synthesis of the following in intestinal mucosa:
   a. Calcium Binding Protein
   b. Alkaline Phosphatase
   c. Calcium-dependent ATPase
   d. All of the above
106. A high plasma calcium level decreases intestinal absorption of calcium by
   a. Stimulating the secretion of parathormone
   b. Inhibiting the secretion of parathormone
   c. Decreasing the synthesis of cholecalciferol
   d. Inhibiting the secretion of thyrocalcitonin
107. Hypercalcaemia can occur in all the following except
   a. Hyperparathyroidism
   b. Hypervitaminosis D
   c. Milk alkali syndrome
   d. Nephrotic syndrome
108. Copper deficiency can cause
   a. Polycythaemia
   b. Leukocytopenia
   c. Thrombocytopenia
   d. Microcytic anaemia

109. All the following statements about ceruloplasmin are correct except
   a. It is a copper-containing protein
   b. It possesses oxidase activity
   c. It is synthesised in intestinal mucosa
   d. Its plasma level is decreased inWilson's disease
110. All the following statements about Wilson's disease are correct except
   a. It is a genetic disease
   b. The defect involves copper-dependent P-type ATPase
   c. Copper is deposited in liver, basal ganglia and around cornea
   d. Plasma copper level is increased in it
111. Which of the following statements about Menke's disease are true.
   a. It is an inherited disorder of copper metabolism
   b. It occurs only in males
   c. Plasma copper is increased in it
   d. Hair becomes steely and kinky in it
112. All the following statements about ceruloplasmin are correct except
   a. It is a copper-containing protein
   b. It possesses oxidase activity
   c. It is synthesised in intestinal mucosa
   d. Its plasma level is decreased inWilson's disease
113. The major calcium salt in bones is
   a. Calcium carbonate b. Calcium chloride
   c. Calcium hydroxide d. Calcium phosphate
114. The correct statement about serum inorganic phosphorous concentration is
   a. It is higher in men than in women
   b. It is higher in women than in men
   c. It is higher in adults than in children
   d. It is higher in children than in adults
115. Serum inorganic phosphorous rises in all the following conditions except
   a. Hypoparathyroidism b. Hypervitaminosis D
   c. Chronic renal failure d. After a carbohydrate-rich meal
116. Aldosterone increases reabsorption of sodium in
   a. Proximal convoluted tubules b. Ascending limb of loop of Henle
   c. Descending limb of loop of Henle d. Distal convoluted tubules
117. Restriction of sodium intake is commonly advised in
   a. Addison's disease b. Diarrhoea
   c. Hypertension d. None of these
118. Serum sodium level rises in all of the following except
   a. Renal failure b. Prolonged steroid therapy
   c. Aldosteronism d. Dehydration

119. All the following statements about endemic goiter are true except
   a. It occurs in areas where soil and water have low iodine content
   b. It leads to enlargement of thyroid gland
   c. It results ultimately in hyperthyroidism
   d. It can be prevented by consumption of iodised salt
120. Zinc is a cofactor for
   a. Acid phosphatase b. Alkaline phosphatase
   c. Amylase d. Lipase
121. Consumption of iodised salt is recommended in
   a. Patients with hyperthyroidism b. Patients with hypothyroidism
   c. Pregnant women d. Goitre belt areas
122. Zinc is involved in storage and release of
   a. Histamine b. Epinephrine
   c. Acetylcholine d. Insulin
123. Zinc deficiency occurs commonly in
   a. Acrodermatitis enteropathica b. Wilson's disease
   c. Xeroderma pigmentosum d. Menke's disease
124. Healing of wounds may be impaired in deficiency of
   a. Selenium b. Copper
   c. Zinc d. Cobalt
125. Hypochromic microcytic anaemia can occur in
   a. Zinc b. Copper
   c. Manganese d. None of these
126. Molybdenum is a cofactor for
   a. Xanthine oxidase b. Aldehyde oxidase
   c. Sulphite oxidase d. All of the above
127. A trace element having antioxidant function is
   a. Selenium b. Tocopherol
   c. Chromium d. Molybdenum
128. Selenium is a constituent of
   a. Glutathione reductase b. Glutathione peroxidase
   c. Catalase d. Superoxide dismutase
129. Selenium decreases the requirement of
   a. Copper b. Zinc
   c. Vitamin D d. Vitamin E
130. Cobalt is essential component of
   a. Vitamin B1 b. Vitamin B12
   c. Vitamin B6 d. All of the above

131. Which of the following is true for Iron
   a. Stored primarily in spleen
   b. Absorbed in the intestine
   c. Absorbed in the ferric, Fe+++ form
   d. Stored in the body in combination with ferritin

132. Iron is absorbed from
   a. Jejunum
   b. Duodenum and
   c. Both
   d. None

133. Transferrin is a type of
   a. Albumin
   b. β1 globulin
   c. α-globulin
   d. γ-globulin

134. Ceruloplasmin shows the activity
   a. As ferroxidase
   b. As ligase
   c. As reductase
   d. As transferase

135. The principal cation of extra cellular fluid:
   a. K+
   b. H+
   c. Na+
   d. Ca2+

136. What is the principal cation of intracellular fluid?
   a. K+
   b. Ca2+
   c. Na+
   d. Mg2+

137. What is the normal level of K+ in the serum?
   a. 137–148 mEq/L
   b. 120–160 mEq/L
   c. 3.9–5.0 mEq/L
   d. 0.3–0.59 mEq/L

138. What are the functions of potassium?
   a. In muscle contraction
   b. Cell membrane function
   c. Enzyme action
   d. All of these

139. What is ceruloplasmin?
   a. Plasma protein
   b. Stored form of copper
   c. Both a and b
   d. None of these

140. Sulphur is made available to the body by the amino acids:
   a. Cystine and methionine
   b. Taurine and alanine
   c. Proline and hydroxyproline
   d. Arginine and lysine

141. Sulphur containing coenzyme is
   a. NAD
   b. FAD
   c. Pyridoxal phosphate
   d. Biotin

142. Microsomal hydroxylase system contains a
   a. Di-oxygenase
   b. Mono-oxygenase
   c. Both a and b
   d. None of these

143. Superoxide radicals can be detoxified by
   a. Cytochrome c b. Cytochrome b
   c. Cytochrome a d. None of these
144. A copper containing cytochrome is
   a. Cytochrome a b. Cytochrome P-450
   c. Cytochrome a3 d. None of these
145. Iron-pophyrin is present as prostheticgroup in
   a. Cytochromes b. Catalases
   c. Peroxidase d. None of these
146. Tetany can occur in
   a. Hypocalcaemia b. Hypercalcaemia
   c. Alkalosis d. Hypocalcaemia and alkalosis
147. Zn is present as prosthetic group in this enzyme:
   a. Carbonic anhydrase b. Carboxy peptidase
   c. Lactate dehydrogenase d. All of the above
148. The major calcium salt in bones is
   a. Calcium carbonatc b. Calcium chloride
   c. Calcium hydroxide d. Calcium phosphate
149. Ferritin is
   a. Coenzyme
   b. One of the component of photophosphorylation
   c. It is the stored form of iron
   d. Non-protein moiety
150. The following are the functions of copper:
   a. Constituent of cytochromes b. Catalase
   c. Tyrosinase d. All of the above

Answer Key

1	d	2	c	3	d	4	b	5	a	6	c	7	b
8	a	9	c	10	a	11	a	12	d	13	a	14	d
15	a	16	d	17	b	18	c	19	a	20	a	21	a
22	d	23	a	24	a	25	a	26	b	27	a	28	a
29	b	30	a	31	a	32	b	33	b	34	a	35	d
36	c	37	a	38	b	39	b	40	b	41	a	42	a
43	a	44	d	45	a	46	c	47	a	48	d	49	a
50	c	51	b	52	c	53	b	54	b	55	a	56	a
57	a	58	c	59	a	60	a	61	b	62	c	63	d
64	d	65	c	66	a	67	d	68	d	69	b	70	d
71	d	72	c	73	b	74	a	75	c	76	a	77	c
78	d	79	a	80	c	81	c	82	d	83	d	84	d
85	a	86	c	87	c	88	c	89	c	90	a	91	c
92	c	93	b	94	b	95	d	96	a	97	c	98	a
99	d	100	d	101	c	102	d	103	a	104	b	105	d
106	b	107	d	108	d	109	c	110	d	111	c	112	c
113	d	114	d	115	a	116	d	117	c	118	a	119	d
120	b	121	d	122	d	123	a	124	c	125	b	126	d
127	a	128	b	129	d	130	b	131	d	132	c	133	b
134	b	135	b	136	a	137	c	138	d	139	c	140	a
141	d	142	b	143	a	144	c	145	d	146	d	147	d
148	d	149	c	150	d								

15

Biochemistry of Energy Metabolism

Divyaprakash Choravada[1], Juli Chakma[2]

[1]Department of Biochemistry, IVSAH, SOA Deemed to be University, Bhubaneshwar

[2]Department of Animal Nutrition, IVSAH, SOA Deemed to be University, Bhubaneshwar

Introduction

Energy metabolism is the complex process by which living organisms convert nutrients into energy for survival, growth, and reproduction. It involves a series of interconnected biochemical reactions that occur within cells.

Key Components of Energy Metabolism

- **Catabolism:** The breakdown of complex molecules (carbohydrates, proteins, and fats) into simpler ones, releasing energy.
- **Anabolism:** The synthesis of complex molecules from simpler ones, requiring energy input.
- **ATP:** The primary energy currency of cells, used to power various cellular processes.
- **Enzymes:** Catalysts that facilitate metabolic reactions.

Major Metabolic Pathways

- **Glycolysis:** The breakdown of glucose into pyruvate, producing ATP and NADH.
- **Citric Acid Cycle (Krebs Cycle):** Oxidizes acetyl-CoA (derived from carbohydrates, fats, and proteins) to produce ATP, NADH, and FADH2.
- **Electron Transport Chain (ETC):** Utilizes NADH and FADH2 to generate ATP through oxidative phosphorylation.
- **Beta-oxidation:** Breaks down fatty acids into acetyl-CoA.
- **Gluconeogenesis:** Synthesis of glucose from non-carbohydrate sources.
- **Glycogenolysis and Glycogenesis:** Breakdown and synthesis of glycogen, respectively.

Regulation of Metabolism

Metabolism is tightly regulated by hormones, enzymes, and allosteric effects to maintain energy balance and adapt to changing conditions.

Overall Goal

The ultimate goal of energy metabolism is to produce ATP, which is essential for various cellular functions, including muscle contraction, nerve impulse transmission, and protein synthesis.

1. Metabolism is:
   a. The process of breaking down food
   b. The sum of all chemical reactions in the body
   c. The process of building up tissues
   d. The conversion of food into energy
2. Catabolism involves:
   a. building up complex molecules
   b. Storing energy
   c. Breaking down molecules to release energy
   d. Creating new cells
3. Anabolism is the process of:
   a. Releasing energy b. Uilding complex molecules
   c. Breaking down food d. Converting glucose to ATP
4. Which of the following is an example of catabolism?
   a. Protein synthesis b. Photosynthesis
   c. Digestion d. Glycogen storage
5. Which of the following is an example of anabolism?
   a. Cellular respiration b. Muscle growth
   c. Breakdown of glucose d. Digestion of fats
6. The energy released during catabolism is primarily stored as:
   a. ATP b. Glucose
   c. Fats d. Proteins
7. Anabolic processes generally require:
   a. Energy input b. Energy output
   c. No energy change d. Oxygen
8. Catabolic and anabolic processes are:
   a. Independent of each other b. Interconnected
   c. Opposites d. Identical
9. Metabolism is essential for:
   a. Growth and repair b. Energy production
   c. Maintaining body temperature d. All of the above
10. Which of the following factors can influence metabolic rate?
    a. Age b. Gender
    c. Physical activity d. All of the above

11. ATP is considered the energy currency of the cell. Which of the following bonds in ATP stores the most energy?
    a. Adenosine-ribose bond
    b. Ribose-phosphate bonds
    c. Phosphate-phosphate bonds
    d. All bonds store equal energy
12. Which enzyme is responsible for the hydrolysis of ATP to ADP and inorganic phosphate?
    a. ATP synthase
    b. ATPase
    c. Kinase
    d. Phosphatase
13. How is ATP regenerated in the cell?
    a. Glycolysis only
    b. Cellular respiration only
    c. Photosynthesis only
    d. Both glycolysis and cellular respiration

Redox Reactions

14. In a redox reaction, the molecule that loses electrons is said to be:
    a. Oxidized
    b. Reduced
    c. Catalyzed
    d. Hydrolyzed
15. Which of the following molecules is a common electron carrier in redox reactions?
    a. NAD+
    b. ATP
    c. Glucose
    d. Oxygen
16. The electron transport chain is a series of redox reactions that occurs in the:
    a. Cytoplasm
    b. Nucleus
    c. Mitochondria
    d. Endoplasmic reticulum

Free Energy

17. Gibbs free energy (ΔG) is a measure of:
    a. The total energy in a system
    b. The energy available to do work
    c. The energy lost as heat
    d. The activation energy of a reaction
18. A reaction with a negative ΔG is considered:
    a. Exergonic
    b. Endergonic
    c. Spontaneous
    d. Both a and c
19. Which of the following factors affects the free energy change of a reaction?
    a. Temperature
    b. Concentration of reactants and products
    c. Pressure
    d. All of the above

20. Coupling of an exergonic reaction to an endergonic reaction allows:
    a. The endergonic reaction to proceed
    b. The exergonic reaction to proceed faster
    c. Both reactions to reverse direction
    d. No change in the overall energy of the system
21. Glycolysis takes place in the:
    a. Nucleus b. Mitochondria
    c. Cytoplasm d. Golgi apparatus
22. The net ATP yield from glycolysis is:
    a. 2 b. 4
    c. 36 d. 38
23. The end product of glycolysis is:
    a. Pyruvate b. Acetyl CoA
    c. Lactic acid d. Ethanol
24. Which enzyme is considered the rate-limiting enzyme of glycolysis?
    a. Hexokinase b. Phosphofructokinase-1 (PFK-1)
    c. Pyruvate kinase d. Enolase
25. Which of the following is an activator of phosphofructokinase-1 (PFK-1)?
    a. ATP b. Citrate
    c. ADP d. Acetyl CoA
26. Under anaerobic conditions, pyruvate is converted to:
    a. Acetyl CoA b. Lactic acid or ethanol
    c. Oxaloacetate d. Glucose
27. Glycolysis is a process of:
    a. Oxidation b. Reduction
    c. Both oxidation and reduction d. Neither oxidation nor reduction
28. How many molecules of NADH are produced in glycolysis?
    a. 1 b. 2
    c. 3 d. 4
29. The energy investment phase of glycolysis requires:
    a. 1 ATP b. 2 ATP
    c. 3 ATP d. No ATP
30. Which of the following is not a product of glycolysis?
    a. Pyruvate b. ATP
    c. NADH d. Oxygen
31. Gluconeogenesis primarily occurs in which organs?
    a. Liver and kidneys b. Muscles and brain
    c. Pancreas and intestines d. Heart and lungs

32. The starting material for gluconeogenesis is:
    a. Glucose
    b. Glycogen
    c. Pyruvate, lactate, glycerol, and amino acids
    d. Fructose
33. The key regulatory enzyme in the gluconeogenic pathway is:
    a. Hexokinase
    b. Pyruvate kinase
    c. Phosphoenolpyruvate carboxykinase (PEPCK)
    d. Glucose-6-phosphatase
34. Gluconeogenesis is stimulated by:
    a. Insulin
    b. Glucagon and cortisol
    c. Adrenaline
    d. Growth hormone
35. Which of the following is NOT a substrate for gluconeogenesis?
    a. Lactate
    b. Alanine
    c. Acetyl-CoA
    d. Glycerol
36. Gluconeogenesis is important for:
    a. Maintaining blood glucose levels during fasting
    b. Providing glucose for the brain
    c. Preventing hypoglycemia
    d. All of the above
37. The process of converting pyruvate to oxaloacetate in gluconeogenesis is called:
    a. Glycolysis
    b. Pyruvate dehydrogenase complex
    c. Pyruvate carboxylation
    d. Gluconeogenesis
38. Which hormone inhibits gluconeogenesis?
    a. Insulin
    b. Glucagon
    c. Cortisol
    d. Growth hormone
39. Gluconeogenesis occurs primarily in the:
    a. Cytosol
    b. Mitochondria
    c. Both a and b
    d. Nucleus
40. Gluconeogenesis is the process of:
    a. Breaking down glucose
    b. Synthesizing glucose from non-carbohydrate precursors
    c. Storing glucose as glycogen
    d. Converting glucose to pyruvate
41. The primary storage form of glucose in animals is:
    a. Starch
    b. Glycogen
    c. Cellulose
    d. Maltose

42. The enzyme responsible for the breakdown of glycogen to glucose-1-phosphate is:
    a. Glycogen synthase
    b. Glycogen phosphorylase
    c. Glucose-6-phosphatase
    d. Hexokinase
43. The process of glycogen synthesis is called:
    a. Glycogenolysis
    b. Gluconeogenesis
    c. Glycogenesis
    d. Glycolysis
44. The hormone that stimulates glycogen breakdown is:
    a. Insulin
    b. Glucagon
    c. Cortisol
    d. Growth hormone
45. The key enzyme in glycogen synthesis is:
    a. Glycogen phosphorylase
    b. Glycogen synthase
    c. Glucose-6-phosphatase
    d. Hexokinase
46. The site of glycogen storage in the body includes:
    a. Liver and muscles
    b. Kidneys and brain
    c. Adipose tissue and heart
    d. Blood and lungs
47. The process of converting glucose-6-phosphate to glucose occurs primarily in the:
    a. Liver
    b. Muscles
    c. Brain
    d. Red blood cells
48. Which of the following is NOT a regulatory mechanism of glycogen metabolism?
    a. Hormonal control
    b. Allosteric regulation
    c. Covalent modification
    d. Vitamin C deficiency
49. The enzyme that transfers glucose residues from UDP-glucose to the growing glycogen chain is:
    a. Glycogen phosphorylase
    b. Glycogen synthase
    c. Branching enzyme
    d. Debranching enzyme
50. Glycogen storage diseases are caused by:
    a. Excess glycogen production
    b. Deficiencies in glycogen metabolism enzymes
    c. Increased glucose intake
    d. Hormonal imbalances
51. The process of breaking down fatty acids into acetyl-CoA units is called:
    a. Glycolysis
    b. Beta-oxidation
    c. Gluconeogenesis
    d. Ketogenesis
52. Where does beta-oxidation primarily occur in the cell?
    a. Cytosol
    b. Mitochondria
    c. Endoplasmic reticulum
    d. Golgi apparatus

53. Each cycle of beta-oxidation produces:
    a. 1 acetyl-CoA, 1 NADH, and 1 FADH2
    b. 2 acetyl-CoA, 2 NADH, and 2 FADH2
    c. 1 acetyl-CoA, 2 NADH, and 1 FADH2
    d. 2 acetyl-CoA, 1 NADH, and 1 FADH2

Energy Yield

54. Fatty acids are a more efficient energy source than carbohydrates because:
    a. They contain more oxygen
    b. They produce more ATP per gram
    c. They are easier to digest
    d. They are stored in larger quantities
55. The total ATP yield from complete oxidation of a 16-carbon fatty acid is approximately:
    a. 100 ATP
    b. 120 ATP
    c. 140 ATP
    d. 160 ATP

Ketogenesis

56. Ketogenesis primarily occurs in the:
    a. Liver
    b. Kidney
    c. Muscle
    d. Adipose tissue
57. The three main ketone bodies produced in the liver are:
    a. Acetone, acetoacetate, and beta-hydroxybutyrate
    b. Pyruvate, lactate, and alanine
    c. Glucose, fructose, and galactose
    d. Cholesterol, bile acids, and steroid hormones
58. Ketogenesis is stimulated under conditions of:
    a. High carbohydrate intake
    b. Low carbohydrate intake
    c. Excessive protein intake
    d. Increased insulin levels
59. Ketone bodies can be used as an alternative energy source by:
    a. The brain only
    b. The heart only
    c. The liver only
    d. The brain, heart, and skeletal muscle
60. Excessive ketone body production can lead to a condition called:
    a. Ketoacidosis
    b. Ketosis
    c. Hyperglycemia
    d. Hypoglycemia
61. The rate-limiting enzyme in fatty acid synthesis is:
    a. Cetyl-CoA carboxylase
    b. Fatty acid synthase
    c. Thioesterase
    d. β-ketoacyl-ACP synthase

62. The primary site of fatty acid synthesis is:
    a. Liver b. Muscle
    c. Kidney d. Brain
63. The immediate precursor for fatty acid synthesis is:
    a. Acetyl-CoA b. Malonyl-CoA
    c. Palmitoyl-CoA d. Citrate
64. Which hormone stimulates fatty acid synthesis?
    a. Insulin b. Glucagon
    c. Epinephrine d. Cortisol
65. The end product of fatty acid synthesis is primarily:
    a. Palmitic acid b. Stearic acid
    c. Oleic acid d. Linoleic acid
66. The enzyme responsible for elongating the fatty acid chain is:
    a. Acetyl-CoA carboxylase b. Fatty acid synthase
    c. Thioesterase d. β-ketoacyl-ACP synthase
67. Which of the following is not a component of fatty acid synthase?
    a. Acetyl-CoA-acyl carrier protein transacylase
    b. Malonyl-CoA-acyl carrier protein transacylase
    c. β-hydroxyacyl-ACP dehydrogenase
    d. Enoyl-ACP reductase
68. Citrate plays a role in fatty acid synthesis by:
    a. Activating acetyl-CoA carboxylase
    b. Inhibiting acetyl-CoA carboxylase
    c. Directly participating in the synthesis process
    d. Transporting acetyl-CoA from mitochondria to cytosol
69. Which of the following conditions favors fatty acid synthesis?
    a. High levels of insulin b. Low levels of glucose
    c. High levels of glucagon d. Fasting state
70. The process of fatty acid synthesis occurs in the:
    a. Mitochondria b. Cytosol
    c. Endoplasmic reticulum d. Golgi apparatus
71. Which of the following is the main component of a lipoprotein core?
    a. Phospholipids b. Cholesterol
    c. Triglycerides d. Proteins
72. Apoproteins are essential components of lipoproteins. What is their primary function?
    a. Structural support
    b. Lipid digestion
    c. Ligand binding for receptor recognition
    d. Energy storage

73. Which lipoprotein is primarily responsible for transporting cholesterol from the liver to peripheral tissues?
    a. Chylomicrons
    b. VLDL
    c. LDL
    d. HDL
74. What is the role of HDL (High-Density Lipoprotein)?
    a. Transports cholesterol from the liver to the tissues
    b. Transports triglycerides from the liver to the tissues
    c. Removes excess cholesterol from the bloodstream and transports it to the liver
    d. Is involved in lipid digestion

Lipoprotein Metabolism and Disease

75. Which lipoprotein is often referred to as "bad cholesterol"?
    a. LDL
    b. HDL
    c. VLDL
    d. chylomicrons
76. Elevated levels of which lipoprotein are associated with an increased risk of atherosclerosis?
    a. HDL
    b. LDL
    c. Chylomicrons
    d. VLDL
77. What is the primary function of lipoprotein lipase (LPL)?
    a. Breaks down triglycerides in chylomicrons and VLDL
    b. Synthesizes cholesterol
    c. Transports cholesterol to the liver
    d. Converts cholesterol to bile acids
78. Which of the following is NOT a risk factor for developing high cholesterol levels?
    a. Physical inactivity
    b. Healthy diet
    c. Smoking
    d. Obesity

Lipoprotein Classification and Testing

79. Lipoproteins are classified based on their density. Which of the following is the correct order of lipoproteins from lowest to highest density?
    a. Chylomicrons, VLDL, LDL, HDL
    b. HDL, LDL, VLDL, Chylomicrons
    c. VLDL, LDL, HDL, Chylomicrons
    d. LDL, HDL, VLDL, Chylomicrons
80. A blood test that measures the levels of total cholesterol, LDL, HDL, and triglycerides is called a:
    a. Lipid profile
    b. Liver function test
    c. Complete blood count
    d. Fasting blood sugar
81. Which process removes the amino group from an amino acid to produce ammonia?
    a. Deamination
    b. Transamination
    c. Urea cycle
    d. Gluconeogenesis

82. The transfer of an amino group from one amino acid to another is called:
    a. deamination b. Transamination
    c. Urea cycle d. Gluconeogenesis
83. The primary organ responsible for the urea cycle is:
    a. Kidney b. Liver
    c. Lung d. Muscle
84. The end product of the urea cycle is:
    a. Ammonia b. Urea
    c. Uric acid d. Creatinine
85. Glutamate dehydrogenase is a key enzyme in:
    a. Deamination b. Transamination
    c. Urea cycle d. Gluconeogenesis
86. Which of the following is not involved in the urea cycle?
    a. Ornithine b. Citrulline
    c. Aspartate d. Pyruvate
87. Transamination reactions require the coenzyme:
    a. NAD+ b. FAD
    c. Pyridoxal phosphate (PLP) d. Coenzyme A
88. Ammonia is converted to a less toxic form called:
    a. Urea b. Uric acid
    c. Creatinine d. Glutamine
89. The urea cycle takes place in both the mitochondria and the cytosol.
    a True b False
90. Which of the following amino acids is often involved in transamination reactions?
    a. Alanine b. Glycine
    c. Serine d. Cysteine
91. Protein synthesis involves two main processes. These are:
    a. Transcription and translation b. Replication and transcription
    c. Translation and replication d. Transcription and replication
92. The site of protein synthesis in the cell is:
    a. Nucleus b. Ribosomes
    c. Mitochondria d. Golgi apparatus
93. The genetic code is:
    a. Triplet b. Doublet
    c. Singlet d. Quadruplet
94. The start codon for protein synthesis is:
    a. AUG b. UAA
    c. UAG d. UGA

95. The molecule that carries amino acids to the ribosomes during protein synthesis is:
   a. mRNA
   b. tRNA
   c. rRNA
   d. DNA

96. The process of transferring genetic information from DNA to mRNA is called:
   a. Translation
   b. Transcription
   c. Replication
   d. Mutation

97. The codon on mRNA that signals the termination of protein synthesis is:
   a. AUG
   b. UAA
   c. UAG
   d. Both b and c

98. The number of amino acids coded by a codon is:
   a. One
   b. Two
   c. Three
   d. Four

99. The genetic code is said to be degenerate because:
   a. a codon codes for more than one amino acid
   b. More than one codon can code for the same amino acid
   c. The code is universal
   d. The code is non-overlapping

100. The enzyme that reads the DNA template and synthesizes mRNA is:
   a. DNA polymerase
   b. RNA polymerase
   c. DNA ligase
   d. Aminoacyl tRNA synthetase

101. Where is the electron transport chain located in the cell?
   a. Cytoplasm
   b. Nucleus
   c. Inner mitochondrial membrane
   d. Golgi apparatus

102. Which molecules donate electrons to the electron transport chain?
   a. Glucose and pyruvate
   b. NADH and FADH2
   c. ATP and ADP
   d. Oxygen and carbon dioxide

103. What is the final electron acceptor in the electron transport chain?
   a. Water
   b. Carbon dioxide
   c. Oxygen
   d. NADH

104. Which process is coupled to the electron transport chain to produce ATP?
   a. Glycolysis
   b. Krebs cycle
   c. Oxidative phosphorylation
   d. Fermentation

105. What is the role of cytochrome c in the electron transport chain?
   a. It is a mobile electron carrier
   b. It is the first electron acceptor
   c. It is the final electron acceptor
   d. It catalyzes the formation of ATP

106. Which complex in the electron transport chain pumps protons into the inter-membrane space?
   a. Complex I, II, and III
   b. Complex I, III, and IV
   c. Complex II, III, and IV
   d. All complexes

107. What is the role of the proton gradient generated across the inner mitochondrial membrane?
    a. To drive ATP synthesis b. To transport electrons
    c. To break down glucose d. To produce oxygen
108. Which of the following is not a component of the electron transport chain?
    a Cytochromes b. Ubiquinone
    c ATP synthase d. Flavoproteins
109. How does cyanide inhibit the electron transport chain?
    a. By blocking complex I
    b. By inhibiting ATP synthase
    c. By binding to cytochrome c oxidase
    d. By preventing glucose breakdown
110. What is the overall goal of the electron transport chain?
    a. To produce glucose b. To break down ATP
    c. To generate a proton gradient d. To produce ATP
111. chemiosmosis primarily involves the movement of:
    a. Sodium ions b. Potassium ions
    c. Hydrogen ions (protons) d. Calcium ions
112. The energy stored in the proton gradient is used to:
    a Directly synthesize glucose
    b. Power the movement of molecules across the membrane
    c Drive the synthesis of ATP
    d. Reduce NADP+
113. The enzyme responsible for ATP synthesis during chemiosmosis is:
    a. ATPase b. ATP synthase
    c. Phosphorylase d. Kinase
114. The proton gradient is established across the:
    a. Outer mitochondrial membrane b. Inner mitochondrial membrane
    c. Cytoplasmic membrane d. Nuclear membrane
115. The F0 part of ATP synthase is involved in:
    a. Synthesis of ATP b. Transport of protons
    c. Binding ADP and Pi d. Regulation of ATP synthesis
116. The energy for rotating the F1 part of ATP synthase comes from:
    a. The flow of electrons b. The movement of protons
    c. The hydrolysis of ATP d. The breakdown of glucose
117. Chemiosmosis occurs in:
    a. Mitochondria only b. Chloroplasts only
    c. both mitochondria and chloroplasts d. None of the above

118. In mitochondria, the proton gradient is generated during:
  a. Glycolysis b. Krebs cycle
  c. Electron transport chain d. Fermentation

119. The final electron acceptor in the electron transport chain is:
  a. Oxygen b. Water
  c. NAD+ d. FAD

120. The process of ATP synthesis coupled to chemiosmosis is called:
  a. Substrate-level phosphorylation b. Oxidative phosphorylation
  c. Photophosphorylation d. Chemiosmotic phosphorylation

121. Which of the following is a common metabolic intermediate shared by glycolysis and gluconeogenesis?
  a. Pyruvate b. Glucose-6-phosphate
  c Acetyl-CoA d. Oxaloacetate

122. The citric acid cycle and urea cycle are linked through:
  a. Acetyl-CoA b. Aspartate
  c. Citrate d. Fumarate

123. Fatty acid synthesis and degradation share which common intermediate?
  a Acetyl-CoA b. Glycerol
  c. Malonyl-CoA d. Palmitate

124. The pentose phosphate pathway and glycolysis are connected by:
  a. Glucose-6-phosphate b. Ribose-5-phosphate
  c. Fructose-6-phosphate d. Glyceraldehyde-3-phosphate

125. Which pathway provides reducing equivalents (NADPH) for fatty acid synthesis?
  a. Glycolysis b Citric acid cycle
  c. Pentose phosphate pathway d. Urea cycle

126. Amino acids can enter the metabolic pathways through:
  a. Transamination b Deamination
  c. Gluconeogenesis d All of the above

127. The Cori cycle involves the interconversion of:
  a. Glucose and lactate b. Glucose and glycogen
  c. Pyruvate and lactate d. Glycogen and lactate

128. Which hormone stimulates both glycogenesis and lipogenesis?
  a. Insulin b. Glucagon
  c. Epinephrine d. Cortisol

129. The glycerol backbone of triglycerides can be converted into:
  a. Glucose b. Fatty acids
  c. Amino acids d. Acetyl-CoA

130. a metabolic pathway that is both catabolic and anabolic is called:
  a. Amphibolic b. Linear
  c. Cyclic d. Convergent

131. Which of the following is NOT a primary function of hormones in metabolic regulation?
   a. Stimulating enzyme synthesis b. Inhibiting enzyme activity
   c. Directly catalyzing metabolic reactions d. Modifying enzyme activity
132. Which hormone is primarily responsible for stimulating glucose uptake by cells?
   a. Insulin b. Glucagon
   c. Cortisol d. Epinephrine
133. The binding of a hormone to its receptor typically initiates a(n) __________ within the cell.
   a. Enzyme cascade b. Gene transcription
   c. Cellular response d. All of the above
134. Hormonal regulation is essential for maintaining:
   a. Blood glucose levels b. Growth and development
   c. Reproduction d. All of the above
135. Allosteric regulation occurs when a molecule binds to a(n) __________ site on an enzyme.
   a. Active b. Regulatory
   c. Catalytic d. Substrate-binding
136. A molecule that enhances an enzyme's activity is called a(n):
   a. Inhibitor b Activator
   c. Effector d. Modulator
137 allosteric regulation is typically associated with:
   a. Feedback inhibition b. Enzyme activation
   c. Both a and b d. Neither A nor B
138 Which of the following is NOT a common feature of allosteric enzymes?
   a. Quaternary structure b. Multiple subunits
   c. Cooperative binding d. Linear structure
139 allosteric regulation is important for:
   a. Maintaining metabolic balance b. Responding to cellular needs
   c. Efficient energy utilization d. All of the above
140 An example of an allosteric effector is:
   a. ATP b. Glucose-6-phosphate
   c. Acetyl-CoA d. All of the above
141 Which of the following vitamins is NOT directly involved in energy metabolism?
   a. Vitamin A b. Vitamin B1
   c. Vitamin B2 d. Vitamin B3

142. Coenzymes are:
   a. Proteins that catalyze chemical reactions
   b. Organic molecules that assist enzyme function
   c. Inorganic substances required for enzyme activity
   d. The end products of metabolic pathways
143. Thiamine (B1) is essential for:
   a. Fat metabolism b. Protein synthesis
   c. Carbohydrate metabolism d. Bone health
144. Which vitamin is involved in the transfer of electrons in the electron transport chain?
   a. Vitamin C b. Vitamin D
   c. Riboflavin (B2) d. Vitamin K
145. A deficiency of niacin can lead to:
   a. Pellagra b. Rickets
   c. Scurvy d. Anemia
146. Coenzymes bind to enzymes at the:
   a. Active site b. Allosteric site
   c. Catalytic site d. Substrate binding site
147. Which of the following is NOT a function of coenzymes?
   a. Activating enzymes b. Carrying electrons
   c. Providing energy directly d. Assisting in substrate binding
148. Pantothenic acid is a precursor to:
   a. Coenzyme A b. NAD
   c. FAD d. Pyridoxal phosphate
149. Vitamin B6 is involved in:
   a. Amino acid metabolism b. Fat digestion
   c. Carbohydrate absorption d. Calcium absorption
150. A deficiency of vitamin B12 can lead to:
   a. Pernicious anemia b. Beriberi
   c. Pellagra d. Rickets

Answer Key

1	b	2	c	3	b	4	c	5	b	6	a	7	a
8	b	9	d	10	d	11	c	12	b	13	d	14	a
15	a	16	c	17	b	18	d	19	d	20	a	21	c
22	a	23	a	24	b	25	c	26	b	27	c	28	b
29	b	30	d	31	a	32	c	33	c	34	b	35	c
36	d	37	c	38	a	39	c	40	b	41	b	42	b
43	c	44	b	45	b	46	a	47	a	48	d	49	b
50	b	51	b	52	b	53	a	54	b	55	c	56	a
57	a	58	b	59	a	60	a	61	a	62	a	63	b
64	a	65	a	66	b	67	d	68	a	69	a	70	b
71	c	72	c	73	c	74	c	75	a	76	b	77	a
78	b	79	a	80	a	81	a	82	b	83	b	84	b
85	a	86	d	87	c	88	a	89	a	90	a	91	a
92	b	93	a	94	a	95	b	96	b	97	d	98	a
99	b	100	b	101	c	102	b	103	c	104	c	105	a
106	b	107	a	108	c	109	c	110	d	111	c	112	c
113	b	114	b	115	b	116	b	117	c	118	c	119	a
120	c	121	a	122	b	123	a	124	a	125	c	126	d
127	a	128	a	129	a	130	a	131	c	132	a	133	d
134	d	135	b	136	b	137	c	138	d	139	d	140	d
141	a	142	b	143	c	144	c	145	a	146	a	147	c
148	a	149	a	150	a								

16

Biochemistry of Blood and Body Fluid

***N.R. Srikanth*[3], *M.K. Vidya*[1], *C.N. Darshan*[2] *and Ramesh Doreswamy*[4]**

[1]*Division of Veterinary Biochemistry, Livestock Research Station, Lam, Guntur Sri Venkateswara Veterinary University*

[2]*Department of Physiology and Biochemistry, Veterinary College, KVAFSU Hassan, Karnataka*

[3]*Department of Animal Husbandry and Veterinary Services, Karnataka*

[4]*Department of Veterinary physiology and biochemistry, Veterinary College Hassan, KVAFSU, Karnataka*

Introduction

Biochemistry of blood is extremely complex. It plays vital role in maintaining homeostasis with in the body. Blood is a specialized connective tissue which is a fluid that circulates all through the body in cardio vascular system. Blood consists of 55 per cent of plasma and 45 per cent of cellular components.

Plasma: A straw coloured liquid component of blood. Understanding the chemical basis of plasma is very crucial for diagnosis and treating various conditions. The compositional breakdown of plasma can be put forth as 90-92 % of water that acts as transport medium for the remaining 8-10 % of the solutes. Solutes further can be classified as electrolytes (salts), proteins, Lipids, other nutrients and waste products.

Plasma electrolytes: These are the minerals found in the blood that are electrically charged. Their role is very crucial in lot of physiological activities like

- Maintaining the balance of fluids interior and exterior to the cells.
- Carries electrical signals all through the body
- Helps in contraction of muscles
- Regulates blood pressure

Prime electrolytes of plasma are sodium, potassium, chloride, calcium, magnesium, bicarbonate and phosphate. Homeostasis is maintained in a normal healthy body. Any change in these electrolytes can lead to different pathological conditions and the alterations in the levels of these electrolytes can be diagnostic importance for physiological derailments. Electrolyte imbalances may occur in a body for trivial reasons like dehydration to most dreadful kidney diseases. So the plasma electrolyte concentrations have profound diagnostic importance in medical and veterinary sciences. These imbalances can be noticed in diarrhoea, vomiting, dehydration, excessive sweating, kidney conditions *etc.*

Symptoms like muscle cramps, fatigue, nausea, vomiting, headache, disorientation, cardiac arrhythmias are often noticed in cases of electrolyte imbalance.

- Fluid balance maintenance: Plasma electrolytes maintain an osmotic gradient across the cell membranes. This gradient create a difference in pressure on either side of the membranes which influences the movement of water molecules. Within the cells and plasma electrolyte gradient is maintained in such a way that the water flows all through and maintains the hydration state in the body.
- Electrical signalling: Electrolytes remain as dissolved ions with electric charge which facilitate generation and propagation of action potentials across cell membranes. Action potentials are the reason that maintain nerve impulses and muscle contractions.
- Muscle function: Electrolyte play a major role in muscle function at cellular level. Calcium ions trigger muscle contraction. When voltage gated calcium channels open calcium influx into the cell happens and activates sarcoplasmic reticulum to release even more calcium which binds to troponin that in turn initiates the muscle contraction. Potassium ions maintain the resting membrane potential of muscle cells. Potassium concentration is high inside and low outside the cell which creates electrochemical gradient. Magnesium acts as a cofactor for many enzymes involved in muscle energy metabolism mainly for those which use ATP. Magnesium also helps in muscle relaxation by antagonising the effects of calcium.
- Cardiac muscle function: Potassium and magnesium are essential for maintaining electrical gradient across the membranes of cardiac muscle cells. Alterations in the concentrations of potassium and magnesium can lead to changes in the action potential of waveform, which affects the cardiac conduction velocity and contractility. In severe form electrolyte imbalances can cause cardiac arrhythmias and even the life threatening form, ventricular fibrillation.
- Regulation of Blood Pressure: Sodium influences the blood pressure by affecting blood volume and vascular tone. Plasma osmolality is maintained by blood plasma sodium concentration. Hypernatremia, an increase in sodium concentration elevates plasma osmolality which draws water out of the cells into the blood stream. This increases blood volume leads into an increase in blood pressure (hypertension). Conversely, hyponatremia causes water to move from the blood stream to cells there by causing hypotension.
- pH Balance: electrolytes maintain pH homeostasis. Electrolytes like bicarbonate and phosphate act as buffers to resist the change in pH.

Plasma proteins: They play critical role in maintaining homeostasis by executing various kinds of essential activities. Albumin, globulin, fibrinogen, to name a few are prime plasma proteins.

- Transport: Plasma proteins act as carrier proteins to carry variety of molecules like lipids, vitamins, hormones, metal ions and minerals. Albumin, the major plasma protein is responsible for transporting steroids, thyroid hormones and fatty acids.
- Buffering: Plasma proteins act as buffers and regulate the blood pH there by maintaining homeostasis.
- Oncotic pressure: Again albumin plays crucial part in maintaining the oncotic pressure, which is also referred to as colloid osmotic pressure of blood. This

pressure pulls the fluid out of tissues there by avoiding the accumulation of fluid in tissues that may lead to edema.

- Immunity: Immunoglobulins which in general terms called as antibodies are nothing but plasma proteins that are produced by B lymphocytes. These immunoglobulins are a type of globulins that protect the body from pathogens like bacteria and viruses.
- Blood clotting: Fibrinogen, one of the important blood clotting factor. When some sort of injury happens to the blood capillaries or vessels, the insoluble fibrin is formed from fibrinogen which forms clot to seal the wound.

Plasma lipids: Lipids have their conspicuous role in energy storage and cellular function. However the lipids are insoluble in water and hence the plasma. Here comes into the picture the lipoproteins. Lipoproteins are spherical particles that carry the plasma lipids from one place to other of the body. The inner greasier portion filled with cholesterol esters and triglycerides, which were enveloped by phospholipid and protein shell, which make the lipoprotein structure in entirety that is has water soluble property and hence can be transported across in the plasmachylomicrons, very-low-density lipoproteins (VLDL), low-density lipoproteins (LDL) and high-density lipoproteins (HDL) are the major lipoproteins that help transport of lipids in the plasma at various stages. Triglycerides, cholesterol and phospholipids are the main plasma lipids. Triglycerides are main storage of energy, cholesterol is an intrinsic part of the cell membranes and hormone synthesis. Phospholipids are amphipathic nature with hydrophilic heads and hydrophobic tails forming the outer shell of the lipoproteins allowing them to be hydrophilic from outside. Maintaining proper balance of the plasma lipids is crucial. High LDL levels and low HDL levels lead to atherosclerosis increasing the risk of cardiac failure and stroke.

Nutrients like blood glucose and fats for energy and amino acids for protein building are part of blood plasma constituents. Urea, a protein breakdown product, creatinine, a muscle breakdown product and uric acid are the waste products often seen in the plasma. Gases like oxygen and carbon dioxide are also found in plasma as part of cellular respiration.

Cellular components of Blood: Red blood cells (RBccarry oxygen to body from the lungs and carbon dioxide to lungs from the body using heme (iron) containing globulin, haemoglobin. White blood cells (WBcare the components of immune system that protect the body against pathogens like bacteria, viruses *etc*. Platelets are tiny cell fragments that help in blood clotting.

Biochemistry of other body fluids: Other than the blood's vital role many other body fluids with diverse biochemical compositions play specific functions in the body.

- Interstitial fluid (ISF): A watery fluid that fills the void between cells. The chemical composition of ISF is similar to plasma but have lesser protein content due to limited permeability. ISF acts as bridge between blood and cells facilitating nutrient and waste exchange.
- Intracellular fluid (ICF): Present with in the cells with higher potassium and lower sodium content compared to plasma, carrying various macro molecules like proteins, carbohydrates and enzymes.
- Cerebrospinal fluid (CSF): The composition is similar to plasma with lower protein content and similar electrolyte content as plasmacSF is a colourless fluid which acts as mechanical shock absorber for brain and spinal cord which regulates intra cranial pressure as well helps in waste removal.

- Synovial fluid: Rich in hyaluronic acid, a thick fluid that lubricates the joints reducing the friction.
- Mucus: Primarily water but varies in composition based on the location. Mucus is made of water, mucins (a glycoprotein), electrolytes and enzymes. Mucus protects by lubricating various passages like respiratory, digestive *etc.* there by trapping the pathogens and aiding their removal.
- Urine: Dissolved in water excretes waste products like urea that are generated by metabolism thereby regulating the blood pressure and volume keeping electrolyte balance in check.

1. The animal body contains
   a. 30 – 40 % water b. 40 – 50 % water
   c. 50 – 60 % water d. 60 – 70 % water
2. In an aqueous solution of NaCl the solute is
   a. Water b. NaCl
   c. Both a & b d. None of these
3. If each 100ml of solution contains 5g of solute. What is the percentage of solution in the solute
   a. 5 % b. 4 %
   c. 3% d. 2%
4. Solutions most frequently encountered are in
   a. Solid state b. Liquid state
   c. Gaseous state d. None of these
5. The substance whose physical state is preserved when solution is formed is know as
   a. Solvent b. Solute
   c. Water d. None of these
6. The substance whose physical state is not preserved when solution is formed is know as
   a. Solute b. Solvent
   c. Water d. None of these
7. A membrane that permits the passage of solvent but not solute is known as
   a. Permeable membrane b. Non Permeable membrane
   c. Semi Permeable membrane d. None of these
8. The membrane that permits the passage not only of solvent but also of selected solutes is known as
   a. Selectively Permeable membrane b. Semi Permeable membrane
   c. Slightly Permeable membrane d. All of the above
9. The properties of solution that are determined by the number of particles rather than by kind of particles is known as
   a. Physical properties b. Physiological properties
   c. Colligative properties d. Dynamic properties

10. Osmotic pressure is measured in
    a. Milliliters of Mercury
    b. Millimeters of Mercury
    c. Milligrams of Mercury
    d. None of these
11. One osmolar solution contains
    a. 1 osm in 10 ml
    b. 1 osm in 100 ml
    c. 1 osm in 1 kg
    d. 1 osm in 1 L
12. The effective osmotic pressure with respect to a selectively permeable membrane is called as
    a. Tone
    b. Tonicity
    c. Both a & b
    d. None of these
13. Tone is not a colligative property because it is not determined by the
    a. Total number of particles in the solution
    b. Total mass of the particles in the solution
    c. Both a & b
    d. None of these
14. Minerals that dissolve to yield a conducting solution is known as
    a. Electrolytes
    b Conductors
    c Both a & b
    d. None of these
15. Positively charged particles is known as
    a. Anion
    b. Cation
    c. Ion
    d. None of these
16. Negatively charged particles is known as
    a. Anion
    b. Cation
    c. Non ion
    d. None of these
17. A mill equivalent is equal to
    a. One tenth of an equivalent
    b. One hundredth of an equivalent
    c. One thousandth of an equivalent
    d. None of these
18. Simple diffusion occurs under the influence of
    a. Brownian motion
    b. Thermal motion
    c. Both a & b
    d. None of these
19. Small particles can diffuse through the membrane by
    a. Postulated spores
    b. Protein channels
    c. Both a & b
    d. None of these
20. Larger particles are transported through the membrane by
    a. Facilitated diffusion
    b. Protein channels
    c. Both a & b
    d. None of these
21. The most abundant substance in the body to diffuse is
    a. Water
    b. Blood
    c. Salts
    d. Electrolytes

22. The amount of a substance diffusing into the cell is usually balanced by
    a. Equal amount of water diffusing out
    b. Equal amount of substance diffusing out
    c. Both a & b
    d. None of these
23. Greater the number of particles
    a. The greater the osmotic pressure b. The lower the osmotic pressure
    c. Same will be the osmotic pressure d. None of these
24. Which of these is simply a number and doesn't have any dimension
    a. Specific gravity b. Colligative property
    c. Tonicity d. All of the above
25. Negative pore charge assists in
    a. Sodium ion movement b. Potassium ion movement
    c Calcium ion movement d All of the above
26. The average animal(neither fat nor lean) has water equivalent to____% of bodyweight
    a. 60 b. 80
    c. 50 d. 90
27. Plasma constitutes ____% of water
    a. 80 b. 70
    c. 92 d. 96
28. Cellular over hydration is known as_______
    a. Water retention b. Water intoxication
    c. Vacuole formation d. Hyper hydration
29. Plasma constitutes ___ % protein
    a. 10 b. 12
    c. 8 d. 5
30. Dye rapidly binds to _____ after injection
    a. Red blood cells b. Leukocytes
    c. Plasma proteins d. serum
31. Plasma volume can be measured by ________ dye
    a. Methyl blue b. Saffranin
    c. Evan's blue d. Giemsa
32. Lush green fodder contains ____% water
    a. 10-15 b. 15-30
    c. 50-60 d. 75-90
33. Oxidation of one gram of carbohydrate leads ___ml of water
    a. 1 b. 2
    c. 0.6 d. 0.1

34. What is the primary method used to measure total body water?
    a. Bioelectrical impedance   b. MRI
    c. CT scan   d. Ultrasound
35. Which of the following is commonly used indicator for measuring extracellular fluid volume
    a. Sodium   b. Potassium
    c. Chloride   d. Urea
36. Which of the following is a direct method to measure total body water
    A. Ibdirect calorimetry   b. D2O dilution
    c. Plasma osmolarity   d. Urine output
37. Following substances is commonly used as a marjer for measuring plasma volume?
    a. Inulin   b. Sodium
    c. Iodine   d. Albumin
38. What principle is used to determine fluid volumes with dye dilution methods?
    a. Radioactive decay   b. Light absorption
    c. Volume conservation   d. Magnetic resonance
39. What is the primary fluid compartment measured using the inulin clearance test ?
    a. Total body water   b. Plasma volume
    c. Extracellular fluid   d. Interstitial fluid
40. If a hypertonic NaCl solution were injected intravenously water would begin to
    a. Shift into plasma
    b. Shift into blood cells
    c. Remains in blood cells
    d. Distribute evenly in extracellular fluid
41. Plasma volume can be measured by injection of a substance such as
    a Cango red   b. Evans blue dye
    c. Methylene blue   d. Acridine dye
42. Which part of the brain is primarily responsible for regulating thirst
    a. Cerebellum   b. Hypothalamus
    c. Medulla ablongata   d. Amygdala
43. What triggers the sensation of thirst
    a. High blood sugar level   b. Low blood oxygen level
    c. High blood osmolality   d. Low body temperature
44. Which ion concentration is most influential in the regulation of thirst
    a. Potassium   b. Sodium
    c. Calcium   d Magnesium
45. What effect does dehydration have on blood pressure
    a. Increases it   b. Decreases it
    c. No effect   d. Stabilizes it

46. Which of the following conditions can lead to excessive thirst
    a. Diabetes mellitus b. Hypertension
    c. Hypothyroidism d. Hyperthyroidsm
47. Which of the following is a symptom of dehydration
    a Clear urine b Dry mouth
    c. Frequent urination d. Increase saliva production
48. For most of domestic animals the oxidative or metabolic water represents only ____ % of total water intake
    a. 5 -10 b. 10-15
    c. 15-20 d. 20-25
49. Which organ is primarily responsible for water reabsorption in body
    a. Heart b. Liver
    c. Kidney d. Lungs
50. Which hormone plays a key role in regulating water balance and blood pressure
    a. Insulim b. Cortisol
    c. Vasopressin d. Thyroxine
51. The excretion of water by kidney is controlled by
    a. AST b. ALT
    c. ADH d. BUN
52. Release of ADH is from
    a. Posterior Pitutary b. Anterior Pitutary
    c. Pineal d. Thyroid
53. Hypertonic saline solution injected into carotid artery _______ in urine flow
    a. Increase b. Decrease
    c. Remain same d. None
54. The maximum urine concentration is highest in which species
    a. Dog b. Cat
    c. Sheep d. Cattle
55. If animal is overhydrated ADH will present in blood will be
    a. Less b. More
    c. Absent d. None
56. Loss of water from body during dehydration
    a. 1-2% b. 2-3%
    c. 2-4% d. 4-5%
57. Anhidrosis is a form of sweat gland exhaustion this condition seen in
    a. Cattle b. Race Horse
    c. Dog d. Sheep
58. Which one of the following is not function of kidney
    a. Regulation of blood pH b. Production of Urine
    c. Metabolism of Carbohydrate d. Regulation of blood volume

59. Which of the following condition can result in failure of kidney to excrete waste products
    a. Metabolic acidosis
    b. Hyperglycemia
    c. Hyperthyroidism
    d. Hypocalcemia
60. Which of the component present in urine
    a. Urea
    b. Glucose
    c. RBC
    d. Protein
61. Immediate source of water lost from the body is
    a. Extracellular fluid
    b. Intracellular fluid
    c. Interstial fluid
    d. Pericardial fluid
62. When animal is deprived of water _______ may act as source of water
    a. Extracellular fluid
    b. Rumen fluid
    c. Adipose tissue
    d. Glycogen
63. During cooler desert night stored heat is dissipated and body temperature is
    a. Increases
    b. Decreases
    c. Normal
    d. Increase followed by decreases
64. The erythrocyte of camel are________ in shape
    a. Circular
    b. Oval
    c. Biconcave
    d. Elliptical
65. The slightly unequal distribution of all diffusible ions across the capillary wall is known as
    a. Gibbs donnan phenomenon
    b. Osmosis
    c. Dialysis
    d. Diffusion
66. The major cations of the fluid of the cell are ___________
    a. Na and K
    b. K and Mg
    c. Na and Al
    d. Zn and Na
67. The osmotic pressure across the capillary wall is created by _________
    a. Cation and anions
    b. GFR
    c. Plasma Protein
    d. None of these
68. For maintaining of blood volume and pressure ____________is responsible
    a. Total Osmotic Pressure
    b. Hydrostatic Pressure
    c. Osmosis
    d. Gravitational force
69. During the formation of urine ultrafiltration takes place in
    a. Bowman's capsule
    b. PCT
    c. DCT
    d. Loop of henle
70. Which ruminant is compared to camel in term of ability to withstand dehydration
    a. Horse
    b. Cow
    c. Donkey
    d. Goat

71. What is the primary reason that camels can survive longer without water compared to humans
    a. They store large amount of water in their rumen
    b. They have the ability to conserve water and tolerate greater dehydration
    c. They produce more metabolic water from fat than other animals
    d. They drink water only once in week
72. What is main purpose of hump in camel
    a. To store water
    b. To Provide a source of energy
    c. To regulate body temperature
    d. To store Oxygen
73. The first sign of dehydration is
    a. Tendency to seek and drink water
    b. Laying Down
    c. More sweating
    d. Sheavering
74. During deprived of water in moderate condition in dog__________
    a. 10% loss
    b. 20% loss
    c. 5% loss
    d. 8% loss
75. The Proximal convulated tubule is lined by the following
    a. Simple cuboidal epithelium
    b. Simple columnar epithelium
    c. Simple cuboidal brush border epithelium
    d. Simple columnar brush border epithelium
76. What are the three classes of blood cells?
    a. Erythrocytes, Leukocytes, Platelets
    b. Erythrocytes, Plasma, Serum
    c. Granulocytes, Agranulocytes, Plasma
    d. Erythrocytes, Granulocytes, Agranulocytes
77. What is the primary difference between plasma and serum?
    a. Plasma is clear, while serum is yellow.
    b. Serum contains clotting factors, while plasma does not.
    c. Plasma contains clotting factors, while serum does not.
    d. Plasma is obtained from coagulated blood, while serum is not.
78. What is the percentage distribution of water and solids in plasma?
    a. 80-85% water, 15-20% solids
    b. 70-75% water, 25-30% solids
    c. 91-92% water, 8-9% solids
    d. 85-90% water, 10-15% solids
79. Which plasma protein functions in the regulation of osmotic pressure?
    a. Globulins
    b. Fibrinogen
    c. Albumin
    d. Hemoglobin
80. Which anticoagulant is preferred for blood studies that involve morphology and quantitative methods?
    a. EDTA
    b. Heparin
    c. Citrate
    d. Sodium fluoride

81. Which anticoagulant is a natural product of basophils and mast cells?
   a. Sodium citrate
   b. EDTA
   c. Heparin
   d. Potassium oxalate
82. What percentage of the red blood cell is typically occupied by hemoglobin?
   a. 25%
   b. 50%
   c. 75%
   d. 95%
83. Which anticoagulant is commonly used for blood transfusions in animals and can cause hypocalcemia if overdosed?
   a. Sodium citrate
   b. EDTA
   c. Heparin
   d. Potassium oxalate
84. What is the usual time required for the development of an erythrocyte from a rubriblast?
   a. 1-2 days
   b. 3-5 days
   c. 7-10 days
   d. 14-21 days
85. Which of the following does NOT describe a function of plasma albumin?
   a. Maintenance of colloidal osmotic pressure
   b. Transport of free fatty acids
   c. Buffering of extracellular fluid
   d. Formation of fibrin for blood clotting
86. What hormone primarily regulates plasma potassium concentration ([K+])?
   a. Insulin
   b. Aldosterone
   c. Cortisol
   d. Atrial natriuretic peptide
87. How does Addison's disease typically affect plasma potassium levels?
   a. It decreases plasma potassium levels
   b. It has no effect on plasma potassium levels
   c. It increases plasma potassium levels
   d. It normalizes plasma potassium levels
88. What is the effect of excess aldosterone secretion on plasma potassium levels?
   a. It increases plasma potassium levels
   b. It decreases plasma potassium levels
   c. It has no effect on plasma potassium levels
   d. It normalizes plasma potassium levels
89. What percentage of the filtered potassium load reaches the distal nephron and collecting ducts?
   a. Approximately 10%
   b. Approximately 25%
   c. Approximately 50%
   d. Approximately 90%
90. Which body fluid compartment contains about 90% of total body potassium?
   a. Extracellular fluid
   b. Plasma
   c. Interstitial fluid
   d. Intracellular fluid

91. Which hormone is most directly involved in regulating plasma potassium concentration ([K+])?

a. Insulin b. Aldosterone

c. Cortisol d. Atrial natriuretic peptide

92. What effect does Addison's disease have on plasma potassium levels?

a. Decreases plasma potassium levels

b. No effect on plasma potassium levels

c. Increases plasma potassium levels

d. Normalizes plasma potassium levels

93. What impact does excess aldosterone secretion have on plasma potassium levels?

a. Increases plasma potassium levels

b. Decreases plasma potassium levels

c. No effect on plasma potassium levels

d. Normalizes plasma potassium levels

94. Approximately what percentage of the filtered potassium load reaches the distal nephron and collecting ducts?

a. 10% b. 25%

c. 50% d. 90%

95. Which body fluid compartment contains about 90% of the total body potassium?

a. Extracellular fluid b. Plasma

c. Interstitial fluid d. Intracellular fluid

96. What is the Intracellular Fluid (ICF) volume in a calf that weighs 50 kg, given that TBW is 580 ml/kg body weight and ECF is 210 ml/kg body weight?

a. 370 ml/kg body weight b. 150 ml/kg body weight

c. 580 ml/kg body weight d. 210 ml/kg body weight

97. If the Extracellular Fluid (ECF) is 210 ml/kg body weight and the Plasma Volume (PV) is 60 ml/kg body weight, what is the Interstitial Fluid (ISF) volume?

a. 150 ml/kg body weight b. 250 ml/kg body weight

c. 120 ml/kg body weight d. 180 ml/kg body weight

98. What percentage of body weight is represented by Total Body Water (TBW) if it is measured as 580 ml/kg body weight in a calf?

a. 58% b. 21%

c. 100% d. 30%

99. If the Packed Cell Volume (PCV) is 40 percent, what is the Blood Volume (BV) in a calf with a body weight of 50 kg, calculated from PV = 60 ml/kg body weight?

a. 100 ml/kg body weight b. 30 ml/kg body weight

c. 120 ml/kg body weight d. 10% of body weight

100. Which method is used to measure Plasma Volume (PV)?

a. Tritium oxide b. Sodium thiosulfate

c. T-1824 d. Potassium

101. What is the main site of erythropoietin (EPO) production in adult mammals?
   a. Liver
   b. Spleen
   c. Bone marrow
   d. Kidney
102. How does excitement affect Packed Cell Volume (PCV) in dogs?
   a. It decreases PCV due to dehydration
   b. It has no effect on PCV
   c. It increases PCV due to splenic contraction releasing stored red blood cells
   d. It decreases PCV due to the release of epinephrine
103. Which of the following is true regarding hemoglobin synthesis?
   a. It is confined only to the rubriblast
   b. It can continue in reticulocytes containing RNA and a portion of the nucleus
   c. It stops as soon as the erythrocyte enters circulation
   d. It occurs only in mature erythrocytes1529.
104. Why is carbon monoxide detrimental to oxygen transport by hemoglobin?
   a. It oxidizes iron in hemoglobin, forming methemoglobin
   b. It binds to myoglobin, preventing oxygen from binding
   c. It binds to hemoglobin with a higher affinity than oxygen, preventing oxygen transport
   d. It reduces the hemoglobin synthesis rate
105. What is the main physiological difference between fetal and adult hemoglobin?
   a. Fetal hemoglobin has a lower affinity for oxygen
   b. Fetal hemoglobin has a higher affinity for oxygen
   c. Fetal hemoglobin lacks heme groups
   d. Fetal hemoglobin is identical to adult hemoglobin
106. What is the primary reason fetal hemoglobin has a higher oxygen affinity than adult hemoglobin in most mammals?
   a. Fetal hemoglobin has a different heme structure than adult hemoglobin.
   b. Fetal hemoglobin has structurally distinct globin chains that increase oxygen affinity.
   c. Fetal red blood cells have lower concentrations of 2,3-bisphosphoglycerate (BPG) than adult red blood cells.
   d. Fetal hemoglobin binds more tightly to BPG, increasing its oxygen affinity.
107. Which of the following animals does NOT have structurally distinct fetal hemoglobins but still maintains higher oxygen affinity in fetal blood?
   a. Ruminants
   b. Dogs
   c. Cats
   d. Horses

108. According to the oxygen-hemoglobin dissociation curve, what does the steeper curve of fetal hemoglobin indicate?
   a. Fetal hemoglobin releases less oxygen to tissues for each increment of oxygen tension decrease.
   b. Fetal hemoglobin releases more oxygen to tissues for each increment of oxygen tension decrease.
   c. Fetal hemoglobin has the same oxygen release rate as adult hemoglobin.
   d. Fetal hemoglobin has a lower oxygen affinity than adult hemoglobin.
109. What is the primary factor that allows oxygen to be transferred from maternal to fetal blood across the placenta?
   a. Active transport
   b. Higher oxygen affinity of maternal hemoglobin
   c. Diffusion based on the oxygen tension gradient
   d. Lower oxygen concentration in maternal blood
110. What happens to fetal hemoglobin levels in calves after birth?
   a. Fetal hemoglobin levels remain constant throughout life.
   b. Fetal hemoglobin is gradually replaced by adult hemoglobin within 2 to 3 months
   c. Fetal hemoglobin is immediately replaced by adult hemoglobin at birth.
   d. Fetal hemoglobin levels decrease but never completely disappear.
111. What is the average life span of erythrocytes in chickens?
   a. 10 to 20 days b. 20 to 30 days
   c. 30 to 40 days d. 40 to 50 days
112. In iron-deficiency anemia, what stage of erythrocyte development is arrested?
   a. Reticulocyte stage b. Rubricyte stage
   c. Proerythroblast stage d. Erythroblast stage
113. What is the primary site of erythrocyte destruction in humans?
   a. Liver b. Spleen
   c. Bone marrow d. Lymph nodes
114. What pigment is heme initially converted into during hemoglobin degradation?
   a. Bilirubin b. Stercobilin
   c. Biliverdin d. Urobilinogen
115. Which condition might result in a yellow color in tissues, known as jaundice?
   a. High levels of urobilinogen in the urine
   b. Complete bile duct blockage
   c. Decreased hemolysis of erythrocytes
   d. Excessive iron storage in MPS cells

116. Which of the following factors can increase hemoglobin concentration in an animal?
   a. Increased dietary iron intake
   b. Excitement due to the release of catecholamines
   c. Decreased partial pressure of oxygen (Po2) in the blood
   d. All of the above
117. What is the normal range for plasma iron concentration in most animals?
   a. 40 to 50 µg/dl b. 100 to 300 µg/dl
   c. 200 to 400 µg/dl d. 50 to 150 µg/dl
118. What is the primary function of myoglobin in muscle tissue?
   a. To carry carbon dioxide from muscles to the lungs
   b. To store oxygen within the muscle fibers for use during contractions
   c. To transport oxygen from the lungs to the muscles
   d. To regulate the production of red blood cells
119. Why is carbon monoxide (CO) particularly dangerous when inhaled?
   a. CO increases the oxygen affinity of hemoglobin, making it harder to release oxygen to tissues.
   b. CO binds to hemoglobin with an affinity more than 200 times greater than oxygen, preventing oxygen transport.
   c. CO causes the oxidation of hemoglobin to methemoglobin, which cannot carry oxygen.
   d. CO causes the immediate destruction of hemoglobin molecules.
120. What distinguishes methemoglobin from oxyhemoglobin?
   a. Methemoglobin contains ferric iron (Fe^{3+}), while oxyhemoglobin contains ferrous iron (Fe^{2+}).
   b. Methemoglobin binds oxygen more tightly than oxyhemoglobin.
   c. Methemoglobin is the oxygenated form of hemoglobin, while oxyhemoglobin is the deoxygenated form.
   d. Methemoglobin has a higher oxygen affinity than oxyhemoglobin.
121. What happens to hemoglobin derived from intravascular hemolysis when it binds with haptoglobin?
   a. It is filtered through the kidney glomeruli
   b. It enters MPS cells and is degraded as in extravascular hemolysis
   c. It causes hemoglobinuria immediately
   d. It is directly excreted in the urine
122. Which of the following is required for the synthesis of DNA in erythrocytes?
   a. Vitamin C and iron
   b. Pyridoxine and riboflavin
   c. Vitamin B (cyanocobalamin) and folic acid
   d. Copper and cobalt

123. What is the condition called when free hemoglobin is filtered at the glomeruli and appears in urine?

a. Hemoglobinemia b. Hemoglobinuria

c. Anemia d. Hemochromatosis

124. Which mineral is essential for the synthesis of hemoglobin and is stored in the protein-bound form in its ferric oxidation state?

a. Copper b. Iron

c. Cobalt d. Zinc

125. What is the primary site of erythropoietin (EPO) production in adult mammals?

a. Liver b. Spleen

c. Bone marrow d. Kidney

126. Erythrocytes in circulating blood of mammals are

a. Non nucleated and non motile b. Non nucleated and motile

c. Nucleated and non motile d. Nucleated and motile

127. Enzyme which catalyses reversible reaction of carbon dioxide and bicarbonate ions

a. Oxidase b. Carbonic anhydrase

c. Transferase d. None

128. RBCs of cold blooded animals are

a. Circular without nuclei b. Elliptical without nuclei

c. Circular with nuclei d. Elliptical with nuclei

129. In early fatal development nucleated RBCs are produced in

a. Bone marrow b. Spleen

d. Yolk sac d. Liver

130. _______ an erythrocyte precursor proliferate from the erythrocytic unipotent CFU

a. Rubriblasts b. Rubricytes

c. Prorubriblast d. Prorubricytes

131. True sentence about RBCs is

a. Younger the cell, Larger it is and larger the nucleus

b. Younger the cell, larger it is and smaller the nucleus

c. Younger the cell smaller it is and larger the nucleus

d. Younger the cell, smaller it is and smaller the nucleus

132. Time taken for rubriblasts to develop into an erythrocyte

a. 1-2 days b. 4-5 days

c. 4-5 weeks d. 10 days

133. Average life span of RBCs of dog

a. 190 days b. 20 days

c. 118 days d. 78 days

134. Erythropoietin, a hormone that regulates red blood cell production, is primarily produced by which organ?

a. Heart b. Lungs

c. Kidneys d. Liver

135. Mode of destruction of RBCs by phagocytosis by MPS cells

a. Extravascular hemolysis b. Intravascular hemolysis

c. Intervascular hemolysis d. Intravenous hemolysis

136. Fate of heme after hemolysis

a Bilirubin (yellow) à biliverdin (green)

b Biliverdin (green) à bilirubin (yellow)

c Bilirubin (green) à biliverdin (yellow)

d Biliverdin (yellow) à bilirubin (green)

137. Free bilirubin, which is water insoluble will bind to ________ after released into plasma

a. Globulin b. Platelet

c. Heme d. Albumin

138. In liver, insoluble bilirubin is made soluble by conjugation with

a. Glycogen b. Glucoronic acid

c. Amino acid d. Uremic acid

139. Precursor for thrombocytes

a. Lymphoblasts b. Myeloblasts

c. Megakaryoblasts d. Monoblasts

140. Precursor for granulocytes

a. Lymphoblasts b. Myeloblasts

c. Megakaryoblasts d. Monoblasts

141. Cytoplasm of rubriblasts contains ________

a. DNA b. RNA

c. Both d. None

142. Normally calculated erythrocyte indices are

a. MCV b. MCH

c. MCHC d. All of the above

143. Iron deficiency in all mammals characterised by

a. Macrochromic Anemia b. Microchromic Anemia

c. Microcytic Anemia d. Macrocytic Anemia

144. Average cell size in cubic micrometre can be provided by

a. MCV b. MCH

c. MCHC d. MCVH

145. Pernicious Anemia is characterized by

a. Macrochromic Anemia b. Microchromic Anemia

c. Microcytic Anemia d. Macrocytic Anemia

146. Factors which affect number of RBCs
   a. Age b. Sex
   c. Pregnancy d. All of the above
147. Unit of MCV
   a. Picogram b. g/dl
   c. femtoliter d. Micrometre
148. Unit of MCH
   a. g/dl b. Picogram
   c. Femtoliter d. Micrometre
149. Unit of MCHC
   a. Picogram b. g/dl
   c. femtoliter d. Micrometre
150. Which is not the developmental stage of erythrocyte
   a. Rubriblasts b. Rubricytes
   c. Prorubricytes d. Prorubriblasts
151. How methemoglobin is formed?
   a. Oxidation of ferric to ferrous state
   b. Oxidation of ferrous to ferric state
   c. Reduction of ferric to ferrous state
   d. Reduction of ferrous to ferric state
152. True oxide of haemoglobin______________
   a. Myoglobin b. Corboxyhaemoglobin
   c. Oxyhaemoglobin d. Methemoglobin
153. The color of methemoglobin___________
   a. Bright red b. Chocolate brown
   c. Bluish red d. Chocolate black
154. Nitrate poisoning in ruminants cause_______formation.
   a. Oxyhemoglobin b. Methemoglobin
   c. Myoglobin d. Corboxyhemoglobin
155. What is the antidote for nitrate poisoning?
   a. Methylene blue b. Charcoal
   c. Carbogen d. Methyl red
156. Leukocytes carry their functions predominantly in the_______
   a. Blood b. Serum
   c. Tissue d. Plasma
157. The approximate ratio of RBC:WBC in the blood stream in different animals given below, select the incorrect one:
   a. Sheep-1000:1 b. Dog-100:1
   c. Swine-400:1 d. Cattle-800:1

158. In which condition leukocytosis is seen?
  a. Viral disease b. Fungal disease
  c. Bacterial disease d. Neoplasms
159. In which condition increases the number of lymphocytes?
  a. Viral disease b. Fungal disease
  c. Neoplasms d. Bacterial disease
160. Leukopenia seen in ____________
  a. Viral disease b. Bacterial disease
  c. Fungal disease d. Neoplasms
161. During excitement, the total WBC in the circulation is increased due to:
  a. Norepineprine b. Epineprine
  c. Exercise d. Both b & c
162. Agranulocytes are___________
  a. Lymphocytes b. Neutrophils
  c. Monocytes d. Both a & c
163. Most abundant granulocytes are______
  a. Basophils b. Neutrophils
  c. Eosiniphils d. Lymphocytes
164. Choose the false sentence among the following:
  a. 3-5 segmented nucleus present in neutrophils
  b. Neutophil have ameboid activity & phagocytocize to defend the body against the foreign particles
  c. Neutrophil have azurophilic granules and acidophilic granules
  d. Azurophilic granules contain lysosomes
165. Heterophil seen in________
  a. Camel b. Horse
  c. Poultry d. dog
166. Cytoplasmic granules of eosinophil stained with _______dye.
  a. Basic dye b. Acid dye
  c. Neutral dye d. None of the above
167. Eosinophilia due to:
  a. Allergic condition b. Anaphylactic condition
  c. Parasitisim d. All of the above
168. The hormones that are responsible eosinophenia________
  a. ACTH b. Epinephrine
  c. GnRH d. Both a & b
169. Basophils and Mast cells have receptors for:
  a. IgE b. IgG
  c. IgA d. IgD

170. Lymphocytes are produced by:
   a. Peyer's patches
   b. Spleen
   c. Tonsils
   d. Both a,b,c

171. Choose the correct sentence among the following:
   a. T-lymphocytes :Cell-Mediated immunity
   b. T-lymphocytes:Produce antibodies
   c. B-lymphocytes:Humoral immunity
   d. Both a & c

172. Choose the false sentence among the following :
   a. Cytotoxic T cells-Attacks cells of transplanted organs
   b. Helper T cells-Involved in recognition of Ag & stimulate B cells to produce Antibodies
   c. Suppressor T cells-Suppress both humoral and cell mediated immunity
   d. Memory T cells -Short lived and allow to T & B cells responds to Ag

173. Which type of T-cells called killer cells?
   a Cytotoxic T cell
   b. Suppressor T cell
   c. Memory T cell
   d. Helper T cell

174. At what % B-lymphocytes present in blood stream?
   a. 25%
   b. 15%
   c. 5%
   d. 35%

175. At what % T -lymphocytes present in blood?
   a. 85%
   b. 75%
   c. 55%
   d. 65%

176. Monocyte cell become after leaving blood circulation -------
   a. Dendrtic cell
   b. Macrophage
   c. Neutrophil cell
   d. Lymphocyte

177. % of neutrophils in traumatic reticulitis in cow
   a. 70%
   b. 80%
   c. 90%
   d. 20%

178. Increase in number of immature neutrophils in blood circulation leads to
   a. Shift to right
   b. Shift to left
   c. Shift to left and then right
   d. None

179. Increase in number of immature neutrophils during
   a. Viral infection
   b. Fungal infection
   c. Bacterial infection
   d. Parasitic imfection

180. Nucleated platelet seen in
   a. Pig
   b. Sheep
   c. Goat
   d. Chicken

181. Normal platelet count in domestic mammal
   a. 450000 – 150000 / µl b. 45000 – 15000 / µl
   c. 15000 – 40000 /µl d. 300000- 150000/µl
182. Half life of platelet
   a. 3-5 day b. 2-3 day
   c. 1-2 day d. 5-7 day
183. Largest lymphoid organ in animal body
   a. Spleen b. Liver
   c. Thymus d. Kidney
184. Blood reservoir organ in bird
   a. Spleen b. Liver
   c. Thymus d. Lung
185. Specific gravity of Blood of cattle
   a. 1.036-1.061 b. 1.041-1.061
   c. 1.046-1.061 d. 1.052-1.055
186. Roulex formation seen in
   a. Cattle b. Sheep
   c. Horse d. Goat
187. Following which is not anticoagulant
   a. Heparin b. EDTA
   c. NaF d. NaCl
188. Sludged Blood means
   a. Increase blood circulation b. Complete stasis of blood
   c. Incomplete stasis of blood d. Blood Coagulation
189. ESR value in Dog
   a. 1-5mm in 30 min b. 1-4mm in 15 sec
   c. 6-7mm in 30 min d. 6-7mm in 15 sec
190. Immunoglobulin present in colostrum
   a. IgE b. IgA
   c. IgD d. IgM
191. Blood glucose level in cattle
   a. 40-80 mg/dl b. 30-50 mg/dl
   c. 40-60 mg/dl d. 40-50 mg /dl
192. Blood Ca measured in
   a. µg/L b. mg/dl
   c. mEq/L d. g/L
193. Following which is not plasma protein
   a. Albumin b. Globulin
   c. Fibrinogen d. Plasminogen

194. Most abundant immunoglobulin in animal
   a. IgG b. IgA
   c. IgM d. IgD
195. Immunoglobulin produced during allergic condition
   a. IgG b. IgA
   c. IgE d. IgM
196. Normal range in albumin level in dog
   a. 3.4 -4.4 g/dl b. 3-5 g/dl
   c. 3.5-4.5g/dl d. 2.3-5.5g/dl
197. Normal level of serum Ca in laying hen
   a. 7.5-8.5mEq/L b. 8.5-19.5mEq/L
   c. 4.5-6mEq/L d. 3-5mEq/L
198. First antibody produced by the activated B cell is
   a. IgE b. IgM
   c. IgD d. IgG
199. Interferon having
   a. Antibacterial activity b. Antifungal activity
   c. Antiparasitic activity d. Antiviral activity
200. Secretory immunoglobulin is
   a. IgA b. IgD
   c. IgM d. IgE
201. What is the total WBC count in week 1st for "Elsie"?
   a. 8000/microliter b. 8000/milliliter
   c. 8000/ liter d. 800/ liter
202. The term reaction of blood usually refers to________ in the intact animal.
   a. pH of blood b. Buffer of blood
   c. Gases of blood d. None
203. The balance of all cations against anions is reflected in the _________.
   a. [OH] ion concentration b. [H] ion concentration
   c. CO gas concentration d. Both A & B
204. The negative logarithmic of [H] ion concentration is _______.
   a. pH b. Kw
   c. [H] ion concentration d. None
205. The pH of blood fluctuates only within ________ limits.
   a. Constant b. Broad
   c. Narrow d. None
206. Arterial blood is slightly ______ alkaline than the venous blood.
   a. More b. Less
   c. Remains constant d. Both a & c

207. Plasma is _____ alkaline than the corpuscles.
 a. More b. Less
 c. Remains constant d. None

208. What is the limit of the pH of blood compatible with life.
 a. 7.0 and 7.8 b. 6.5 and 7.0
 c. 8.0 and 7.0 d. 7.8 and 6.8

209. Which is the volume that use for interpretation and understanding PCV, Hemoglobin, RBC, WBC etc.
 a. Water b. Plasma
 c. Serum d. Blood

210. An increase in blood volume is termed as _______.
 a. Hypertonic b. Hypervolemia
 c. Hypertension d. Hyperthermia

211. An decrease in blood volume is termed as ________.
 a. Hypotonic b. Hypotension
 c. Hypovolemia d. Hypothermia

212. ______& _______ mechanism retain a large amount of blood in the vessels.
 a. Clotting & vasoconstriction b. Buffer & vasoconstriction
 c. Vasodilation and clotting d. Both a & b

213. In analytical work , the term accuracy refers to_________.
 a. Tightness of actual value b. Closeness to actual value
 c. Farness to actual value d. None

214. In analytical work,the term precision concerns _____.
 a. Repeatability of value b. Closeness to value
 c. Both a & b d. None

215. Methods based on ______ procedure have greater accuracy and precision
 a. Dilution b. Concentration
 c. Wet mount d. None

216. What are the numerous methods of estimating blood volume in the living animals.
 a. Evans blue dye b. Radioactive Iodine
 c. Thallium d. Both a & b

217. ______ method require less blood and is used most frequently for coagulation of blood.
 a. Lee method b. White method
 c. Capillary tube method d. Both a & b

218. Normal coagulation time of most animals between ___& ____ in capillary tube method.
 a. 1 & 5 minutes b. 10 & 20 minutes
 c. 6 & 10 minutes d. None

219. A larger quantity of blood is used in _____&_____ method of coagulation.
   a. Lee method
   b. White method
   c. Capillary tube method
   d. Both a & b
220. What is the coagulation time in Lee and white method of blood coagulation.
   a. 2-5 minutes
   b. 5- 10 minutes
   c. 5- 8 minutes
   d. 10 – 15 minutes
221. Plasma albumin, fibrinogen , some of the globulin and prothrombin are formed in_______.
   a. Kidney
   b. Liver
   c. Bone marrow
   d. Thymus
222. The balance of globulins including gamma globulins are formed in ____&_____ tissue.
   a. Liver and kidney
   b. Lymph nodes and mucosal tissue
   c. Bone marrow and liver
   d. None
223. Which one of the following most closely approximate the number of erythrocytes in domestic animals.
   a. 7000000/microliter
   b. 7000000/ milliliter
   c. 7000/liter
   d. None
224. The % of total body water is similarly _______ as the body fat increases.
   a. Increase
   b. Decrease
   c. Remains constant
   d. None
225. Erythropoiesis associated with iron deficiency results in_______.
   a. Microcytic, hypochromic, anemia
   b. Microcytic, hyperchromic, anemia
   c. Both a and b
   d. None

Answer Key

1	d	2	b	3	a	4	b	5	a	6	a	7	c
8	a	9	c	10	b	11	d	12	c	13	a	14	a
15	b	16	a	17	c	18	c	19	c	20	c	21	a
22	b	23	a	24	a	25	a	26	a	27	c	28	a
29	c	30	c	31	c	32	d	33	c	34	a	35	a
36	b	37	d	38	c	39	d	40	a	41	b	42	b
43	c	44	b	45	b	46	a	47	b	48	a	49	c
50	c	51	c	52	a	53	b	54	b	55	a	56	a
57	b	58	c	59	a	60	a	61	a	62	b	63	c
64	b	65	a	66	b	67	c	68	a	69	a	70	c
71	b	72	b	73	b	74	a	75	c	76	a	77	c
78	c	79	c	80	a	81	c	82	d	83	a	84	b
85	d	86	b	87	c	88	b	89	a	90	d	91	b
92	c	93	b	94	a	95	d	96	a	97	a	98	a
99	a	100	c	101	d	102	c	103	b	104	c	105	b
106	c	107	b	108	b	109	c	110	b	111	b	112	b
113	b	114	c	115	b	116	b	117	b	118	b	119	b
120	a	121	b	122	c	123	b	124	b	125	d	126	a
127	b	128	d	129	c	130	a	131	a	132	b	133	c
134	c	135	a	136	b	137	d	138	b	139	c	140	b
141	b	142	d	143	c	144	a	145	d	146	d	147	c
148	b	149	b	150	d	151	b	152	d	153	b	154	b
155	a	156	c	157	b	158	c	159	c	160	a	161	d
162	d	163	b	164	c	165	c	166	b	167	d	168	d
169	a	170	d	171	d	172	d	173	a	174	b	175	a
176	b	177	a	178	b	179	c	180	d	181	a	182	b
183	a	184	a	185	c	186	c	187	d	188	b	189	a
190	b	191	a	192	c	193	d	194	a	195	c	196	a
197	b	198	b	199	d	200	a	201	a	202	a	203	b
204	a	205	c	206	a	207	a	208	a	209	d	210	b
211	c	212	a	213	b	214	a	215	a	216	d	217	c
218	a	219	d	220	a	221	b	222	b	223	a	224	b
225	a												

17

Biochemistry of Tissues

Sasmita Barik[1] and Shiv Kumar Yadav[2]*

[1]Department of Veterinary Physiology and Biochemistry, College of Veterinary Sciences and Animal Husbandry, Guru Angad Dev Veterinary and Animal Scienes Univeristy, Ludhiana, Punjab

[2]KVK, Shahjahanpur, Uttar Pradesh

Introduction

Human and animal body comprises of various tissues that are the functional unit of organ functioning and coordination. The tissues are further consisting of well differentiated cells that makes the tissue to behave in a special way for a particular purpose. The animal tissues are divided into epithelial, connective, muscular and nervous tissues. Epithelial tissues form the protective covering and inner lining of the body and organs. Connective tissues develop from the mesodermal cells of the embryo. they support and bind other tissues in the body. The muscular tissue develops from the mesoderm of the embryo and meant for movement and locomotion. Nervous tissue makes up the peripheral and the central nervous system and is responsible for initiation and transmission the nerve impulse. The tissues are biochemically composed of water, lipid, protein, ash, and carbohydrate along with other mineral and vitamins that are needed for its basic functioning. The extracellular matrix (ECM) forms a major component of connective tissue that forms layer and surrounds the cells or tissues meant for protection, signalling and communication. The protein component of ECM basically includes collagen, elastin, keratins, fibrillin, fibronectin, laminin and proteoglycans. Collagen is the major protein component of connective tissue that provides tensile strength, shape and fixes the organ in its position. Collagen is not homogenous rather consists of around 19 different types of proteins. There are around 30 variants of protein found in collagen. collagens type I and type II are respectively found in skin and bone. Collagen is triple helical polymer of highly elongated fibrils consisting of around 1000 amino acids majority of which consists of glycine along with proline and hydroxyproline. The forces like hydrogen bonds, covalent bonds, electrostatic, hydrophobic, and van der Waals are responsible for stabilizing the structure of collagen. Crosslinking of lysine and hydroxylysine provides the required strength to the collagen for maintenance of shape structure and function of connective tissue. The protein collagen is synthesized as primitive form as prepro- collagen in ribosome in cytosol and then transported to Er for post translational modifications like hydroxylation, glycosylation and sulfation to form procollagen and then to functional collagen. Abnormal synthesis and modification of collagen associated with aging, neuronal degeneration and other genetic clinical conditions like Ehlers-Danlos syndrome, Alport syndrome, Osteogenesis imperfecta, Epidermolysis bullosa, Scurvy, lathyrism etc.

Elastin is the second major protein found in connective tissue that maintains the extensibility and elasticity of tissues and organs (liver, kidney, lungs, blood vessels, heart etc.) and is responsible for unstoppable action. Elastin in ribosome is synthesized as pre-elastin and hydroxy proline was added during posttranslational modification. However, Elastin differs from collage in absence of hydroxylysine, no triple helix and no repeat sequence of Gly-X-Y. Defective synthesis of elastin due to mutation is associated with Williams syndrome.

Fibrillin, fibronectin and laminin are the three other proteins found in connective tissue that are responsible for maintaining shape, strength and functioning of organs. Genetic mutation and defective synthesis in fibrillin are responsible for Marfan syndrome associated with hyperextensibility of joints and skeletal system. Fibronectin in connective tissue is responsible for interaction of cells with extra cellular matrix and the deficiency of which results in tumour development as the cells lose adhesion properties causing metastasis. Laminin has specific role in nerve growth and regeneration deficiency of which is often associated with Alzheimer's disease. Keratin is another structural protein associated with hair, nail, horn and exoskeleton of insects, crustaceans and other sea animals. Like collagen it contains three polypeptide chains in alpha-helical structure which are bonded by disulphide bonds that provides the tensile strength.

Contractile proteins are present in muscles in organs like heart, lungs, skeleton etc which are responsible for continuous function. The basic unit of muscle is fibre which is elongated, multinucleated and surrounded by a membrane known as sarcolemma. The cytoplasm of fibre is known as sarcoplasm that carries the myofibrils embedded in it which are the basic functional unit of muscle contraction. The myofibrils are formed of alternate A and I band depending upon their protein content. A band refers to anisotropic band which is dark because of thick filaments. Whereas I band is isotropic band and is light because of thin filaments. The central region of thick and thin filament is H and Z line respectively. Whereas the unit between two Z lines is referred as sarcomere. The ultimate functioning of the muscle fibre depends on sliding of thick and thin filaments along each other for which ATP is needed as source of energy. The ATP along with other metabolic intermediates are present in sarcoplasm for immediate supply. Biochemically the thick filament consists the protein myosin in A band. Similarly, the thin filaments contain three kinds of protein namely actin, tropomyosin and troponin in it. The process of muscle contraction includes sliding of myosin over actin filaments. Out of different types of myosin proteins myosin II is the prime one to be present in muscle that is responsible for contraction. It is a hexamer of six polypeptide chains with one pair of heavy chains, and two pairs of light chains. Light chains form the helical part to coil around each other whereas the heavy chain forms the globular head part of myosin that reacts with actin during muscle contraction. Twi forms of actin present in thin filament known as G and F. F actin generally reacts with myosin during muscle contraction. Other two proteins namely tropomyosin and troponin serve as crosslinking agents.

Tropomyosin is a dipeptide attached to F actin whereas, troponin is a tripeptide in T, I and C form. T form binds tropomyosin, I form inhibit F-actin myosin interaction and C form is the calcium binding polypeptide. Apart from these proteins namely titin, nebulin, dystrophin, calcineurin and desmin are also reported to be present in muscle. For muscle contraction continuous supply of energy is needed in the form of ATP that is generated in sarcoplasm in the process of glycolysis, TCA cycle and oxidative phosphorylation. Creatine phosphate is a storage form of energy in muscle. In heavy exercise when all the

ATP exhausted, anaerobic glycolysis occurs alongwith creatine phosphate is used as instant source of energy.

1. Tissues are composed of
   a. Lipid b. Protein
   c. Carbohydrate d. All of the above
2. The major component of tissue is
   a. Lipid b. Protein
   c. Carbohydrate d. Water
3. Types of tissue present in human body
   a. Epithelial b. Connective
   c. Nervous d. All of the above
4. Which of the following tissue provides strength to organ
   a. Epithelial b. Connective
   c. Nervous d. All of the above
5. The major protein in connective tissue is
   a. Collagen b. Elastin
   c. Troponin d. Neuramin
6. The major protein in muscular tissue is
   a. Collagen b. Elastin
   c. Troponin d. Neuramin
7. The major protein in nervous tissue is
   a. Collagen b. Elastin
   c. Troponin d. Neuramin
8. Which of the following tissue is responsible transmission of impulse
   a. Epithelial b. Connective
   c. Nervous d. All of the above
9. Which kind of protein is collagen?
   a. Homogenous b. Heterogenous
   c. Both d. None
10. The level of organisation in collagen protein is
    a. Primary b. Secondary
    c. Tertiary d. Quaternary
11. The function of collagen is
    a. Cell Proliferation b. Cell Differentiationt
    c. Cell Migration d. All of the above
12. The type of collagen found in skin collagens type I and type II
    a. Type I b. Type L1
    c. Both d. None

13. The type of collagen found in skin collagens type I and type ll
    a. Type I   b. Type Ll
    c. Both   d. None
14. The structure of collagen is
    a. Double helical   b. Triple Helical
    c. Both   d. None
15. Collagen protein is rich in which type of aminoacids
    a. Glycine   b. Alanine
    c. Serine   d. Threonine
16. The average length of collagen molecule in tissues is
    a. 100 nm   b. 200 nm
    c. 300 nm   d. 400 nm
17. The average diameter of collagen molecule in tissues is
    a. 0.4 nm   b. 1.4 nm
    c. 2.4 nm   d. 3.4 nm
18. The repetitive amino acid sequence of collagen is
    a. GIy-X-Y   b. AlA-X-Y
    c. Ser-X-Y   d. None
19. Which of the following protein is glycine rich?
    a. Collagen   b. Elastin
    c. Keratin   d. Fibrillin
20. The triple helical structure of collagen is stabilized by which type of forces.
    a. Covalent   b. Electrostatic
    c. Hydrophobic   d. All of the above
21. Collagen synthesis occurs in which type of cells
    a. Fibroblasts   b. Chondroblasts
    c. Odontoblasts   d. All of the above
22. Collagen is rich in which amino acids
    a. Valine   b. Lysine
    c. Hydroxylysine   d. All of the above
23. Collagen is rich in which amino acids
    a. Pre-collagen   b. Pro-collagen
    c. Prepro-collagen   d. None
24. Collagen protein is synthesized in
    a. Cytosol   b. Nucleus
    c. Ribosomes   d. ER
25. The type of posttranslational modifications occurring in collagen
    a. Hydroxylation   b. Glycosylation
    c. Disulfide formation   d. All of the above

26. Prepro Collagen protein is synthesized in
    a. Cytosol b. Nucleus
    c. Ribosomes d. ER
27. Procollagen protein is synthesized in
    a. Cytosol b. Nucleus
    c. Ribosomes d. ER
28. Which vitamin is needed for formation of collagen?
    a. Vit A b. Vit B
    c. Vit C d. Vit D
29. Why vitamin C is needed in the synthesis of collagen
    a. Hydroxylation of proline b. Hydroxylation of lysine
    c. Both d. None
30. Which of the biochemical reaction occurs in Collagen synthesis?
    a. Sulfation b. Phosphorylation
    c. Hydroxylation d. Reduction
31. Mutation in collagen gene is associated with which genetic condition
    a. Sulfation b. Phosphorylation
    c. Hydroxylation d. Reduction
32. Defect in collagen synthesis is related to which of the following conditions
    a. Lathyrism b. Epidermolysis bullosa
    c. Scurvy d. All of the above
33. Which of the following condition is associated with mutation in collagen?
    a. Ehlers-Danlos syndrome b. Alport syndrome
    c. Osteogenesis imperfecta d. All of the above
34. What are the symptoms of Ehlers-Danlos syndrome
    a. Hyperextensibilityof skin b. Abnormal tissue fragility
    c. Both d. None
35. Collagen is required for which process
    a. Epithelial maintainance b. Membrane integrity
    c. Both d. None
36. Alport syndrome is associated with which system
    a. Renal b. Hepatic
    c. Visual d. Dental
37. Which of the following are the symptoms of Alport syndrome?
    a. Haematuria b. Defective glomeruli.
    c. Both d. None
38. Osteogenesis imperfecta is associated with which of the following
    a. Defective albumin synthesis b. Defective collagen synthesis
    c. Both d. None

39. Which of the following are the symptoms of Osteogenesis imperfecta?
    a. Fragility of Bones
    b. Decreased formation of collagen.
    c. Both
    d. None
40. Epidermolysis bullosa is associated with which of the following
    a. Defective albumin synthesis
    b. Defective collagen synthesis
    c. Both
    d. None
41. Which of the following are the symptoms of Epidermolysis bullosa?
    a. Skin breaks
    b. Blisters formation
    c. Both
    d. None
42. Alport syndrome is associated with which type of collagen
    a. Collagen I
    b. Collagen II
    c. Collagen III
    d. Collagen IV
43. Epidermolysis bullosa is associated with which type of collagen
    a. Collagen IV
    b. Collagen V
    c. Collagen VI
    d. Collagen VII
44. Scurvy is basically associated with
    a. Deficiency of vit C
    b. Defective collagen
    c. Both
    d. None
45. Scurvy is characterized by
    a. Bleeding of gums
    b. Poor wound healing
    c. Subcutaneous hemorrhages
    d. All
46. The toxic compound found in keshari dal is
    a. p-oxalyl amino alanine
    b. p-oxalyl amino valine
    c. p-oxalyl amino leucine
    d. None
47. Lathyrism is associated with which food
    a. Carb
    b. Legume
    c. Cereal
    d. none
48. Defective cross-linking of lysine in collegen is due to
    a. Inhibition of lysyl oxidase
    b. Activation of lysyl oxidase
    c. Regulation of lysyl oxidase
    d. None
49. Lathyrism is characterised by
    a. Bone Deformities
    b. Defective Membrane
    c. Both
    d. None
50. Which of the following is found in kesari dal?
    a. BOAA
    b. COAA
    c. DOAA
    d. AOAA
51. Deformity in collagen in lathyrism is due to
    a. Defective cross-linking of lysine
    b. Inhibition of enzyme lysyl oxidase
    c. Both
    d. None

52. Enzyme lysyl oxidase is associated with
    a. Collagen synthesis
    b. Elastin synthesis'
    c. Keratin synthesis
    d. All of the above
53. Protein responsible for elasticity of tissues and organs
    a. Collagen
    b. Elastin
    c. Keratin
    d. All of the above
54. Elastin is synthesized as_________in ribosomes
    a. Pre-elastin
    b. Pro-elastin
    c. Prepro-elastin
    d. None
55. Which aminoacid derivative is required for elastin synthesis
    a. Hydroxylysine
    b. Hydroxyproline
    c. Both
    d. None
56. Which aminoacid derivative is required for collagen synthesis
    a. Hydroxylysine
    b. Hydroxyproline
    c. Both
    d. None
57. Hydroxylysine is found in which protein
    a. Collagen
    b. Elastin
    c. Both
    d. None
58. Hydroxyproline is found in which protein
    a. Collagen
    b. Elastin
    c. Both
    d. None
59. Triple helix is found in which protein
    a. Collagen
    b. Elastin
    c. Both
    d. None
60. Repeat sequence of Gly-X-Y is found in which protein
    a. Collagen
    b. Elastin
    c. Both
    d. None
61. Collagen contains which of the following
    a. Triple helix
    b. Repeat sequence of Gly-X-Y
    c. Both
    d. None
62. Elastin contains which of the following
    a. Triple helix
    b. Repeat sequence of Gly-X-Y
    c. Both
    d. None
63. Elastin differs from collage in which of the following
    a. Absence of Hydroxylysine
    b. Absence of Triple Helix
    c. Absence of Repeat Sequence of Gly-X-Y
    d. All of the above

64. Elastin contains which of the following
    a. Double helix
    b. Triple helix
    c. Quadruple helix
    d. None
65. Defective synthesis of elastin is associated with
    a. Williams syndrome
    b. Ehlers-Danlos syndrome
    c. Alport syndrome
    d. Osteogenesis imperfecta
66. Williams syndrome is associated with
    a. Defective synthesis of elastin
    b. Defective synthesis of collagen
    c. Both
    d. None
67. Williams syndrome affects which system
    a. Connective tissue
    b. Central nervous system
    c. Both
    d. None
68. Which of the following is observed in pulmonary emphysema?
    a. Defective synthesis of elastin
    b. Defective synthesis of collagen
    c. Both
    d. None
69. Aging of skin is associated with
    a. Defective synthesis of elastin
    b. Defective synthesis of collagen
    c. Both
    d. None
70. Marfan syndrome is associated with defective synthesis of which protein
    a. Fibrillin
    b. Fibronectin
    c. Laminin
    d. All of the above
71. Marfan syndrome associated with which of the following symptoms
    a. Hyperextensibility of Joints
    b. Hyperextensibility of skeletal system
    c. Both
    d. None
72. Defective synthesis of fibrillin is associated with
    a. Williams syndrome
    b. Ehlers-Danlos syndrome
    c. Alport syndrome
    d. Marfan syndrome
73. Biochemically fibronectin is
    a. Protein
    b. Phosphoprotein
    c. Glycoprotein
    d. Sulphoprotein
74. Fibronectin is involved in which of the following action
    a. Cell-cell communication
    b. Cell-cell interaction
    c. Cell- matrix interaction
    d. None
75. Tumor cells are deficient in which of the following connective tissue protein
    a. Fibrillin
    b. Fibronectin
    c. Laminin
    d. All

76. Fibronectin is associated with which of the following action
a. Cell adhesion
b. Cell migration
c. Cell-cell interaction
d. All

77. Fibronectin is observed in which tissues
a. Blood
b. Connective tissue
c. Muscular tissue
d. None

78. Fibronectin is absent in which condition
a. Diabetes
b. Ketosis
c. Tumour
d. None

79. Tumor cells loss which function due to lack of fibronectin
a. Adhesion
b. Proliferation
c. Migration
d. All of the above

80. Tumor cells loss Adhesion function due to lack of which protein
a. Elastin
b. Fibronectin
c. Laminin
d. Collagen

81. Which of the following protein is synthesized during embryogenesis?
a. Elastin
b. Fibronectin
c. Laminin
d. Collagen

82. The protein found in basal lamina of glomerular membrane
a. Elastin
b. Fibronectin
c. Laminin
d. Collagen

83. Defective synthesis of laminin is associated with which condition
a. Tumour
b. Alzheimers desease
c. Both
d. None

84. Triple helical structure is present in which protein
a. Keratin
b. Collegen
c. Both
d. None

85. Triple helix in connective tissue protein is attached by which bonds
a. H bond
b. Covalent bond
c. Sulphide bond
d. Hydride bind

86. Uncoiling of hair is due to ------of sulphuide bond present in keratin
a. Oxidation
b. Reduction
c. Hydroxylation
d. All of the above

87. The main component of exoskeleton of insects is
a. Elastin
b. Fibronectin
c. Laminin
d. Keratin

88. Which protein is majorly found in animal hoof?
a. Elastin
b. Fibronectin
c. Laminin
d. Keratin

89. Which protein is majorly found in human nail?
   a. Elastin b. Fibronectin
   c. Laminin d. Keratin
90. Which protein is majorly found in crustaceans' surface?
   a. Elastin b. Fibronectin
   c. Laminin d. Keratin
91. Hair wauing (curling) through artificial means is possible with suitable alterations in which protein
   a. Elastin b. Fibronectin
   c. Laminin d. Keratin
92. The strength of keratins is directly related to the
   a. Number of disulfide bonds b. Number of cysteines aminoacids
   c. Both d. None
93. The amount of glycine in collagen is
   a. 1/3rd b. 2/3rd
   c. 1/4th d. 3/4th
94. 1/3rd of aminoacids in collagen is
   a. Glycine b. Serine
   c. Cysteine d. Lysine
95. Collagen forms what part of the total body proteins.
   a. $1/3^{rd}$ b. $2/3^{rd}$
   c. $1/4^{th}$ d. $3/4^{th}$
96. The most abundant body protein is
   a. Elastin b. Collagen
   c. Fibronectin d. Laminin
97. Type I mature collagen contains what no of polypeptides
   a. 1 b. 2
   c. 3 d. 4
98. Type I mature collagen present in which form
   a. Double helical b. Triple helical
   c. Both d. None
99. Second most abundant body protein is
   a. Elastin b. Collagen
   c. Fibronectin d. Laminin
100. Triple helical structure is found in which connective tissue protein
   a. Elastin b. Collagen
   c. Both d. None
101. Contractile proteins are present in
   a. Connective tissue b. Blood
   c. Muscle d. Nerves

102. The basic unit of muscle is
    a. Sarcom b. Neoron
    c. Fibre d. Fibril
103. The unit of muscle responsible for contraction is
    a. Sarcomere b. Neuron
    c. Fibre d. Fibril
104. The basic functional unit of muscle contraction is
    a. Sarcoplasm b. Sarcolemma
    c. Sarcomere d. Fibre
105. Energy required for muscle contraction in the form of
    a. GTP b. UTP
    c. ATP d. None
106. Myofibrils consists of which of the following
    a. Dark band b. Light band
    c. Both d. None
107. A band is present in
    a. Connective tissue b. Muscle
    c. Neuron d. All of the above
108. I band if present in
    a. Fibre b. Fibrils
    c. Neuron d. Collagen
109. ATP for muscle contraction is present in
    a. Sarcolemma b. Sarcomere
    c. Sarcoplasm d. Fibre
110. Unit between two Z lines is known as
    a. Fibre b. Fibrils
    c. Sarcolemma d. Sarcomere
111. Myosin is a protein related to
    a. Neurotransmision b. Muscle contraction
    c. Both d. None
112. Thick filament contains which protein
    a. Actin b. Myosin
    c. Troponin d. Tropomyosin
113. Thin filament contains which protein
    a. Actin b. Troponin
    c. Tropomyosin d. All of the above
114. Which of the following protein is absent in thin filament
    a. Actin b. Troponin
    c. Myosin d. Tropomyosin

115. H band in muscle fibre is known as
    a. Dark band
    b. Myosin band
    c. Anisotropic band
    d. All of the above
116. I band in muscle fibre is known as
    a. Light band
    b. Isotropic band
    c. Actin band
    d. All of the above
117. Number of polypeptides present in myosin protein
    a. 3
    b. 4
    c. 5
    d. 6
118. Myosin protein in H band is a
    a. Tetramer
    b. Pentamer
    c. Hexamer
    d. None
119. Which muscular protein has ATPase activity
    a. Myosin
    b. Actin
    c. Troponin
    d. None
120. Which part of myosin has ATPase activity
    a. Head
    b. Tail
    c. Fibre
    d. None
121. Which type of myosin reacts with actin
    a. Heavy
    b. Light
    c. Both
    d. None
122. Muscular dystrophy occurs due a mutation in the gene coding for the protein
    a. Myosin
    b. Actin
    c. Titin
    d. Dystrophin
123. Immediate source of energy for muscle contraction
    a. UTP
    b. GTP
    c. ATP
    d. All of the above
124. Storage form of energy in muscle is
    a. ATP
    b. GTP
    c. Creatine phosphate
    d. None
125. ATP in muscle is generated from which of the following process
    a. Glycolysis
    b. TCA cycle.
    c. Both
    d. None
126. Which of the following is the marker of muscle degeneration
    a. Creatine phosphate
    b. Creatine kinase
    c. Both
    d. None
127. In muscle tearing which enzyme concentratioOn increases in serum
    a. Creatine phosphate
    b. Creatine kinase
    c. Both
    d. None

128. The forms of troponin are
   a. T form b. I form
   c. C form d. All of the above
129. Which form of troponin binds tropomyosin
   a. I form b. T form
   c. C form d. All of the above
130. Which form of troponin is inhibitory in nature
   a. T form b. I form
   c. C form d. All of the above
131. Which forms of troponin is calcium binding in nature
   a. T form b. I form
   c. C form d. All of the above
132. Type I mature collagen present in which form
   a. Double helical b. Triple helical
   c. Both d. None
133. Second most abundant body protein is
   a. Elastin b. Collagen
   c. Fibronectin d. Laminin
134. Triple helical structure is found in which connective tissue protein
   a. Elastin b. Collagen
   c. Both d. None
135. The type of collagen found in skin collagens type I and type II
   a. Type I b. Type II
   c. Both d. None
136. The type of collagen found in skin collagens type I and type II
   a. Type I b. Type II
   c. Both d. None
137. The structure of collagen is
   a. Double helical b. Triple helical
   c. Both d. None
138. Which vitamin is needed for formation of collagen?
   a. Vit A b. Vit B
   c. Vit C d. Vit D
139. Why vitamin C is needed in the synthesis of collagen
   a. Hydroxylation of proline b. Hydroxylation of lysine
   c. Both d. None
140. Which of the biochemical reaction occurs in Collagen synthesis?
   a. Sulfation b. Phosphorylation
   c. Hydroxylation d. Reduction

141. Elastin contains which of the following
    a. Triple helix
    b. Repeat sequence of Gly-X-Y
    c. Both
    d. None
142. Elastin differs from collage in which of the following
    a. Absence of Hydroxylysine
    b. Absence of Triple Helix
    c. Absence of Repeat Sequence Of Gly-X-Y
    d. All of the above
143. Elastin contains which of the following
    a. Double helix
    b. Triple helix
    c. Quadruple helix
    d. None
144. Tumor cells loss Adhesion function due to lack of which protein
    a. Elastin
    b. Fibronectin
    c. Laminin
    d. Collagen
145. Which of the following protein is synthesized during embryogenesis?
    a. Elastin
    b. Fibronectin
    c. Laminin
    d. Collagen
146. The protein found in basal lamina of glomerular membrane
    a. Elastin
    b. Fibronectin
    c. Laminin
    d. Collagen
147. A band is present in
    a. Connective tissue
    b. Muscle
    c. Neuron
    d. All of the above
148. I band if present in
    a. Fibre
    b. Fibrils
    c. Neuron
    d. Collagen
149. ATP for muscle contraction is present in
    a. Sarcolemma
    b. Sarcomere
    c. Sarcoplasm
    d. Fibre
150. Unit between two Z lines is known as
    a. Fibre
    b. Fibrils
    c. Sarcolemma
    d. Sarcomere

Answer Key

1	d	2	d	3	d	4	b	5	a	6	c	7	d
8	c	9	b	10	d	11	d	12	a	13	b	14	b
15	a	16	c	17	b	18	a	19	a	20	d	21	d
22	d	23	c	24	c	25	d	26	c	27	d	28	c
29	c	30	c	31	c	32	d	33	d	34	c	35	c
36	a	37	c	38	b	39	c	40	b	41	c	42	d
43	d	44	c	45	d	46	a	47	b	48	a	49	c
50	a	51	c	52	a	53	b	54	a	55	c	56	c
57	c	58	c	59	a	60	a	61	c	62	d	63	d
64	d	65	a	66	a	67	c	68	a	69	c	70	d
71	c	72	d	73	c	74	c	75	c	76	d	77	b
78	c	79	a	80	b	81	c	82	c	83	c	84	c
85	c	86	b	87	d	88	d	89	d	90	d	91	d
92	c	93	a	94	a	95	a	96	b	97	c	98	b
99	a	100	c	101	c	102	c	103	d	104	c	105	c
106	c	107	b	108	a	109	c	110	d	111	b	112	b
113	d	114	c	115	d	116	d	117	d	118	c	119	a
120	a	121	a	122	d	123	c	124	c	125	c	126	b
127	b	128	d	129	b	130	b	131	c	132	b	133	a
134	c	135	a	136	b	137	b	138	c	139	c	140	c
141	d	142	d	143	d	144	b	145	c	146	c	147	b
148	a	149	c	150	d								

18

Cellular Biology

***Ramesh D.*[1] *and Barkha Gupta*[2]**

[1]*Department of Veterinary Physiology and Biochemistry, Veterinary College, Hassan (KVAFSU), Karnataka-573202*

[2]*Department of Veterinary Physiology and Biochemistry, Post Graduate Institute of Veterinary Education and Research (PGIVER), Jaipur (RAJUVAS), Rajasthan-302031*

Introduction

Robert Brown discovered the nucleus in some plant cells in 1831. After analyzing tissues from a range of animals and plants, T. Schwann (1839) declared, "All living organisms are composed of cells."

The fundamental elements of Prokaryotic and Eukaryotic cells

The simplest cells, called prokaryotic cells, have a straightforward structural arrangement. There is only one membrane system in it. They contain rickettsia, spirochete, mycoplasma, virus, blue-green algae, and bacteriablue-green algae, or cyanobacteria are the largest and most intricate prokaryotes, where higher plant photosynthesis occurs and have changed throughout time.

Prokaryotic cells

Prokaryotic cells range in size from 1 to 10 µm. They take place in a range of formats.

A bacterial cell is made up of three basic parts:

I. **External layer:** It is composed of the inner cell or plasma membrane, middle cell wall and outer slimy capsule.

   a. **Cell membrane:** The thin, flexible membrane of the cell, composed of proteins and lipids, regulates the flow of chemicals throughout the cell. It carries respiratory enzymes for reactions that release energy.

      Respiratory enzymes are found in mesosomes, which are folded regions of the plasma membrane that are compared to the mitochondria in eukaryotic cells. Similarly, the pigments and enzyme molecules found in photosynthetic cells are linked to the in-folds of the plasma membrane known as photosynthetic lamella, which is responsible for absorbing light and converting it into chemical energy.

   b. **The cell wall**: It is the non-living, semi-rigid layer that encloses the cell membrane, with a thickness that varies from 1.5 to 100 µm. It is chemically made up of peptidoglycans. Certain bacteria, such as mycoplasma, don't have cell walls.

c. **Slimy capsule:** The slimy capsule is a viscous coating that exists outside of the cell wall. It is primarily made up of polysaccharides, while it occasionally contains polypeptides as well other chemicals as well. It shields the cell from viral attacks, desiccation, antibiotics and phagocytosis.

II. **Cytoplasm:** The cytoplasm of prokaryotes is composed of proteins, lipids, glycogen, and inorganic ions, ribosomes, tRNA, and enzymes involved in biosynthetic processes and mRNA in the production of proteins. Certain unique characteristics of prokaryotic cytoplasm include as follows:

a. It is devoid of cell organelles such as the microtubules, mitochondria, Golgi apparatus, centrosomes, vacuoles, lysosomes, microfilaments, and intermediate filaments.

b. Ribosomes are the only cytoplasmic organelle present in prokaryotic cells. They are free to roam around in the cytoplasm and are smaller than eukaryotic ribosomes, or 70S. At the time of protein synthesis, they organize into poly-ribosomes. They are the sites of protein synthesis.

c. Prokaryotic cells lack cyclosis and streaming movement in their cytoplasm, in contrast to eukaryotic cells where these movements are present.

d. Certain prokaryotic cells can also generate gas vacuoles.

e. Substances enter and exit the cell through the cell membrane. Phagocytosis, pinocytosis, and exocytosis are not present in the cell.

f. Polysaccharide or inorganic phosphate deposits may be present.

III. **Nucleoid:** Prokaryotic cells lack a nuclear envelope, and their genetic material is deposited straight into the cytoplasm. A nucleoid is a type of nuclear substance. A highly coiled single pro-chromosome makes up a nucleoid.

a. **Plasmid:** In some prokaryotic cells, in addition to nucleoid, a small circular double-stranded DNA molecule is present. It is called a plasmid. Plasmids typically include 1000–30,000 base pairs and encode proteins that the organism needs to withstand antibiotics and other harmful substances.

IV. **Flagellum:** Several bacteria have this whip-like locomotory feature. It has a 10–15 μm length and is 150Å thick. As the flagellum does not have any surrounding membrane, it grows at the tip. The basal body and filament are the two main components.

a. **Filament:** Filament extends from cells into the media. It is composed of many intertwined spiral chains of the subunits of a protein called flagellin. Actins and tubulins are not the same as flagellin.

b. **Basal Body:** The flagellum is attached to the cell by the basal body, which also produces the force that rotates it. It is composed of a large number of proteins and components. It has two parts: shaft and hook.

V. **Pili:** Found on many bacteria, they are brief, rod-like, non-motile structures, also known as fimbriae. The protein pilin forms them. Typically, their thickness is less than 10 nm. They facilitate the attachment of bacteria to food, surfaces, or to one another. Tubular sex Pili are present in some bacteria.

Eukaryotic Cells

Size: The majority of eukaryotic cells are tiny, with sizes ranging from 10 to 100 μm. *Plasmodium vivax* sporozoites are some of the smallest cells in the world, measuring only 2 μm in length. The dimensions of an Ostrich egg are 175 x 120 mm. The longest cells are nerve cells, with a fiber that can reach several meters in length. Human cells typically measure between 20 and 30 μm.

Cell membrane: Also known as a plasma membrane or plasmalemma, the cell membrane is a thin, elastic layer that surrounds the cell, giving it structure, controlling material transfer through it, and holding its contents in place. It consists of a combination of lipids and proteins. It lacks respiratory enzymes. It permits both endocytosis and exocytosis in a variety of protists and mammalian cells.

The cell membrane is shielded and supported by a thick, inflexible, non-living cell wall in all plant cells, many fungi, and certain protists. Prokaryotes differ from eukaryotes in that the cell wall surrounding the plasma membrane is structurally different.

Cytoplasm: The cytoplasm or the cytosome is a semi-fluid, homogeneous, translucent ground substance known as cytoplasmic matrix or cytosol which is present between the cell membrane and the nucleus. The inner layer around the central fluid mass of a protozoan cell is known as endoplasm, while the outside, solid covering of cytoplasm is known as ectoplasm. "Cyclosis," or the flowing movement, is observed in the cytosol. The characteristics of the Eukaryotic cytoplasm are as follows:

Organelles: Organelles are arranged structures with specialized roles and, in some situations, the ability to grow and multiply. The organelles that are visible under a light microscope are Mitochondria, centrosomes, Golgi bodies, plastids, and vacuoles; on the other hand, endoplasmic reticulum, ribosomes, microfilaments, microtubules, intermediate filaments, and microbodies are only visible with an electron microscope. These organelles are often described as protoplasmic structures. The basal bodies of cells containing cilia or flagella are located in the cytoplasm, while the remaining portion of the structure extends out of the cytoplasm. These organelles are described as follows:

i. **Mitochondria:** They are globular or rod-shaped structures, dispersed throughout the cytoplasm, and can be found alone or in clusters. A double lipoprotein membrane surrounds them. Cristae, a finger-like structure seen in the inner membrane, can divide the mitochondria's inner chamber to some extent. On the interior surface, there are cristae, which resemble mushrooms, and oxysomes that are related to Phosphorylation. The space between the membranes and its lumen is filled with mitochondrial matrix. The matrix and membranes both have a lot of oxidative coenzymes as well as enzymes. Since mitochondria contain DNA molecules and ribosomes, they synthesize certain proteins. They produce the energy and reserve it in the form of adenosine triphosphate (ATP).

ii. **Centrosomes** (9+0): A distinct region of cytoplasm known as centrospheres is present in the clear zone around centrioles, close to the nucleus. Its matrix is called kinoplasm that bears two rounded bodies the "centrioles". Each centriole consists of nine fibrillar units and each of them is found to contain three microtubules arranged in a circle. The placement of both centrioles is perpendicular to one another. During cell division, centrioles create the microtubule spindles. Plant cells lack centrioles, and the spindle forms without their assistance.

iii. **Golgi bodies:** These are the stack of flattened parallel-arranged sacs and vesicles found in association with endoplasmic reticulum. Numerous lamellae, tubules, vesicles, and vacuoles make up their structure. Their membranes, which are made of lipoproteins, are thought to have originated in the ER. During cell division, the Golgi complex, also known as the dictyosome, secretes components necessary for the formation of the cell wall in plant cells. It aids in the release of hormones, enzymes, and other synthetic materials as well as the development of the sperm acrosome.

iv. **Cilia:** They are tiny structures that cover the surface of some cells, together with basal bodies and flagellaboth cilia and flagella originate from the basal bodies or blepharoplast lying in the cytoplasm. They consist of nine outer fibrils with two larger fibrils in the centre. Each fibril consists of two microtubules or has a 9+2 arrangement. Certain cells give birth to structures called cilia and flagella. They are comprised of tubulin-containing microtubules. They have a 9 + 2 plan of microtubule. Both grow at the base. They move by their beats or undulations, acting as locomotory organelles, because they obtain their energy from the breakdown of ATP molecules.

v. **Microtubules:** The incredibly thin tubulin protein tubules that run through the cytoplasm of plant and animal cells, giving the cell its structural support and dictating its overall cytoplasmic structure and shape, are referred to as microtubules. Each tubule is composed of thirteen separate filaments. Microtubules are involved in the production of spindles during cell division, cytoplasmic streaming (cyclosis), and the movement of ions and water.

vi. **Basal granules:** The spherical structures known as basal bodies are located at the base of flagella and cilia. They are all made up of nine fibrils, each of which has three microtubules, two of which enter the cilia or flagella.

vii. **Ribosomes:** Ribosome is the minute spherical structures that originate in nucleolus and are found attached with the membrane of endoplasmic reticulum and in the cytoplasm. They are mainly composed of ribonucleic acids (RNaand proteins. Their primary function is the production of proteins.

viii. **Nucleus:** The genetic material of a eukaryotic cell is surrounded by a unique nuclear envelope, which forms the "Nucleus," a conspicuous spherical organelle. The cytoplasm and nucleoplasm can exchange materials through pores in the nuclear envelope.

Cell Biology

1. Glycocalyx is associated with which of the following

    a. DNA   b. Plasma membrane

    c. Ribosomes   d. Nucleus

2. Which of the following describes an ATP binding cassette (ABC) transport protein that moves lipids the opposite way?

    a. ATPase   b. Scramblase

    c. Flippase   d. Floppases

3. The cell's resting phase, during which it grows and replicates its DNA, is referred to as
   a. Mitosis phase
   b. Interphase
   c. G1 phase
   d. M phase
4. In ribosomes, there are
   a. Only RNA
   b. RNA with proteins
   c. Proteins and DNA
   d. Proteins, fats, and nucleic acids
5. Which of the following describes an organizing hub for microtubules?
   a. Kinetochore
   b. Centrosome
   c. G2 phase
   d. Centrioles
6. The creation of chiasmata occurs during which phase of cell cycle
   a. Metaphase I
   b. Anaphase I
   c. Telophase I
   d. Prophase I
7 Identify the protein that holds two sister chromatids during cell division
   a. Securin
   b. Cohesin
   c. Serotonin
   d. Actin
8 It is possible to artificially produce polyploidy by
   a. Self-pollination
   b. Colchicine
   c. Inbreeding
   d. Line breeding
9. Identify the family of monomeric G-proteins that control cell proliferation
   a. Ras
   b. Rab
   c. Ran
   d. Rho
10. What kind of permeability does the plasma membrane have
   a. Selectively permeable
   b. Impermeable
   c. Single phase flow
   d. Highly permeable
11. Identify the greatest cell surface receptor family
   a. Nuclear receptor
   b. Ion-channel receptor
   c. G protein-coupled receptors (GPCR)
   d. Enzyme-linked receptor
12. Which of the following does not function as an ATP-dependent lipid transporter in a membrane?
   a. V-type ATPase
   b. Flippase
   c. Scramblase
   d. Na-K ATPase
13. Which chromatin region lacks transcription?
   a. Heterochromatin
   b. Nucleoid
   c. Centromere
   d. Euchromatin
14 Which of the following signaling pathways does T-cells follow when stimulated by an antigen?
   a. Juxtracrine signaling
   b. Autocrine signaling
   c. Paracrine signaling
   d. Endocrine signaling

15. Which method is used to see how the protein is distributed throughout the membrane?
    a. Patch clamp technique
    b. Freeze-fracture technique
    c. Freeze-etching
    d. FRAP
16. Which of the following transport proteins enables the movement of a single solute across a membrane in one direction?
    a. Active transport
    b. Co-transporter
    c. Uniporters
    d. Facilitated transport
17. Identify the structure that moves macromolecules from the nucleus to the cytoplasm.
    a. Microtubules
    b. Cilia
    c. Nuclear pores
    d. Centrioles
18. Identify the signal that facilitates a protein's entry or exit from the nucleus
    a. Notch signal
    b. Nuclear localization signal
    c. Paracrine signal
    d. Chemical signals
19. F0–F1Particles can be found on
    a. Thylakoids
    b. EPR
    c. Golgian vacuoles
    d. The inner mitochondrial membrane
20. Lysosomes are found in all except
    a. Erythrocytes
    b. Hepatocytes
    c. Muscle cells
    d. Acinar cells
21. Which of these signal mechanisms does not function as an extracellular signal?
    a. Autocrine
    b. Endocrine
    c. Cyclic AMP
    d. Paracrine
22. Identify the location where xenobiotic compound detoxification occurs
    a. Cytosol
    b. Rough EPR
    c. Ribosome
    d. Smooth EPR
23. What is the name of the cell membrane of muscle cells?
    a. Sarcoplasm
    b. Sarcolemma
    c. Perimysium
    d. Endomysium
24. The nucleus's non-membrane bound body, which vanishes in late prophase and reappears in telophase
    a. Chromosome
    b. Nucleolus
    c. Nucleoplasm
    d. Nuclear pore
25. Identify the drug that triggers microtubules to depolymerize into tubulin subunits.
    a. Cytochalasin D
    b. Latrunculin
    c. Nocodazole
    d. Phalloidin

26. Which of these describes the occluding junction?
    a. Adherence junction
    b. Tight junction
    c. Desmosomes
    d. Gap junction
27. Which of the subsequent cell organelles does the fluid mosaic model describe
    a. Nucleus
    b. Ribosome
    c. Plasma membrane
    d. Golgi complex
28. What part do vinblastine and vincristine play in microtubule growth?
    a. Causes depolymerization
    b. Prevent polymerization
    c. Prevent nucleation
    d. Prevent depolymerization
29. Specify the method that is utilized to see how lipids migrate laterally
    a. Microscopy
    b. Chromatography
    c. Spectrometry
    d. FRAP- Fluorescence recovery after photobleaching
30. Which microbe among the following has two nuclei?
    a. Slime molds
    b. Paramecium
    c. Cyanobacteria
    d. Amoeba
31. Which of these does not belong in the nucleus?
    a. Chromosome
    b. Nucleolus
    c. EPR
    d. Nuclear envelope
32. Cell mobility and shape are controlled by the
    a. Centrioles
    b. Intermediate filament
    c. Microfilaments
    d. Microtubule
33. Appendages of motile cells, such as cilia and flagella, are created by
    a. Doublet microtubule
    b. Singlet microtubule
    c. Triplet microtubule
    d. None
34. How do the tiny molecules get past the mitochondria's outer membrane?
    a. ATP pump
    b. Carrier protein
    c. Mitochondrial porins are voltage-dependent anion-selective channels (VDAC)
    d. Channels
35. Which of the following division methods is shared by bacteria and mitochondria?
    a. Binary fission
    b. Budding
    c. Binary fusion
    d. Meiosis
36. Identify the element that is not a member of the lipid bilayer
    a. Glycerol or Sphingosine
    b. Fatty acids
    c. Nucleic acids
    d. Phosphate

37. Note the nuclear lamina assertion that is incorrect
    a. Filaments found in the nucleus' inner membrane
    b. Composed of lamin proteins
    c. It has ribosome boundaries
    d. Give the nucleus mechanical support
38. Which of the following statements about the endosymbiotic theory is incorrect
    a. Mitochondria are self-replicating structures that resemble microscopic creatures
    b. They have unique DNA
    c. Their ribosomes and enzymes like those of bacteria.
    d. The sizes of mitochondria and bacteria are different
39. Which kind of leucoplast is in the role of storing fat?
    a. Amyloplast b. Elaioplasts
    c. Aleuroplasts d. Proteinoplasts
40. Identify the plant organelle that serves as a key location for an oxidative process.
    a. Mitochondria b. Chloroplast
    c. Thylakoid d. Peroxisomes
41. Identify the organelle that Entamoeba uses for ATP production and aerobic respiration.
    a. Hydrogenosome b. Mitosome
    c. Mitochondria d. Peroxisome
42. Which of the following is in charge of creating and storing pigments?
    a. Leucoplast b. Chromoplast
    c. Etioplast d. Chloroplast
43. Identify the scientists who initially found the cell in the cork piece
    a. Louis Pasteur b. Anton van Leeuwenhoek
    c. Rudolf Virchow d. Robert Hooke
44. Which of the following does not belong in the theory of modern cells?
    a. A cell is a functional and structural unit of life
    b. energy flow occurs within the cell
    c. No two cells are chemically identical
    d. All living things are composed of one or more cells
45. Ankyrin and Spectrin are examples of the following
    a. Nucleoprotein b. Monotopic
    c. Integral protein d. Peripheral protein
46. Which of the following organelles uses hydrolytic enzymes to regulate the intracellular digestion of macromolecules?
    a. Plasmasome b. Peroxisome
    c. Ribosome d. Lysosome

47. Which one of the following processes mediates the release of melanosomes from melanocytes?
    a. Autophagy
    b. Exocytosis
    c. Pinocytosis
    d. Endocytosis
48. Identify the one membrane that encircled each vacuole.
    a. Contractile vacuole
    b. Meninges
    c. Sarcolemma
    d. Tonoplast
49. Which of the following organelles functions in plants as a lysosome?
    a. Contractile vacuole
    b. Plastid
    c. Vacuole
    d. Peroxisome
50. Octameric histones comprise of
    a. 4 types of histones
    b. 8 histones of four different types
    c. 6 types of histones
    d. 5 types of histones
51. The cell's chemical products are transported and dispersed by
    a. Golgi apparatus
    b. ER compartments
    c. Cytoplasm
    d. Ribosomes
52. In what kind of glycosylation does the Golgi apparatus participate?
    a. T-linked glycosylation
    b. O-linked glycosylation
    c. G-glycosylation
    d. N-linked glycosylation
53. Which one of these removes extra water from the cell?
    a. Lysosome
    b. Peroxisome
    c. Vacuoles
    d. Contractile vacuole
54. Amphisome: What is it?
    a. Early endosome
    b. Vacuole
    c. Fusion of endosome and autophagosome
    d. The bigger size of lysosome
55. Which of these do not belong to the lysosome's hydrolytic enzymes?
    a. Lipases
    b. Aldolase
    c. Phosphatases
    d. Sulfatases
56. Digestion of a cell's constituent part is referred to as
    a. Phagocytosis
    b. Heterophagy
    c. Autophagy
    d. Pinocytosis
57. Centrioles participate in the development of which of the following
    a. Cell plate
    b. Nucleus
    c. Spindle
    d. Actin filaments
58. Which coated protein is transported from the ER to the Golgi via a coated vesicle?
    a. Clathrin
    b. COP I
    c. COP II
    d. COP III

59. Which of the following theories describes the fusion of vesicles?
    a. Lipid raft hypothesis
    b. Adhesion hypothesis
    c. SNARE hypothesis
    d. Cell kill hypothesis
60. What is the name of the lipid bilayer that covers the hollow sphere?
    a. Bilayer
    b. Lipid raft
    c. Liposome
    d. Micelle
61. Which coated vesicle that moves proteins from the endosome to the plasma membrane.
    a. COP I
    b. Clathrin
    c. COP II
    d. COP IV
62. Identify the GTPase that regulates the identification of v-SNARE and t-SNARE interactions
    a. Rac protein
    b. Ras protein
    c. Rho protein
    d. Rab protein
63. Which ATPase is responsible for separating SNARE?
    a. N-ethylmaleimide-sensitive fusion protein/ NEM sensitive factor
    b. V-ATPase
    c. F-ATPase
    d. P-ATPase
64. The marker enzyme of Golgi apparatus is
    a. Acetyl -CoA synthetase
    b. Galactosyl transferase
    c. Pyruvate kinase
    d. Cytochrome oxidase
65. Identify the sequence of amino acids that keeps the resident protein in the ER lumen
    a. KDEL
    b. KKXX
    c. KXXK
    d. KLDE
66. Comprising of Golgi cisternae, the Golgi stack is also called as
    a. Microsome
    b. Dictyosome
    c. Ribosome
    d. None
67. Which of the organelles participates in the subsequent secretion process?
    a. Cytoplasm
    b. ER compartments
    c. Golgi apparatus
    d. Ribosomes
68. In what kind of glycosylation does the EPR participate
    a. T-linked glycosylation
    b. O-linked glycosylation
    c. G-glycosylation
    d. N-linked glycosylation
69. Cristae are associated with which of the following cell organelles
    a. Mitochondria
    b. Cytoplasm
    c. Peroxisomes
    d. Ribosomes
70. Name the researcher who made the Golgi apparatus discovery
    a. Robert Remake
    b. Camillo Golgi
    c. Rudolf Virchow
    d. Theodor Schwann

71. Sodium and potassium pumps are examples of
   a. Active transport   b. Passive transport
   c. Symport   d. Facilitated transport
72. Identify the antibiotic that prevents oligosaccharide production
   a. Tunicamycin   b. Cephalosporin
   c. Penicillin   d. Ofloxacin
73. Amyloplasts are things that store which of the following
   a. Nucleic acids   b. Lipid
   c. Protein   d. Starch
74. Which of the following steps of cell division is stopped by colchicine?
   a. Anaphase   b. Metaphase
   c. Interphase   d. Telophase
75. Which of the following is the largest single membrane-bound intracellular compartment
   a. Ribosome   b. Golgi apparatus
   c. Endoplasmic reticulum   d. Nucleus
76. The protein undergoes which modifications in ER before reaching its final destination
   a. Glycosylation   b. Phosphorylation
   c. Proteolysis   d. Esterification
77 In the ER, detoxification of cholesterol medications and other dangerous substances is completed by
   a. Cytochrome P450   b. Cytochrome b
   c. Cytochrome D   d. Cytochrome F
78. Spindle fibers consist of which of the following
   a. Actin   b. Flagella
   c. Tubulin   d. Myosin
79. Chromosomes are separated during which phase of cell division
   a. Prophase   b. Anaphase
   c. Metaphase   d. Telophase
80. Centriole replication takes place in which phase of the cell cycle
   a. Interphase   b. Prophase
   c. Anaphase   d. Metaphase
81. Characteristics of a microsome are
   a. Compartment of Golgi   b. Small vesicles of fragmented ER
   c. Small ER compartments   d. Smaller ribosomes
82. Which of the following does not constitute a glycosylation function?
   a. Helps in proper folding of the protein   b. Confer stability in proteins
   c. Synthesis of membrane lipid   d. Helps in cell-cell adhesion

83. The membrane found in the endoplasmic reticulum that is connected to ribosomes is called
    a. EPR lumen
    b. Endosome
    c. Rough endoplasmic reticulum
    d. Smooth endoplasmic reticulum
84. In the meiotic phase of cell division, when does synapsis happen?
    a. Zygotene
    b. Leptotene
    c. Pachytene
    d. Diplotene
85. Cell drinking is also called as
    a. Endocytosis
    b. Phagocytosis
    c. Pinocytosis
    d. Exocytosis
86. Which glucose transporter is functional in the liver?
    a. GLUT-1
    b. GLUT-2
    c. GLUT-5
    d. GLUT-3
87. Which of the following ATPases keeps lysosomes and other vesicles at an acidic pH?
    a. P-ATPases
    b. ABC transporters
    c. F-ATPases
    d. V-ATPases
88. Which kind of thing is referred to as a mitoplast
    a. Mitochondria without inner membrane
    b. Mitochondria without outer membrane
    c. Another name for mitochondria
    d. Mitochondria without membranes
89. Which of the following transport processes does not require energy from metabolism?
    a. Secondary active transport
    b. Facilitated transport
    c. Passive transport
    d. Active transport
90. What are antiporters used for?
    a. Transfer of the second solute in the same direction
    b. Transfer of single solute
    c. Transfer of the second solute in the opposite direction
    d. Transfer of solute through pores
91. Cellular digestive enzymes are present in which of the cell organelle
    a. Liposomes
    b. Lysosomes
    c. Mitochondria
    d. Ribosome
92. r-RNA is synthesized in which part of the cell
    a. Cytoplasm
    b. Golgi body
    c. Nucleolus
    d. Lysosome
93. Polytene chromosomes are found due to
    a. Mitosis
    b. Endocytosis
    c. Meiosis
    d. Endomitosis

94. Which of the following processes is referred to as "cell eating"

a. Pinocytosis
b. Endocytosis
c. Phagocytosis
d. Caveolae-mediated endocytosis

95. Which of the following amino acids is the most basic?

a. Glycine
b. Phenyl Alanine
c. Tyrosine
d. Aspergillus

96. Which stage of the cell cycle does the synthesis of proteins and RNA occur?

a. M phase
b. S phase
c. G1 Phase
d. G2 phase

97. Identify the transport protein family that permits water to pass through the membrane

a. Facilitated diffusion
b. Aquaporins
c. Active transport
d. Ion channels

98. Animal cells are connected through

a. Desmosomes
b. Membrane plasma
c. Cell membrane
d. Plasmodesmata

99. Which of the following is a major single-pass transmembrane protein of RBC

a. Histones
b. Glycophorin
c. Tubulin
d. Glycoprotein

100. Cell theory is not relevant for which of the following

a. Virus
b. Microorganisms
c. Algae
d. Fungi

Answer Key

1	b	2	d	3	b	4	b	5	b	6	d	7	b
8	b	9	a	10	a	11	c	12	c	13	a	14	b
15	b	16	c	17	c	18	b	19	d	20	a	21	c
22	d	23	b	24	b	25	c	26	b	27	c	28	b
29	d	30	b	31	c	32	d	33	a	34	c	35	a
36	c	37	c	38	d	39	b	40	d	41	b	42	b
43	d	44	c	45	d	46	d	47	b	48	d	49	c
50	b	51	a	52	b	53	d	54	c	55	b	56	c
57	c	58	c	59	c	60	c	61	b	62	d	63	a
64	b	65	a	66	b	67	c	68	d	69	a	70	b
71	a	72	a	73	d	74	b	75	c	76	a	77	a
78	c	79	b	80	a	81	b	82	c	83	c	84	a
85	c	86	b	87	d	88	b	89	a	90	c	91	b
92	c	93	d	94	c	95	a	96	c	97	b	98	a
99	b	100	a										

19

Molecular Biology

Roshan Mohiddin[1] and Mohammed Hasif Ganimattoullah[2]

[1]*Division of Biochemistry, ICAR-NDRI, Karnal, Haryana*

[2]*Institute of Veterinary Science and Animal Husbandry, Siksha O Anusandhan University, Bhubneshwar, Odisha*

Introduction

Nucleic acids, primarily DNA and RNA, are essential for the storage and expression of genetic information. Under physiological conditions, the amino and oxo tautomers of purines and pyrimidines predominate. Adenine a., guanine (G), cytosine c., thymine (T), and uracil (U) are the main building blocks of nucleic acids. Other building blocks include 5-methylcytosine, 5-hydroxymethylcytosine, pseudouridine, and N-methylated heterocycles. A -glycosidic bond connects D-ribose or 2-deoxy-D-ribose to the N-1 of a pyrimidine or the N-9 of a purine, with the syn conformers being the most common.

Nucleotides are the monomeric units of nucleic acids that contain a phosphate group attached to the sugar's 3' or 5' hydroxyl. Extra phosphate groups form nucleoside diphosphates and triphosphates. These have high group transfer potential and help make covalent bonds. Cyclic phosphodiesters cAMP and cGMP act as second messengers. 3′ 5′ phosphodiester bonds link nucleotides to form polynucleotides, which have a directional 5′ and 3′ end. Four bases—A, G, C, and T—compose DNA, and hydrogen bonds (A to T, G to C) hold them together to form a double helix. Human DNA consists of approximately 3 billion base pairs organized into 23 chromosomes, encoding around 25,000 protein-coding genes and various non-coding RNAs (ncRNAs).

RNA, typically single-stranded, includes mRNA, rRNA, tRNA, small nuclear RNAs (snRNAs), and regulatory ncRNAs. At the 5′ end, 7-methylGTP caps mRNA, and at the 3′ end, a poly-A tail says what amino acid sequences go into proteins. tRNA, with a cloverleaf structure, delivers amino acids for protein synthesis. Some RNAs function as enzymes (ribozymes), and they likely played catalytic roles before protein enzymes evolved.

Structure of DNA and RNA

Hydrogen bonds between complementary bases stabilize the organization of DNA into two antiparallel strands that form a double helix. Association with histone proteins compacts the helical structure to form nucleosomes, each of which wraps DNA around an octamer of histones. Nucleosomes further compact into higher-order structures, forming chromatin.

DNA replication occurs during the S phase of the cell cycle, following base-pairing rules. In Okazaki fragments, DNA polymerase replicates each strand, synthesizing the leading strand continuously and the lagging strand discontinuously. Multiple origins initiate replication, leading to the formation of replication bubbles.

RNA synthesis (transcription) involves DNA-dependent RNA polymerases. Bacteria have one RNA polymerase, while eukaryotes have three: RNA polymerase I (rRNA), RNA polymerase II (mRNA, miRNAs, siRNAs, lncRNAs), and RNA polymerase III (tRNA, 5S rRNA). For transcription to start, preinitiation complexes (PICs) made up of general transcription factors (GTFs) and promoter regions need to come together. Transcription has three phases: initiation, elongation, and termination, regulated by distinct DNA elements and protein factors. Nucleosomes can modulate transcription by enhancing or occluding transcription factor binding. Gene Expression and Regulation

Eukaryotic gene expression involves extensive RNA processing. Primary RNA transcripts contain introns and exons, with introns removed during splicing to produce mature mRNA This process includes capping, splicing, and polyadenylation. Regulation occurs at multiple levels, including the transcriptional, post-transcriptional, and translational stages.

Gene cloning and genetic engineering involve isolating, amplifying, and manipulating DNA. Techniques like PCR and endonucleases can create recombinant DNA. These methods are critical for studying gene function and regulation, as well as developing gene therapies.

Nucleotide Metabolism

Nucleotide synthesis involves de novo pathways and salvage pathways. Inosinic acid (IMP) synthesizes purines (A and G), while aspartate and glutamine derive AMP and GMP from IMP. Aspartate and carbamoyl phosphate synthesize pyridinoids (C, T, and U). Feedback mechanisms tightly regulate nucleotide pools, ensuring balanced synthesis for nucleic acid production.

Purine catabolism produces uric acid, which excretes as sodium urate. Urate crystal deposition causes gout and other disorders. Pyrimidine catabolites are water-soluble and do not typically cause clinical abnormalities. However, pyrimidine precursor excretion can occur due to enzyme deficiencies, such as ornithine transcarbamoylase.

DNA Damage and Repair

DNA repair mechanisms correct damage caused by chemical and physical mutagens. Unrepairable DNA triggers programmed cell death. Repair processes involve excision repair, mismatch repair, and recombinational repair. Enzymes such as DNA polymerases, ligases, and endonucleases play critical roles in these pathways. Modern Techniques in Genomics

Advancements in genomics enable precise manipulation of mammalian genomes. Techniques such as CRISPR-Cas allow for targeted gene editing, including gene knockouts, knock-ins, and conditional gene modifications. These tools facilitate the study of gene function, regulation, and the development of genetic therapies.

Conclusion

Nucleic acids are fundamental to genetic information storage and expression. Cellular function depends on the intricate coordination of DNA and RNA structures, nucleotide metabolism, and gene regulation processes. Modern genomic techniques offer powerful tools for studying and manipulating genetic material, driving advancements in biotechnology and medicine.

1. What is the chemical basis of heredity?
   a. RNA b. Proteins
   c. DNA d. Lipids
2. Which types of RNA are produced by DNA?
   a. mRNA, tRNA, rRNA b. mRNA, tRNA, pRNA
   c. mRNA, cRNA, rRNA d. mRNA, rRNA, sRNA
3. Nucleic acids are polymers of which monomers?
   a. Amino acids b. Nucleotides
   c. Monosaccharides d. Fatty acids
4. What type of bond links nucleotides in nucleic acids?
   a. Peptide bonds b. Glycosidic bonds
   c. Phosphodiester bonds d. Hydrogen bonds
5. A nucleotide consists of a base, a sugar, and what else?
   a. Phosphate b. Protein
   c. Lipid d. Carbohydrate
6. Which bases are purines found in both DNA and RNA?
   a. Adenine and Thymine b. Guanine and Cytosine
   c. Adenine and Guanine d. Thymine and Uracil
7. What sugar is found in RNA?
   a. D-deoxyribose b. D-ribose
   c. Sucrose d. Glucose
8. Which model describes the structure of DNA?
   a. Griffith model b. Hershey-Chase model
   c. Watson-Crick model d. Meselson-Stahl model
9. What type of bonds hold the two DNA strands together?
   a. Ionic bonds b. Covalent bonds
   c. Hydrogen bonds d. Metallic bonds
10. What does Chargaff's rule state about the content of DNA bases?
    a. $A = T, G \equiv C$ b. $A = G, T = C$
    c. $A + T = G + C$ d. $A = C, G = T$
11. Which unusual DNA structure consists of three strands?
    a. Double helix b. Bent DNA
    c. Triple-strand DNA d. Four-strand DNA
12. RNA is typically what type of stranded polyribonucleotide?
    a. Double-stranded b. Single-stranded
    c. Triple-stranded d. Quadruple-stranded

13. What is the function of mRNA?
    a. Structural support
    b. Catalysis
    c. Delivering amino acids
    d. Specifying amino acid sequence in protein synthesis
14. What is the cloverleaf structure found in?
    a. mRNA b. rRNA
    c. tRNA d. DNA
15. Which RNA molecules can function as enzymes?
    a. mRNA b. rRNA
    c. tRNA d. Ribozymes
16. What is the DNA-protein structure in eukaryotic cells called?
    a. Chromatin b. Ribosome
    c. Nucleosome d. Spliceosome
17. What proteins form the core of a nucleosome?
    a. Actin b. Myosin
    c. Histones d. Tubulins
18. Which regions of DNA are exceptionally sensitive to nuclease attack?
    a. Hypersensitive sites b. Resistant sites
    c. Structural genes d. Introns
19. In transcription, what regions of DNA are transcribed into RNA?
    a. Exons b. Introns
    c. Histones d. Nucleosomes
20. During which phase of the cell cycle is DNA replicated?
    a. G1 phase b. S phase
    c. G2 phase d. M phase
21. Which enzyme is responsible for DNA synthesis?
    a. RNA polymerase b. DNA ligase
    c. DNA polymerase d. Topoisomerase
22. Which phase involves the formation of replication bubbles in DNA replication?
    a. Initiation b. Elongation
    c. Termination d. Regulation
23. What happens to cells with DNA damage that cannot be repaired?
    a. They divide rapidly
    b. They undergo programmed cell death
    c. They become cancerous
    d. They repair the damage themselves
24. What enzyme synthesizes RNA from a DNA template?
    a. DNA polymerase b. RNA polymerase
    c. Helicase d. Ligase

25. In bacteria, which RNA polymerase is involved in transcription?
    a. RNA polymerase I
    b. RNA polymerase II
    c. RNA polymerase III
    d. A single RNA polymerase
26. Which eukaryotic RNA polymerase transcribes rRNA?
    a. RNA polymerase I
    b. RNA polymerase II
    c. RNA polymerase III
    d. RNA polymerase IV
27. Which transcription factor is required for RNA polymerase II PIC formation?
    a. TFIIB
    b. TFIIA
    c. TFIIH
    d. All of the above
28. What are the three phases of transcription?
    a. Initiation, elongation, termination
    b. Initiation, replication, termination
    c. Binding, synthesis, release
    d. Assembly, elongation, translation
29. What influences transcription by modulating the binding of trans-factors?
    a. Ribosomes
    b. Histones
    c. Nucleosomes
    d. Telomeres
30. What is generated after intron removal and exon ligation in RNA processing?
    a. pre-mRNA
    b. Mature mRNA
    c. rRNA
    d. tRNA
31. What process forms functional mRNA from pre-mRNA?
    a. Replication
    b. Translation
    c. RNA splicing
    d. Transcription
32. What key element in cloning involves changing the sequence of DNA?
    a. Protein synthesis
    b. Genetic engineering
    c. RNA splicing
    d. Chromatin remodeling
33. Which technique identifies genes responsible for diseases?
    a. RNA interference
    b. DNA sequencing
    c. Gene cloning
    d. CRISPR-Cas9
34. What is the role of synthetic analogs of purine and pyrimidine bases?
    a. Antibiotics
    b. Anticancer drugs
    c. Antiviral agents
    d. Antifungal medications
35. Which drugs inhibit purine biosynthesis?
    a. Antifolate drugs
    b. Antibiotics
    c. Antiviral drugs
    d. Antifungal drugs
36. Which enzyme converts AMP to ADP?
    a. DNA polymerase
    b. RNA polymerase
    c. Kinase
    d. Ligase

37. What is the final catabolite of purines in humans?
    a. Urea b. Ammonia
    c. Uric acid d. Creatinine
38. What condition is associated with urate crystals?
    a. Gout b. Diabetes
    c. Hypertension d. Osteoporosis
39. What disease results from purine catabolism disorder?
    a. Lesch-Nyhan syndrome b. Huntington's disease
    c. Cystic fibrosis d. Sickle cell anemia
40. Which RNA polymerase transcribes mRNA in eukaryotes?
    a. RNA polymerase I b. RNA polymerase II
    c. RNA polymerase III d. DNA polymerase
41. What is the cloverleaf structure of tRNA involved in?
    a. DNA replication b. Protein synthesis
    c. RNA splicing d. Transcription
42. What is the precursor of both AMP and GMP in purine biosynthesis?
    a. IMP b. CMP
    c. TMP d. UMP
43. Which amino acid provides the 2-amino group of GMP?
    a. Glutamine b. Aspartate
    c. Glycine d. Serine
44. What molecule primarily converts ADP to ATP?
    a. DNA polymerase b. RNA polymerase
    c. Oxidative phosphorylation d. Glycolysis
45. What regulates hepatic purine nucleotide biosynthesis?
    a. PRPP pool size b. Glucose levels
    c. ATP concentration d. NADH levels
46. Which cyclic phosphodiester functions as an intracellular second messenger?
    a. CAMP b. CGMP
    c. Both CAMP and CGMP d. CIMP
47. What type of bond is found between the base and sugar in a nucleoside?
    a. β-Glycosidic bond b. Phosphodiester bond
    c. Hydrogen bond d. Ionic bond
48. What are the segments of genes that code for proteins called?
    a. Introns b. Exons
    c. Promoters d. Enhancers

49. What happens during the elongation phase of transcription?
  a. RNA polymerase binds to the promoter
  b. RNA strand is synthesized
  c. RNA polymerase detaches from DNA
  d. Transcription factors bind to DNA
50. Which DNA repair mechanism is employed after mutagen exposure?
  a. Replication b. Transcription
  c. DNA repair systems d. Translation
51. What is the functional form of RNA produced after splicing?
  a. rRNA b. tRNA
  c. mRNA d. pre-mRNA
52. What initiates the synthesis of RNA in bacteria?
  a. RNA polymerase binding to the promoter
  b. DNA polymerase binding to the promoter
  c. Ligase binding to the promoter
  d. Helicase binding to the promoter
53. What do eukaryotic RNA polymerases require to initiate transcription?
  a. Sigma factors b. General transcription factors
  c. Helicase d. Topoisomerase
54. What enzyme complex is involved in the regulation of transcription in eukaryotes?
  a. Sigma factor b. Mediator complex
  c. RNA polymerase d. DNA polymerase
55. What is the role of enhancer regions in eukaryotic DNA?
  a. Initiate DNA replication b. Terminate transcription
  c. Increase transcription rates d. Bind to histones
56. Which process involves the removal of introns from pre-mRNA?
  a. DNA replication b. RNA splicing
  c. Translation d. Transcription
57. Which RNA molecule carries amino acids to the ribosome?
  a. mRNA b. tRNA
  c. rRNA d. siRNA
58. Which type of RNA polymerase transcribes tRNA in eukaryotes?
  a. RNA polymerase I b. RNA polymerase II
  c. RNA polymerase III d. DNA polymerase
59. What are the basic units of chromatin called?
  a. Histones b. Nucleotides
  c. Nucleosomes d. Ribosomes
60. Which RNA is a major component of ribosomes?
  a. mRNA b. tRNA
  c. rRNA d. snRNA

61. Which enzyme unwinds the DNA double helix during replication?
    a. Ligase
    b. Helicase
    c. DNA polymerase
    d. Primase
62. Which enzyme synthesizes the RNA primer during DNA replication?
    a. DNA polymerase
    b. RNA polymerase
    c. Primase
    d. Helicase
63. Which enzyme links Okazaki fragments during DNA replication?
    a. Helicase
    b. Ligase
    c. DNA polymerase
    d. Primase
64. What structure ensures the proper replication of chromosome ends?
    a. Centromere
    b. Telomere
    c. Histone
    d. Nucleosome
65. Which RNA molecule is involved in splicing and gene regulation?
    a. mRNA
    b. tRNA
    c. rRNA
    d. snRNA
66. Which molecule provides the energy for DNA synthesis?
    a. ATP
    b. GTP
    c. CTP
    d. DNTPs
67. What type of mutation involves the substitution of one base for another?
    a. Insertion
    b. Deletion
    c. Point mutation
    d. Frameshift mutation
68. Which cellular structure is the site of ribosome assembly?
    a. Nucleus
    b. Nucleolus
    c. Cytoplasm
    d. Mitochondrion
69. What are the components of the ribosome?
    a. Proteins and rRNA
    b. DNA and RNA
    c. mRNA and tRNA
    d. Polysaccharides and proteins
70. Which of the following statements about β,γ-methylene and β,γ-imino derivatives of purine and pyrimidine triphosphates is accurate?
    a. They have potential use as anticancer drugs.
    b. They serve as precursors for B vitamins.
    c. They easily undergo hydrolytic cleavage of the terminal phosphate group.
    d. They can indicate the involvement of nucleotide triphosphates by mechanisms other than phosphoryl transfer.

71. Which of the following statements about nucleotide structures is incorrect?
   a. Nucleotides function as polyfunctional acids.
   b. The structural difference between caffeine and theobromine is solely the number of methyl groups on their nitrogen atoms.
   c. Purines are heterocyclic aromatic molecules made up of a pyrimidine ring fused with an imidazole ring.
   d. NAD+, FMN, S-adenosylmethionine, and coenzyme A are all ribonucleotide derivatives.

72. Which of the following statements about purine nucleotide metabolism is incorrect?
   a. Formation of PRPP (phosphoribosyl 1-pyrophosphate) is an early step in purine biosynthesis.
   b. Orotic acid is an intermediate in pyrimidine nucleotide biosynthesis.
   c. Humans degrade uridine and pseudouridine through similar reactions.
   d. Ribonucleotide reductase converts nucleoside diphosphates into the corresponding deoxyribonucleoside diphosphates.

73. Which of the following statements is incorrect?
   a. Metabolic disorders are infrequently linked to defects in purine catabolism.
   b. Immune dysfunctions are associated with defective adenosine deaminase and purine nucleoside phosphorylase.
   c. Lesch-Nyhan syndrome is due to a defect in hypoxanthine-guanine phosphoribosyl transferase.
   d. Xanthine lithiasis can result from a severe defect in xanthine oxidase.

74. Which of the following components are found in DNA? Choose the most complete answer.
   a. A phosphate group, adenine, and ribose
   b. A phosphate group, guanine, and deoxyribose
   c. Cytosine and ribose
   d. Thymine and deoxyribose

75. The backbone of a DNA molecule consists of which of the following?
   a. Alternating sugars and nitrogenous bases
   b. Nitrogenous bases alone
   c. Phosphate groups alone
   d. Alternating phosphate and sugar groups

76. Which of the following bonds connects the nucleotides of RNA and DNA?
   a. N-glycosidic bonds
   b. 3′-5′ phosphodiester linkages
   c. Phosphomonoesters
   d. 2′ phosphodiester linkages

77. Which component of the DNA duplex gives the molecule a net negative charge at physiological pH?
   a. Deoxyribose
   b. Ribose
   c. Phosphate groups
   d. Chlorine ion

78. Which feature ensures that duplex DNA maintains a nearly constant width along its long axis?
    a. A purine nitrogenous base always pairs with another purine nitrogenous base.
    b. A pyrimidine nitrogenous base always pairs with another pyrimidine nitrogenous base.
    c. A pyrimidine nitrogenous base always pairs with a purine nitrogenous base.
    d. Repulsion between phosphate groups keeps the strands a uniform distance apart.
79. According to Watson and Crick's model, what is true about newly replicated double-stranded daughter DNA molecules?
    a. They are composed of the two original parent DNA strands.
    b. They contain only the two newly synthesized DNA strands.
    c. They consist of two strands that are random mixtures of new and old DNA within each strand.
    d. They have one strand from the original parental DNA and one newly synthesized strand.
80. What mechanism synthesizes RNAs from DNA?
    a. Replicational duplication b. Translation
    c. Transesterification d. Transcription
81. Which interactions predominantly drive RNA secondary and tertiary structure formation?
    a. Hydrophilic repulsion
    b. Formation of complementary base pair regions
    c. Hydrophobic interaction
    d. van der Waals interactions
82. Which enzyme synthesizes RNA from a double-stranded DNA template?
    a. RNA-dependent RNA polymerase
    b. DNA-dependent RNA convertase
    c. RNA-dependent replicase
    d. DNA-dependent RNA polymerase
83. What is the most notable difference in gene expression between eukaryotes and prokaryotes?
    a. Ribosomal RNA lengths
    b. Presence of mitochondria
    c. Presence of lysosomes and peroxisomes
    d. Genomic material is sequestered in the nucleus in eukaryotes
84. Approximately how many base pairs of DNA are there in a typical diploid human cell, and into how many chromosomes is it divided?
    a. 64 billion, 23 b. 6.4 trillion, 46
    c. 64 billion, 46 d. 6.4 billion, 46

85. How many base pairs are associated with a single nucleosome?

a. 146
b. 292
c. 73
d. 1460

86. Which histone is not located within the superhelix formed between DNA and the histone octamer?

a. Histone H2B
b. Histone H3
c. Histone H1
d. Histone H4

87. Which subclass of chromatin is specifically inactivated at certain times within an organism's life or in particular sets of differentiated cells?

a. Constitutive euchromatin
b. Facultative heterochromatin
c. Euchromatin
d. Constitutive heterochromatin

88. Which hypothesis suggests that the physical and functional status of genomic chromatin regions depends on specific histone posttranslational modifications and/or DNA methylation status?

a. Morse code
b. PTM hypothesis
c. Nuclear body hypothesis
d. Epigenetic code

89. What is the repeated stretch of DNA located at the tips of eukaryotic chromosomes called?

a. Kinetochore
b. Telomere
c. Centriole
d. Chromomere

90. What serves as the primer for DNA polymerases during DNA replication?

a. Five carbon sugars
b. Deoxyribose alone
c. A short RNA molecule
d. Proteins with free hydroxyl groups

91. What term describes the discontinuous DNA replication that produces small DNA segments?

a. Okazaki fragments
b. Toshihiro pieces
c. Onishi oligonucleotides
d. Crick strands

92. What supplies the energy for the relief of mechanical strain by DNA gyrase?

a. Pyrimidine to purine conversion
b. Hydrolysis of GTP
c. Hydrolysis of ATP
d. Glycolysis

93. What is the phase of the cell cycle between the end of cell division and the start of DNA synthesis?

a. G1
b. S
c. G2
d. M

94. At which point in the cell cycle are crucial protein kinases, such as cyclin-dependent kinases, activated?

a. Just before mitosis
b. At the start of the S phase
c. Near the end of the G1 phase
d. At the conclusion of the G2 phase
e. All of the above

95. Which disease is frequently linked to a failure in a cell's ability to regulate its own division?
    a. Kidney disease
    b. Cancer
    c. Emphysema
    d. Diabetes

96. What molecular mechanism leads to the rapid decline in Cdk activity, prompting exit from the M phase and entry into G1?
    a. Decrease in mitotic cyclin levels
    b. Reduction in G1 cyclin levels
    c. Increase in G2 cyclin levels
    d. Increase in mitotic cyclin levels

97. Where does RNA polymerase bind on the DNA template to start transcription?
    a. Intron/exon junction
    b. Open reading frame DNA
    c. Terminator
    d. Promoter

98. Which RNA polymerase transcribes large eukaryotic rRNA genes like 18S and 28S?
    a. RNA polymerase III
    b. RNA-dependent RNA polymerase δ
    c. RNA polymerase I
    d. RNA polymerase II

99. What are the accessory proteins called that assist eukaryotic RNA polymerases in binding to promoters and forming functional transcription complexes?
    a. Basal or general transcription factors
    b. Activators
    c. Accessory factors
    d. Elongation factors

100. What is the term for the DNA segment from which the primary transcript is synthesized?
    a. Coding strand
    b. Initiator methionine domain
    c. Translation unit
    d. Transcriptome

101. What type of DNA sequences do eukaryotic genes encoding rRNAs belong to?
    a. Single-copy DNA
    b. Highly repetitive DNA
    c. Moderately repetitive DNA
    d. Mixed sequence DNA

102. When do modifications to the nucleotides of pre-tRNAs, pre-rRNAs, and pre-mRNAs occur?
    a. Postprandially
    b. Postmitotically
    c. Pretranscriptionally
    d. Posttranscriptionally

103. Where are RNA polymerase II promoters located relative to the transcription unit?
    a. 3′ downstream
    b. Nearest to the C-terminus
    c. Nearest to the N-terminus
    d. 5′ upstream

104. Which of the following is not a typical characteristic of eukaryotic mRNAs?
    a. They have special modifications at their 5′ (cap) and 3′ (poly (a) tail) ends.
    b. They are attached to ribosomes during translation.
    c. They are found within peroxisomes in the cytoplasm.
    d. Most have a significant noncoding segment that does not direct amino acid assembly.

105. What type of bond connects the initiation nucleotide of mRNA with the 5me-G Cap structure?
   a. 3′-5′ phosphodiester bond
   b. 5′-5′ triphosphate bond
   c. 3′-3′ triphosphate bond
   d. 3′-5′ triphosphate bond
106. Which feature of mature mRNAs is thought to protect them from degradation?
   a. Special posttranslational modifications
   b. 3′ Polyc.n tail
   c. 5me-G Cap
   d. Introns
107. What might be the consequences of inaccurate mRNA splicing?
   a. a single base error at a splice junction will cause a large deletion.
   b. a single base error at a splice junction will cause a large insertion.
   c. a single base error at a splice junction will cause a large inversion.
   d. both C and E.
   e. a single base error at a splice junction will change the reading frame and result in mRNA mistranslation.
108. What is the macromolecular complex that associates with introns during mRNA splicing?
   a. Splicer
   b. Dicer
   c. Nuclear body
   d. Spliceosome
109. What reaction is catalyzed by reverse transcriptase?
   a. Translation of RNA to DNA
   b. Transcription of DNA to RNA
   c. Conversion of ribonucleotides into deoxyribonucleotides
   d. Transcription of RNA to DNA
110. What process does RNA interference (RNAi) or dsRNA-mediated RNA interference facilitate?
   a. RNA ligation
   b. RNA silencing
   c. RNA inversion
   d. RNA restoration
111. Despite having 64 codons, there are only 20 amino acids found in nature. Therefore, some amino acids are coded by multiple codons. This characteristic of the genetic code is referred to as which of the following?
   a. Degenerative
   b. Duplicative
   c. Nonoverlapping
   d. Overlapping
112. How many stop codons are present in the genetic code?
   a. 3
   b. 21
   c. 61
   d. 64
113. If a tRNA has the sequence 5′-CAU-3′, which codon will it recognize (assuming no wobble base pairing)?
   a. 3′-UAC-5′
   b. 3′-AUG-5′
   c. 5′-ATG-3′
   d. 5′-AUG-3′

114. What sequence is found at the 3′ end of all functional, mature tRNAs?
   a. The cloverleaf loop b. The anticodon
   c. The sequence CCA d. The codon

115. What activity, also found in DNA polymerases, is possessed by most aminoacyl-tRNA synthetases?
   a. Proofreading b. Hydrogenase
   c. Proteolytic d. Helicase

116. What is the correct order for the phases of protein synthesis?
   a. Initiation, termination, elongation
   b. Termination, initiation, elongation
   c. Initiation, elongation, termination
   d. Elongation, initiation, termination

117. Which amino acid typically initiates protein synthesis?
   a. Cysteine b. Threonine
   c. Tryptophan d. Methionine

118. During protein synthesis, where is the initiator tRNA positioned within the active 80S ribosome complex?
   a. E site b. I site
   c. P site d. A site

119. Identify the enzyme responsible for forming peptide bonds during protein synthesis and its chemical nature.
   a. Pepsynthase, protein b. Peptidyl transferase, RNA
   c. Peptidase, glycolipid d. Peptidyl transferase, protein

120. What term is used for mutations within an open reading frame that create a stop codon?
   a. Frameshift mutation b. Missense mutation
   c. Point mutation d. Nonsense mutation

121. In which direction does polypeptide synthesis proceed?
   a. C-terminal to N-terminal b. N-terminal to 3′
   c. N-terminal to C-terminal d. 3′ to 5′

122. Which cis-acting element is typically located adjacent to or overlapping many prokaryotic promoters?
   a. Regulatory gene b. Structural gene(s)
   c. Repressor d. Operator

123. What term describes a segment of a bacterial chromosome where genes for enzymes of a particular metabolic pathway are clustered and controlled together?
   a. Operon b. Operator
   c. Promoter d. Terminal controller

124. What term is used for the complete set of proteins present in a specific cell type?
   a. Genome b. Peptide collection
   c. Transcriptome d. Proteome

125. How does nucleosome formation on genomic DNA impact transcription initiation and elongation?
a. Nucleosomes block access to enzymes needed for all transcription phases.
b. Nucleosomes recruit enzymes that modify histones and DNA, affecting transcription protein access to DNA.
c. Nucleosomes cause DNA degradation where it contacts histones.
d. Nucleosomes do not significantly affect transcription.

126. Which molecules interact with eukaryotic mRNA gene core promoters to aid RNA polymerase II association?
a. Termination factors
b. Sequence-specific transcription factors (transactivators)
c. Elongation factors
d. General or basal transcription factors (GTFs)

127. Most eukaryotic transcription factors have at least two domains. What are these domains?
a. RNA-binding domain and repression domain
b. Activation domain and repression domain
c. DNA-binding domain and activation domain
d. DNA-binding domain and ligand-binding domain

128. Transcription factors at enhancers promote transcription initiation at the core promoter through intermediaries called what?
a. Coactivators
b. Cotranscription proteins
c. Corepressors
d. Receptors

129. What interactions among transcription proteins significantly increase the diversity of regulatory factors from a limited number of polypeptides?
a. Recombination
b. Homodimerization
c. Heterozygosity
d. Heterodimerization

130. What term describes the gene region containing the TATA box and extending to the transcription start site (TSS)?
a. Polymerase home
b. Initiator
c. Start selector
d. Core promoter

131. Which mechanism correctly explains how enhancers can stimulate transcription from long distances?
a. Enhancers excise the intervening DNA between enhancers and promoters.
b. RNA polymerase II binds strongly to enhancer sequences.
c. Enhancers search through DNA to bind directly to the core promoter.
d. Enhancers and core promoters are brought close together by DNA loop formation mediated by DNA-binding proteins.

132. Which histone amino acids are typically acetylated?
a. Lysine
b. Arginine
c. Asparagine
d. Histidine

133. Which method in transcription factor research identifies all genomic sites bound by a specific transcription factor under certain conditions?
  a. Systematic deletion mapping
  b. DNAse I sensitivity
  c. Chromatin immunoprecipitation-sequencing (ChIP-seq)
  d. FISH

134. What sequences lie between the 5′-methylguanosine cap and the AUG initiation codon on eukaryotic mRNAs?
  a. Last exon
  b. Last intron
  c. 3′ UTR
  d. 5′ UTR

135. Which eukaryotic mRNA features are important for message stability?
  a. 5′ UTR sequences
  b. The promoter
  c. The operator
  d. 3′ UTR and poly (a) tail

136. Which statement about nucleotides is accurate?
  a. Nucleotides like ATP are involved in the in vivo synthesis of nucleic acids.
  b. Nucleotides consist only of a pentose sugar and a nitrogenous base, either a purine or pyrimidine.
  c. GTP substitutes ATP in RNA synthesis.
  d. Nucleotides contain deoxyribose in RNA and ribose in DNA.

137. Which of the following statements about nucleotide structure are correct?
  a. Removing the 5’-phosphate from GMP results in guanine.
  b. Removing the 5’-phosphate from AMP results in adenosine.
  c. Removing the ribose 5-phosphate from TMP yields uracil.
  d. Removing the ribose 5-phosphate from CMP yields cytidine.

138. Purine nucleotides are components of which molecules?
  a. FAD
  b. NAD+
  c. NADP+
  d. All of the above

139. Which high-energy bond is found in ATP?
  P) Phosphoester bond
  Q) Ether bond
  R) Phosphoanhydride bond
  S) Phosphodiester bond
  a. Only P
  b. Only R
  c. Both P and Q
  d. Both P and S

140. Deoxyribose in a nucleotide is what type of alcohol?
  a. Primary alcohol
  b. Secondary alcohol
  c. Tertiary alcohol
  d. Phenol

141. The sugar-phosphate backbone in nucleic acids is characterized by which properties?
  P) Hydrophobic in nature
  Q) Hydrophilic in nature
  R) Negatively charged
  S) Shows polarity
  a. P and Q
  b. Q and S
  c. Q, R, and S
  d. P, R, and S

142. Where is the genetic information in nucleic acids stored?

a. Number of nucleotides
b. Types of nucleotides
c. Sequence of nucleotides
d. All of the above

143. The melting temperature (Tm) of a DNA duplex is the temperature at which half the molecules are single-stranded. Under which conditions is Tm maximized?

a. Low ionic strength and high DNA concentration
b. High ionic strength and high DNA concentration
c. High ionic strength and low DNA concentration
d. Low ionic strength and low DNA concentration

144. The helical structure of DNA is determined by which technique?

a. Electron diffraction measurement
b. Neutron diffraction measurement
c. X-ray diffraction measurement
d. Diffraction of visible light

145. Which statement about the structure of B-DNA is incorrect?

a. There are 10 bases per turn within the double helix.
b. Separation of the two strands requires untwisting of the helix.
c. The molar amount of adenine plus thymine equals the molar amount of guanine plus cytosine.
d. The double helix contains antiparallel chains.

146. What lines the major groove of DNA?

a. N3 of purine and N1 of pyrimidine
b. N7 of purine and O2 of pyrimidine
c. N7 of purine and C4 of pyrimidine
d. None of the above

147. Which feature does not differ between A-form and B-form double helix DNA?

a. appearance of the major and minor grooves
b. Thickness of the helix
c. Tilt of the bases
d. Polarity of the two complementary strands

148. What promotes the Z-DNA conformation?

a. 2'-OH steric hindrance
b. Anti-G and C2'-endo sugar
c. Syn-G and O'-endo sugar
d. G4-DNA quartet

149. What makes DNA more stable to alkaline hydrolysis compared to RNA?

a. Greater stability of ribose over deoxyribose
b. DNA having β-glycosidic bonds and RNA having α-glycosidic bonds
c. DNA being more insoluble in water than RNA
d. Absence of a 2'-hydroxyl in DNA to aid in hydrolysis

150. Which statement is incorrect regarding tRNA?

a Nucleotide bases in tRNA are extensively modified after transcription.
b One amino acid may have multiple tRNA species as adaptors.
c. Each tRNA is specific to one amino acid.
d. The size of tRNA generally varies from 600 to 1000 bases.

Answer Key

1	a	2	a	3	b	4	c	5	a	6	c	7	b
8	c	9	c	10	a	11	c	12	b	13	d	14	c
15	d	16	a	17	c	18	a	19	a	20	b	21	c
22	a	23	b	24	b	25	d	26	a	27	d	28	a
29	c	30	b	31	c	32	b	33	b	34	a	35	a
36	c	37	c	38	a	39	a	40	b	41	a	42	a
43	a	44	c	45	a	46	c	47	a	48	b	49	b
50	c	51	c	52	a	53	b	54	b	55	c	56	b
57	b	58	c	59	c	60	c	61	b	62	c	63	b
64	b	65	d	66	d	67	c	68	b	69	a	70	d
71	c	72	d	73	a	74	b	75	d	76	b	77	c
78	c	79	d	80	d	81	b	82	d	83	d	84	d
85	a	86	c	87	b	88	d	89	b	90	c	91	a
92	c	93	a	94	e	95	a	96	a	97	d	98	c
99	a	100	a	101	c	102	d	103	d	104	c	105	b
106	c	107	e	108	d	109	d	110	b	111	a	112	a
113	d	114	c	115	a	116	c	117	d	118	c	119	b
120	d	121	c	122	d	123	a	124	d	125	a	126	d
127	c	128	a	129	d	130	d	131	d	132	a	133	c
134	d	135	d	136	a	137	b	138	d	139	b	140	a
141	c	142	c	143	b	144	c	145	c	146	b	147	d
148	c	149	d	150	d								

20

Recombinant DNA Technology

N.R. Srikanth[1], M.K. Vidya[2] and C.N. Darshan[3]

[1]Scientist-Veterinary Biochemistry, Livestock Research Station, Lam, Guntur Sri Venkateswara Veterinary University

[2]Department of Physiology and Biochemistry, Veterinary College, KVAFSU, Hassan

[3]Department of Animal Husbandry and Veterinary Services, Karnataka

Introduction

In a historic landmark, Genentech, a young Californian Company pioneering in gene splicing (which includes recDNA technology, genetic engineering, gene transplantation, gene cloning), saw its stock price skyrocket form $35 to a staggering $89 within just 20 minutes of the New York Stock Exchange's opening bell on October 15, 1980. This was marked as the fastest stock price growth ever witnessed on that exchange. The company's success was attributed to the ground-breaking work it had been involved in producing human insulin through genetic engineering that offered a revolutionary alternative for diabetics allergic to the then traditional insulin of porcine origin. Genentech's pioneering work in gene splicing has its roots in the early 1970s. In 1972, Stanley Cohen and Herbert Boyer were credited with creating the first recombinant DNA molecule. Their experiments demonstrated the ability to create recombinant DNA molecules that could be introduced into bacteria like *E. coli*, offering a foundation for future advancements in genetic engineering.

Rec DNA Technology involves 5 different stages

1. Selection of "Gene of interest or Gene insert or DNA insert"
2. Creation of rec DNA or chimeric DNA using a cloning vector
3. Introduction of the rec vectors into the host cells – Transformation
4. Multiplication and selection of clones with rec. molecule
5. Expression of the gene of interest

The development of recombinant DNA (rec. DNA) technology has been a revolution in understanding the molecular basis of life.

Mapping and dissection of Chromosomes: RecDNA technology allows scientists to isolate and manipulate specific regions of complex chromosomes. This has been crucial for creating genetic maps, pinpointing the location of genes, and understanding how genes are organized.

Gene and cDNA analysis: By analysing DNA and its complementary form, cDNA (Complementary DNA), researchers can identify unknown genes. This presents exciting avenues to explore the function of these genes and the proteins they encode.

Protein isolation and purification: Once the gene is identified, recDNA techniques can be used to produce the corresponding protein in large quantities. This allows scientists to isolate and purify the protein for further study of its structure and function.

Protein engineering: By making targeted changes (mutations) to genes using techniques like site-directed mutagenesis, scientists can create new types of proteins with altered properties. This allows to unravel the relationship between a protein's structure and its function.

Overall, recDNA technology has revolutionized the ability to

Understand Genes and genomes – Due to recDNA technology we are now able to map, analyse and manipulate genes with much greater precision.

Studying of proteins – recDNA made possible the ways to isolate, purify, and engineer proteins to gain insights into their structure, function, and interaction with other molecules.

This technology has numerous applications in various fields like medicine, agriculture and biotechnology.

It offers rational, scientific approach to understand diseases at the molecular level, focusing on how changes in molecules like DNA, proteins, and enzymes contribute to the development of specific diseases like familial hypercholesterolemia, sickle cell disease, thalassemia, cystic fibrosis, muscular dystrophy etc. Targeted therapies can be envisioned that involve in correcting the underlying genetic defect, replacing the missing proteins or interfering with pathways by the disease process.

RecDNA technology has revolutionized protein production for therapeutic purposes. It allows scientists to introduce the gene coding for a desired protein into a host organism, such as bacteria or yeast. These host cells then become little protein factories, churning out large quantities of specific protein. This technique has been instrumental in the development of numerous life-saving therapies with proteins *viz.,* insulin, growth hormone, tissue plasminogen activator (tPA) etc.

Vaccines and diagnostics: recDNA technology altered the course for obtaining proteins used in vaccines and diagnostic tests. Traditionally, certain vaccines were developed by employing extracted proteins from the concerned pathogens which could be potentially proven risky and was an inefficient process. With recDNA technology, the gene encoding the desired protein within the pathogen can be identified and isolated (ex: Surface protein of the Hepatitis-B virus) and can be inserted into the host organism such as bacteria or yeast, making them produce large quantities of the specific protein for the vaccine. This method employing recDNA technology for production of vaccines is by far safe and reliable source of the antigen to produce a vaccine. Similarly, recDNA technology helps produce specific proteins needed for diagnostic tests. In HIV/AIDS tests, for example, recDNA can be used to create the viral proteins that antibodies in the test bind to if the virus is present. This approach presents highly sensitive and specific tests that improves accuracy in diagnosis.

RecDNA is a powerful tool in diagnosing existing disease and even in predicting the risk of developing certain diseases. RecDNA technology allows to identify and analyse specific genetic variations associated with diseases. As an example, in diagnosing cystic fibrosis, a genetic test can look for mutations in the CTFR gene known to cause the disease. Also, recDNA techniques can be employed to detect infectious agents by identifying their unique DNA sequences. This is used in tests for viruses like HIV or bacteria causing tuberculosis. In addition to diagnosing an existing diseases, recDNA technology can reveal a subject's predisposition to certain diseases. By analysing specific genes or genetic markers, doctors can estimate a person's risk of developing diseases like Peste des petits ruminants (PPR), a viral disease affecting sheep and goats.

Specific adaptations in recDNA technology led to remarkable advances in forensic medicine. Short Tandem Repeat (STR) analysis is the pillar stone of modern forensic DNA analysis. It employs recDNA techniques to amplify and analyse specific highly variable regions of DNA called STRs. By comparing STR profiles investigators can establish strong links in parental verifications and crime scenes. Another important analysis related that utilizes the adaptations from recDNA technology is mitochondrial DNA (mtDNaanalysis. mtDNA is present in much higher numbers per cell compared to nuclear DNA. This makes it easier to analyse even in samples where nuclear DNA is damaged or scarce. Since mtDNA passes down unchanged from mother to offspring, it allows tracing an individual's maternal ancestry. mtDNA analysis is a valuable tool in various fields; in forensics, when crime scene is old or damaged, mtDNA analysis can help identify suspects through maternal lineage; in genealogy, by comparing mtDNA sequences, researchers can understand historical population movements and mternal ancestry; in medical diagnosis, analysis of mutations in mtDNA that may lead to certain inherited diseases can be diagnosed. RecDNA methods have been refined to analyse miniscule amounts of DNA with limited or touch DNA transfer by DNA profiling for low Template DNA (LTD). RecDNA advancements are leading to the possibility of predicting physical characteristics like hair and eye colour from DNA evidence, potentially aiding suspect identification by DNA phototyping.

1. African clawed frog Xenophs laevis gene and pSC101 DNA were recombined using ___________ to develop a recombined plasmid DNA

    a. Restriction endonuclease b. DNA ligase
    c. Exonuclease d. DNA gyrase

2. Desired piece of DNA is referred to as

    a. Gene of interest b. Gene insert
    c. DNA insert d. All of the above

3. Insertion of the selected DNA into a cloning vector creates

    a. Plasmid b. rec DNA
    c. Chimeric DNA d. Both b & c

4. Recombinant DNA is named after a monster in Greek mythology that has lion's head, goat's body and a snake's tail which is

    a. Midas b. Pandora
    c. Chimera d. Hector

5. Introduction of the recDNA into the host cell is referred to as

    a. recDNA technology b. Transformation
    c. Transduction d. Ligation

6. Sickle cell disease is caused by mutation of a single base out of the 3 × 109 in the genome which is a __________ DNA substitution

    a. C to G b. G to C
    c. A to U d. T to A

7 Sickle Cell Disease is ________ change in the mRNA corresponding to the sixth codon of the β-globin gene

a. A to U
b. T to A
c. U to A
d. C to G

8. The altered codon specifies __________ rather than glutamic acid and this causes a structural abnormality of the β-globin molecule in sickle cell disease

a. Isoleucine
b. Glutamine
c. Alanine
d. Valine

9. Method that aim to cure an inherited disease by providing the patient with a correct copy of the defective gene

a. Gene cloning
b. Gene therapy
c. recDNA technology
d. Transformation

10. Transgenic animals are generated by incorporation of genes into

a. Somatic cell
b. Young animal
c. Adult animal
d. Embryo

11. Enzymes that produce internal cuts or cleavages in the DNA molecules are referred to as

a. Ligases
b. Endonucleases
c. Exonucleases
d. Gyrases

12. A class of endonucleases cleaves DNA only within or near those sites which have specific base sequences

a. Restriction
b. Reserved
c. Specific
d. DNA

13. The sites recognised by restriction endonucleases are referred to as

a. Identified sites
b. Noticed sequences
c. Recognition sites
d. Registered sites

14. Restriction enzymes were named after the phenomenon

a. Of restriction by phages
b. Of host restriction of phages
c. Exhibited by phages
d. Created in an in lab procedure

15. The purpose of restriction enzymes in host is

a. To help in recDNA technology
b. To help in transgenics
c. To recognize and cleave foreign DNA
d. To form chimeric DNA

16. The DNA of a cell is protected from its own endonucleases by

a. Acetylation
b. Carbonation
c. Carboxylation
d. Methylation

17. The presence of restriction enzymes was postulated by

a. W. Arber
b. S Cohen
c. H. Boyer
d. R. Hook

18. Smith, Nathans and Arber were awarded the Nobel Prize for Physiology and Medicine in 1978 for the discovery of

    a. Ligases b. Gyrases
    c. Plasmid d. Endonucleases

19. The tools for cutting DNA molecules at predetermined site

    a. Exonucleases b. Restriction endonucleases
    c. DNA ligases d. DNA gyrases

20. Type I restriction endonucleases have recognition sequences of about

    a. 3 bp b. 100 bp
    c. 15 bp d. 1000 bp

21. Type I restriction endonucleasescleavethe DNA about __________ away from the 5'-end of the sequence

    a. 15 bp b. 100 bp
    c. 1000 bp d. 2000 bp

22. Type II restriction endonucleases require ________ ions for cleavage

    a. Ca2+ b. Mn2+
    c. Na+ d. Mg+2

23. The first type II enzyme to be isolated was

    a. EcoRI b. HindIII
    c. HindII d. BamHI

24. Only type of endonucleases used for restriction mapping and gene cloning in view of their cleavage only at specific sites is _______

    a. Type II b. Type III
    c. Type I d. Type IV

25. EcoP1, EcoP15 and HinfIII are examples of which type of restriction endonucleases

    a. Type II b. Type III
    c. Type I d. Type IV

26. In 2003, the International Union of Pure and Applied Chemistry (IUPAC) updated the recommendations for enzyme nomenclature before that the restriction endonucleases are written in which of the following manner.

    a. EcoRI b. ECORI
    c. EcoRI d. EcoRI

27. The recognition sequences for Type II endonucleases form

    a. Palindrome
    b. Rotational symmetry
    c. Double helix
    d. Palindromes with rotational symmetry

28. In a palindrome with rotational symmetry, the base sequence in the first half of one strand of a DNA double helix is the mirror image of
    a. The second half of its complementary strand
    b. Reverse of the second half of the complementary strand
    c. First half of the complementary strand
    d. Of the sequence of itself in entirety
29. Most of the type II restriction endonucleases are rich in
    a. A-U b. A-T
    c. G-C d. A-G
30. Protruding (3' or 5') ends are generated by the action of restriction endonucleases that make ___________
    a. Even cuts b. Staggered cuts
    c. Parallel cuts d. Random cuts
31. The two protruding ends generated by a cleavage given by restriction endonuclease have complementary base sequence and form _________
    a. Cohesive ends b. Even ends
    c. Sticky ends d. Both a & c
32. A DNA molecule that has the ability to replicate in a host cell, into which DNA insert can be integrated forcloning.
    a. Phage b. Module
    c. Gene of interest d. Vector
33. Examples for extra-chromosomal genomes
    a. Plasmid b. Phage
    c. Virus d. All of the above
34. The vector replicon must be under ___________replication control so that it can generate multiple copies of itself in a single host cell
    a. Relaxed b. Restricted
    c. Self d. Host
35. The vector should have suitable __________ genes that allow easy detection and/or selection of the transformed host cells
    a. Complementary b. Non-coding
    c. Marker d. Coding
36. Expression of the DNA insert requires which of the following
    a. Ribosome binding site b. Promoter
    c. Operator d. All of the above
37. Vectors used for propagation of DNA inserts in a suitable host are called
    a. Expression b. Plasmid
    c. Phasmid d. Cloning

38. Production of protein by a vector with gene of interest in the host is referred to as
    a. Chimerization b. Cloning
    c. Expression d. Translation
39. When eukaryotic genes are isolated as ______________ hence they are intron-free
    a. Exon b. cDNA
    c. Single strand DNA d. tRNA
40. Eukaryotic genes are isolated as cDNA and hence they are ______ free
    a. Intron b. Exon
    c. RNA d. Error
41. Expression of prokaryotic genes in eukaryotes without introns is possible by using ____________
    a. cDNA b. Exon
    c. RNA d. tRNA
42. Construction of vectors allowing the synthesis of fusion proteins comprising amino acids coded by a sequence in the vector and those encoded by the DNA insert is referred to as __________ fusion
    a. Replicational b. Transcriptional
    c. Translational d. Chimeric
43. Development of vectors permitting the synthesis of pure proteins encoded exclusively by the DNA inserts is referred to as ________ fusion
    a. Translational b. Replicational
    c. Transcriptional d. Chimeric
44. Which of the following is a natural vector
    a. Cosmid b. Phasmid
    c. Bacteriophage d. Shuttle
45. Which of the following are natural vectors
    a. Plasmid & bacteriophage b. Phasmid & cosmid
    c. Cosmid & bacteriophage d. Plasmid & shuttle vectors
46. The DNA molecule that is capable of independent replication and transmission
    a. Bacteriophage b. Nucleosome
    c. Plasmid d. Viral chromosome
47. The following are man-made vectors
    a. Cosmids b. Phasmids
    c. Shuttle vectors d. All of the above
48. *F* plasmids are responsible for the following action
    a. Killing coli b. Antibiotic resistance
    c. Conjugation d. Excretion

49. R plasmids are responsible for the following action
    a. Killing coli b. Antibiotic resistance
    c. Conjugation d. Excretion
50. *Col* plasmids are responsible for the following action
    a. Killing coli b. Antibiotic resistance
    c. Conjugation d. Excretion
51. These plasmids mediate DNA transfer through conjugation
    a. Conjugative b. Transmissible
    c. *F* plasmids d. All of the above
52. Which among the following is non-conjugative plasmid
    a. *F* plasmid b. Transmissible
    c. R plasmid d. Bacteriophage
53. The replication control of single copy plasmids is __________ that of their bacterial host
    a. Larger than b. Smaller than
    c. Same as d. Non-identical to
54. The replication control of single copy plasmids is the same as that of their bacterial host cells so that they replicate and segregate with the bacterial chromosome; this is called___________ replication
    a. Stringent b. Relaxed
    c. Tight d. Stress-free
55. The replication control of multicopy plasmids is
    a. Stringent b. Relaxed
    c. Tight d. Stress-free
56. Elements which enable transposition of the modules flanked by them
    a. Transpositional modules b. Genes
    c. Insertion sequences d. Plasmids
57. *p*SC101 has ____________________ regulation of replication
    a. Relaxed b. Stringent
    c. Conjugative d. Non-conjugative
58. B and R in the plasmid pBR322represent
    a. Plasmid b. Scientists
    c. Genus d. Species
59. In pUC, UC stand for
    a. University of Carnegie Mellon b. University of Caltech
    c. University of California d. University of Carleton

60. Which of the following is not a feature of pBR322?
   a. Origin of replication
   b. Ampicillin resistance gene
   c. Tetracycline resistance gene
   d. Single restriction enzyme cutting site

61. *p*BR322 is an example of
   a. Natural bacterial chromosome
   b. Modified bacterial plasmid
   c. Viral vector
   d. Transposon

62. The presence of restriction sites within the markers tet and amphelp in
   a. Transformation
   b. Selection of transformed cells
   c. Transfection
   d. Selection of vectors

63. The nic-bom region interferes with replication efficiency of extra-chromosomal DNA in monkey cells; such prokaryotic sequences are called ________________ sequences
   a. Poison
   b. Killer
   c. Suicide
   d. Hijack

64. The poison sequence of pBR322 has been deleted to yield
   a. pBR327
   b. pAT153
   c. pUC7
   d. Both a & b

65. Which of the following statement is wrong
   a. pUC7 is a derivative of pBR322
   b. pBR327 is a derivative of pBR322
   c. pAT153 is a derivative of pBR322
   d. pBR322 is a derivative of pUC7

66. β-galactosidase hydrolyses X-gal (5-Bromo-4-chloro-3-indolyl-β-D-galactoside) to yield a
   a. Red dye
   b. Green dye
   c. Blue dye
   d. Black dye

67. In __________ cycle, the phage chromosome integrates into the bacterial chromosome and multiplies with the latter as prophage
   a. Lytic
   b. Lambda
   c. Viral
   d. Lysogenic

68. Phage vectors are more efficient than plasmids for cloning of ____________ fragments
   a. Large DNA
   b. Small DNA
   c. RNA
   d. Protein

69. The sealed cohesive ends are called ____________ which are the sites of cleavage
   a. Terminal proteins
   b. Cos ends
   c. Toxin genes
   d. Phage ends

70. During annealing and ligation of the DNA insert with the λ vector, two or more recombinant vectors may join end to end, producing a

a. Conglomer b. Concatemer
c. Ligation d. Recombination

71. __________is the proper precursor for packaging of λ genome into phage heads

a. Conglomer b. Concatemer
c. Ligation d. Recombination

72. Best vector used for obtaining single-strand copies of cloned DNA which is especially suited for DNA sequencing

a. Shuttle b. Plasmid
c. Bacteriophage d. Phage M13

73. Cosmid vectors are constructed using

a. RecDNA technology b. Replication
c. Transformation d. Transfection

74. Yeast cell wall is enzymatically digested to produce spheroplasts which can take up DNA following treatment with ____________

a. NaCl b. CaCl2
c. MgCl2 d. CsCl

75. In yeast chromosomes, origin of replication is specified by about 100 bp sequences called

a. Ori C b. SV 40
c. ARS d. T-DNA

76. The first animal vector was devised from the ______, a primate papova virus

a. SV40 b. LPV
c. IBR d. Rhabdo

77. These do not replicate

a. SV-40 non-replicating vectors b. SV-40 replicating vectors
c. Both a & b d. None of the above

78. SV 40 Non-replicating vectors only serve as vehicles for transfecting DNAs which become integrated into the host DNA; such vectors are therefore called __________ transfecting vectors.

a. Active b. Non-passive
c. Passive d. Non-active

79. SV 40 Non-replicating vectors only serve as _____ for transfecting DNAs

a. Motors b. Vehicles
c. Template d. Complementary

80. SV 40 Non-replicating vectors only serve as vehicles for transfecting DNAs which become integrated into ____________

a. The vector b. The virus
c. Into the host DNA d. Into the plasmid DNA

81. SV 40 plasmid vectors are used to study the __________ of DNA inserts in monkey cells

a. Expression
b. Cloning
c. Transformation
d. Transfection

82. The DNA copy of retro virusintegrates into the host genome to become

a. Phasmid
b. Provirus
c. Phage
d. Retrovirus

83. The DNA copy of retro virusintegrates into the host genome to becomea provirus which causes _______________ of the cells

a. Temporary transfection
b. Permanent transformation
c. Temporary transfection
d. Permanent transfection

84. Plasmids pTi and pRi of bacteria Agrobacterium tumefaciens andA. rhizogenes, respectively transfer a part of their DNA, called ___________, into the genomes of most plants.

a. P-DNA
b. T-DNA
c. R-DNA
d. i-DNA

85. Plasmids pTi and pRi of bacteria Agrobacterium tumefaciensand A. rhizogenes, respectively transfer a part of their DNA, called T-DNA into the genomes of most plants. This is referred to as _________________

a. Man-made wonder transformation
b. Root transformation
c. Naturally occurring transformation
d. Tandem repeat single stranded DNA

86. The vectors containing DNA inserts are __________________

a. Plasmids
b. Phages
c. Chimaeric
d. Phasmids

87. Treatment with CaC12 makes E.coli____________________ to DNA

a. Resistant
b. Persistent
c. Precipitant
d. Permeable

88. The chimaeric vectors are introduced into a suitable host, this process is termed as

a. Transfection
b. Transformation
c. Cloning
d. Expression

89 In general, the frequency of transformed cells is per __________μg of plasmid DNA

a. 1010 – 1011
b. 1/(1010 – 1011)
c. 106 - 107
d. 1/(106 - 107)

90. In general, the transformation frequency is _______________plasmid molecules

1. 1/100
2. 1/1000
3. 1/10000
4. 1/100000

91. In transient transfection, the introduced gene(s) is (are) gradually lost from the __________ cells of transfected cells

a. Host | b. Vector
c. Transfected | d. Daughter

92. In ________________ transfection, the introduced gene(s) is (are) gradually lost from the daughter cells of transfected cells

a. Stable | b. Transient
c. Permanent | d. Viral

93. In _____________ transfection, the introduced gene(s) is (are) retained and expressed in all the cells derived from the transfected cells

a. Stable | b. Transient
c. Transferred | d. Viral

94. These transfections are ordinarily due to the integration of introduced gene(s) into the cell genome

a. Stable | b. Transient
c. Transferred | d. Viral

95. Stable transfections are ordinarily due to the integration of introduced gene(s) into the ___________

a. Mitochondria | b. Plasmid
c. Genome | d. Nucleus

96. The delivery of DNA into cells using liposomes is called

a. Lipolysis | b. Lipofection
c. Liposomification | d. Lipoformation

97. Transfection mixture containing cells and DNA is exposed to very brief period to a very high voltage gradient. This process is called _______

a. Power exposure | b. Electrofection
c. Electroporation | d. Electroporosis

98. DNA solution is injected directly into the nucleus of a cell or into the male pronucleus of a fertilized one- to two-cell ovum in this process

a. Microfection | b. Microjection
c. Microinjection | d. Microformation

99. In microinjection DNA solution is injected directly into the nucleus of a cell or into the male pronucleus of a fertilized one- to two-cell ovum

a. Nucleus
b. Male pronucleus of a fertilized ovum
c. None
d. Both a & b

100. From which stage of development, Mouse embryonic stem (ES) cells are produced

a. Blastocyst | b. Gastrulation
c. Fetal | d. Neural tube

101. Key property of mouse ES cells
   a. Only differentiate into muscle cells
   b. Differentiate into any cell type in the body
   c. Divide indefinitely without losing their ability to divide
   d. Forming complete organism on their own
102. Targeted gene transfer aims to accomplish one of the following
   a. Amplification of a specific gene in the genome
   b. Silencing of a specific gene in the genome
   c. Replacement of a specific gene with a desired version
   d. Random integration of a transgene into the genome
103. Homologous recombination, used in targeted gene transfer, involves
   a. The transgene and target gene sharing very similar flanking regions
   b. The transgene and target gene having completely different sequences
   c. The transgene directly replacing the target gene without any cellular processes
   d. The transgene integrating into the genome at a random location
104. Alternative method for targeted gene editing with potentially higher efficiency is
   a. DNA methylation
   b. Restriction enzyme digestion
   c. Southern blotting
   d. CRISPR-Cas9
105. Potential risk of targeted gene transfer
   a. Unwanted mutations
   b. No potential off-target effects
   c. Off target integration may disrupt the function of other genes
   d. Risk only in germline editing
106. Which of the statement below is incorrect about plasmids
   a. Extrachromosomal DNA molecules
   b. Replicate independently of chromosomal DNA
   c. Carry genes for antibiotic resistance
   d. Found in the nucleus of eukaryotic cells
107. Which of the following is the advantage of plasmids that helps in genetic engineering
   a. Plasmids are the main genetic material of the cell
   b. Plasmids contain essential genes for survival
   c. Plasmids are too large to be manipulated
   d. Plasmids can be easily transferred between organisms
108. Ori on a plasmid is responsible for
   a. Antibiotic resistance
   b. Initiation of replication of plasmid DNA
   c. Protein synthesis
   d. Attachment of plasmid to the bacterial chromosome

109. How a restriction enzyme recognizes and cuts the DNA?
   a. By overall length of the DNA
   b. Presence of specific chemical modifications on the bases
   c. Random interaction with DNA back bone
   d. Identifying the palindrome and making hydrogen bonds with DNA
110. Restriction endonucleases are believed to have evolved in bacteria as a defence mechanism against
   a. Mutations in their own DNA
   b. Antibiotic production by other bacteria
   c. Viral infection
   d. Predation by other organisms
111. How the sticky ends can be best defined
   a. Blunt ends with no overhangs
   b. Covalently linked DNA segments
   c. Single stranded overhangs on complementary DNA ends
   d. Inactive fragments of the enzyme
112. How Type II restriction endonucleases differ from Type I?
   a. Require ATP for activity
   b. Generate fragments with blunt ends
   c. These are multi sub-unit enzyme complexes
   d. Cut DNA at a distance from recognition sequence
113. pBR322 contains genes for resistance to
   a. Kanamycin b. Ampicillin and tetracycline
   c. Chloramphenicol d. Streptomycin
114. pBR322 is a/an
   a. Original bacterial plasmid b. Modified bacterial plasmid
   c. Viral genome d. Transposon
115. Which one of the following is NOT a feature of pBR322?
   a. Relaxed ori b. Resistance to tetracyclin
   c. Resistance to ampicillin d. High Moleular weight DNA
116. The sticky ends produced by EcoRI are with
   a. Blunt ends b. 5' overhangs
   c. 3'overhangs d. None of the above
117. pUC7 is
   a. Restriction endonuclease b. Cloning vector
   c. Antibiotic resistance gene d. Natural plasmid
118. Purpose of the 'lacZ' alpha fragment in pUC7
   a. Replication of the plasmid b. Expression of the inserted gene
   c. Blue/white color screening d. Both b & c

119. Primary function of terminase
    a. Replication of DNA
    b. Package of DNA into phage capsid
    c. Transcription of RNA
    d. Restriction of foreign DNA
120. Mutation in the terminase gene causes
    a. Increased viral replication rate
    b. Production of non-functional phage particles
    c. Enhanced host immune response
    d. Earlier lysis of the host cell
121. Genetic material of Phage M13 vectors
    a. dsDNA   b. ssDNA
    c. ssRNA   d. dsRNA
122. M13 infects bacterial cells through
    a. Cos site   b. R pilus
    c. F pilus   d. Endocytocis
123. M13 vectors replicate in the host cellvia
    a. Lytic cycle only   b. Lysigenic cycle only
    b. Both a & b   c. Neither a nor b
124. Cosmids are a hybrid of
    a. Plasmid and bacteria   b. Plasmid and virus
    c. Plasmid and bacteriophage   d. Plasmid and yeast
125. Advantage of cosmids are the ability to hold __________DNA fragments
    a. Very small   b. Any size
    c. Extremely large   d. Extremely large
126. Recombinant cosmid clones are identified by
    a. Electron microscopy   b. DNA fingerprinting
    c. Plaque formation   d. Antibiotic resistance screening
127. Function of cos sites in cosmids
    a. Origin of replication
    b. Restriction endonucleases recognition sites
    c. Antibiotic resistance site
    d. Packaging of DNA into phase caspids
128. Compared to Bacterial Artificial Chromosomes (BACs), cosmids offer the advantage of
    a. Higher insert capacity   b. Greater stability of the insert
    c. Easy library construction   d. More manipulation techniques
129. pSC101 belongs to the class of replicons known as
    a. Cosmids   b. Transposons
    c. Plasmids   d. Episomes

130. Marker gene of pSC101 confers resistance to
   a. Ampicillin
   b. Kanamycin
   c. Tetracycline
   d. Chloramphenicol
131. Type III restriction endonucleases are known for
   a. Playing role in DNA repair
   b. Randomly cleaving DNA molecules
   c. Generated blunt DNA after DNA cleavage
   d. Mediating DNA target methylation
132. Effect of poison sequence in a cell
   a. Decreases protein production
   b. Disrupts DNA repair
   c. Disrupts cell division
   d. Triggers cell death
133. Concatemers are most commonly formed from ___________ DNA
   a. Nucleolar
   b. Cytoplasmic
   c. Chromosomal
   d. Plasmid
134. The approximate size of foreign DNA a cosmid vector can accept is
   a. 2-5 kb
   b. 10-20 kb
   c. 35-45 kb
   d. 50-100 kb
135. In the process of transformation, the competent cells are treated with which of the following
   a. Detergents to weaken cell wall
   b. Heat shock
   c. Antibiotics to kill non-transformed cells
   d. Enzymes to degrade plasmid
136. The primary function of a cloning site in a vector used for transformation?
   a. Replication of the vector inside the host cell
   b. Selection of transformed cells
   c. Insertion of foreign DNA
   d. Packaging of vector into viral particles
137. Gene therapy involves
   a. Tailoring genes of a patient to treat a disease
   b. Treating a patient with genetic mutations with antibiotics
   c. Curtailing the gene mutations by effected part removal
   d. Transferring the blood of patient with non-mutated blood
138. Find the odd man out regarding gene therapy
   a. Adeno virus
   b. Retro virus
   c. Plasmid
   d. Antibiotics
139. First ailment successfully treated with gene therapy
   a. Sickle cell anemia
   b. SCID
   c. Down syndrome
   d. Cystic fibrosis

140. Who among the following did not receive Nobel Prize for Physiology and Medicine in 1978 for the discovery of endonucleases
   a. Smith
   b. Bayer
   c. Nathan
   d. Arber

141. Why are restriction endonucleases indispensible for gene cloning
   a. They amplify the desired gene insert
   b. They degrade unwanted DNA in gene cloning process
   c. They create sticky ends that facilitate joining of DNA fragments
   d. They identify specific gene sequences which need repair

142. Restriction endonucleases recognize and cut DNA at
   a. A-T rich regions
   b. Random places on DNA
   c. Long repetitive sequences
   d. Short specific sequences

143. What property of restriction endonucleases is exploited to isolate a specific gene
   a. Ability to lyse the DNA randomly
   b. Ability to recognize specific DNA sequences
   c. Ability to clear RNA from the desired site
   d. Ability to amplify DNA at random

144. Restriction endonucleases are produced by
   a. Bacteriophages to get protection against viruses
   b. Yeast cells to get protected from bacteria
   c. Bacteria to get protected from viruses
   d. Animal cells to get protected from bacteriophages

145. Staggered of restriction endonucleases are characterized by
   a. Perfect blunt end DNAs
   b. Single cut on a strand with utmost specificity
   c. Multiple random cuts all through the template
   d. Single stranded overhangs on both DNA fragments

146. Which of the following is NOT a major application of recombinant DNA technology?
   a. Production of insulin
   b. Development of pest resistant crops
   c. Gene therapy for treating genetic diseases
   d. Forensic analysis

147. Feature of lambda phage that makes it a useful vector
   a. Can integrate its DNA into host bacterial chromosome
   b. Single stranded DNA genome
   c. Very large genome size
   d. Replicates slowly inside the host

148. When a plasmid and foreign DNA are cut with the same restriction enzyme, what process allows them to join together?
   a. Replication b. Transformation
   c. Ligation d. rec DNA technology

149. In gene therapy, a modified virus might be used to deliver a therapeutic gene to a patient's cells. What part of the virus would most likely be used?
   a. Entire viral genome b. Viral capsid
   c. Envelope d. Tail

150. After a plasmid and a foreign DNA fragment are cut with compatible restriction enzymes, DNA ligase is used to
   a. Separate the cut fragments by size
   b. Reattach the sticky ends of the plasma
   c. Denature the DNA strants
   d. Translation to proteins

Answer Key

1	b	2	d	3	d	4	c	5	b	6	d	7	a
8	d	9	b	10	d	11	b	12	a	13	c	14	b
15	c	16	d	17	a	18	d	19	b	20	c	21	c
22	d	23	c	24	a	25	b	26	d	27	d	28	a
29	c	30	b	31	d	32	d	33	d	34	a	35	c
36	d	37	d	38	c	39	b	40	a	41	a	42	c
43	c	44	c	45	a	46	c	47	d	48	c	49	b
50	a	51	d	52	c	53	c	54	a	55	b	56	c
57	b	58	b	59	c	60	b	61	b	62	b	63	a
64	d	65	d	66	c	67	d	68	a	69	b	70	b
71	b	72	d	73	a	74	b	75	c	76	a	77	a
78	c	79	b	80	c	81	b	82	b	83	d	84	b
85	c	86	c	87	d	88	b	89	c	90	c	91	s
92	b	93	a	94	a	95	c	96	b	97	c	98	c
99	d	100	a	101	b	102	c	103	a	104	d	105	c
106	d	107	d	108	b	109	d	110	c	111	c	112	d
113	b	114	b	115	d	116	c	117	b	118	d	119	b
120	b	121	b	122	c	123	a	124	c	125	c	126	d
127	d	128	c	129	d	130	a	131	d	132	c	133	d
134	c	135	b	136	c	137	a	138	d	139	d	140	b
141	c	142	d	143	b	144	c	145	d	146	b	147	a
148	c	149	b	150	b								

21

Molecular Biology Techniques

Roshan Mohiddin[1] and Mohammed Hasif Ganimattoullah[2]

[1]Division of Biochemistry, ICAR-NDRI, Karnal, Harayana.

[2]Institute of Veterinary Science and Animal Husbandry, Siksha O Anusandhan University, Bhubneshwar, Orissa

Introduction

Biochemical techniques are fundamental tools that allow scientists to investigate the molecular intricacies of biological systems, including DNA, RNA, and proteins. These techniques are essential for understanding cellular processes, genetic functions, and disease mechanisms. By employing biochemical methods, researchers can dissect complex biological systems at the molecular, cellular, and genomic levels, paving the way for advances in basic biology and therapeutic interventions.

Key Techniques and Their Applications

1. **Enzyme Reverse Transcriptase and cDNA Synthesis**
   a. Function: Converts RNA into complementary DNA (cDNA).
   b. Applications include reverse transcription PCR (RT-PCR), gene expression studies, viral diagnostics, and RNA virus research.
2. **Polymerase Chain Reaction (PCR)**
   a. Function: amplifies specific DNA sequences.
   b. Applications include genetic profiling, mutation analysis, forensic science, and infectious disease diagnostics.
3. **Protein Separation and SDS-PAGE**
   a. Function: Separates proteins by size and charge.
   b. applications include protein purity analysis, molecular weight determination, and post-translational modification studies.
4. **Southern Blotting for DNA Detection**
   a. Function: Detects specific DNA sequences within complex samples.
   b. Applications include genetic mapping, mutation detection, and genetic variability studies.
5. **Editing the CRISPR-Cas9 genome**
   a. Function: Precisely modifies DNA sequences.
   b. Applications include gene therapy, genetic engineering, and functional genomics.

6. **Quantitative Real-Time PCR (qRT-PCR)**
   a. Function: Measures gene expression levels.
   b. Applications include gene regulation studies, disease biomarker identification, and drug efficacy testing.
7. **Sanger Sequencing for DNA Analysis**
   a. Function: Determines DNA's nucleotide sequence.
   b. Applications include genetic analysis, variant confirmation, and validation of high-throughput sequencing results.
8. **Chromatin Immunoprecipitation (ChIP)**
   a. Function: Explores protein-DNA interactions within chromatin.
   b. Applications: mapping transcription factor binding sites and histone modifications; studying gene regulation mechanisms.
9. **Next-Generation Sequencing (NGS)**
   a. Function: high-throughput sequencing of DNA and RNA.
   b. Applications include comprehensive genomic, transcriptomic, and epigenomic analyses.
10. **Northern Blotting for RNA Analysis**
    a. Function: Detects and quantifies specific RNA molecules.
    b. Applications include gene expression pattern analysis and mRNA abundance studies.
11. **Western Blotting for Protein Detection**
    a. Function: Detects specific proteins based on size and antigenicity.
    b. Applications include protein characterization, studying protein-protein interactions, and assessing post-translational modifications.
12. **Lateral Flow Immunoassays for Rapid Diagnostics.**
    a. Function: Detects specific biomolecules quickly.
    b. Applications include point-of-care diagnostics, environmental monitoring, and food safety testing.
13. **Enzyme-Linked Immunosorbent Assay (ELISA)**
    a. Function: Detects and quantifies proteins, antibodies, and other analytes.
    b. Applications include clinical diagnostics, biomarker discovery, and drug development.
14. **RNA sequencing (RNA-Seq) for transcriptome analysis**
    a. Function: Analyzes the transcriptome for gene expression profiles.
    b. Applications include developmental biology, cancer research, and personalized medicine.
15. **Protein Interaction Studies: Co-Immunoprecipitation (Co-IP)**
    a. Function: Investigates protein-protein interactions.
    b. Applications include deciphering signaling pathways and protein trafficking mechanisms.

16. ***In Situ* Hybridization (ISH) for Spatial Gene Expression Analysis**
    a. Function: visualizes and localizes specific nucleic acid sequences in tissues or cells.
    b. Applications: developmental biology, neuroscience, and pathology.
17. **Assay for Transposase-Accessible Chromatin Using Sequencing (ATAC-Seq)**
    a. Function: Profile chromatin accessibility across the genome.
    b. Applications include studying regulatory elements, enhancer activity, and gene regulation dynamics.
18. **Bisulfite sequencing for DNA methylation analysis**
    a. Function: Analyzes DNA methylation patterns.
    b. Applications include studies of epigenetic regulation, development, aging, and disease processes.
19. **Fluorescence in Situ Hybridization (FISH) for Genome Visualization**
    a. Function: visualizes and localizes specific DNA or RNA sequences.
    b. Applications include chromosomal abnormality studies, gene expression pattern analysis, and the spatial organization of genomes.
20. **Molecular Interaction Analysis using Surface Plasmon Resonance (SPR)**
    a. Function: Investigates biomolecular interactions in real time.
    b. Applications include drug discovery, protein engineering, and structural biology.
21. **Yeast Two-Hybrid Screening for Protein Interaction Networks**
    a. Function: Identifies protein-protein interactions within living cells.
    b. Applications include high-throughput analysis of protein interaction networks and elucidating cellular pathways.

Conclusion

In conclusion, biochemical techniques are indispensable for exploring the intricate mechanisms governing biological molecules and cellular processes. These methods help us learn a lot about molecular biology, genetics, and disease pathology. They do things like amplifying DNA sequences, finding RNA transcripts, studying protein interactions, and looking at chromatin architecture. By integrating diverse biochemical techniques, researchers continue to push the boundaries of scientific knowledge, paving the way for innovative diagnostics, personalized medicine, and biotechnological advancements that impact human health and well-being.

1. Enzyme reverse transcriptase is used to synthesize:
   a. DNA from cDNA b. RNA from DNA
   c. DNA from RNA d. cDNA from DNA
2. Polymerase Chain Reaction (PCR) is used for?
   a. Sequencing DNA b. Amplifying DNA
   c. Degrading RNA d. Synthesizing proteins
3. Protein can be seperated based on their size and charge by which of the following technique?
   a. SDS Gel electrophoresis b. Southern blotting
   c. Northern blotting d. Western blotting
4. Which technique involves transferring of DNA fragments from gel to membrane followed by probe hybridization?
   a. PCR b. Southern blotting
   c. Northern blotting d. Western blotting
5. Editing of genome by introducing indels can be achieved by which tool?
   a. PCR b. CRISPR-Cas9
   c. Gel electrophoresis d. Sanger sequencing
6. The expression levels of specific genes can be measured using?
   a. PCR b. Western blotting
   c. QRT-PCR (quantitative Real-Time PCR)
7. The reference genes used in Real-Time PCR is also known as?
   a. Coding genes b. Housekeeping genes
   c. Target genes d. Non-coding genes
8. Method used for determining the nucleotide sequence of DNA is known as?
   a. Western blotting b. Gel electrophoresis
   c. Sanger sequencing d. Northern blotting
9. Protein-DNA interactions can be studied by using?
   a. Western blotting b. Southern blotting
   c. Chromatin immunoprecipitation (ChIP) d. Northern blotting
10. Why next-generation sequencing (NGS) is preferred over Sanger sequencing?
    a. Lower cost per base sequenced b. Faster sequencing speed
    c. Higher throughput d. All of the above
11. Typical RNA-Seq workflow doesNOT involves which step?
    a. RNA extraction b. cDNA synthesis
    c. DNA methylation d. Sequencing
12. Cells of a particular characteristic phenotype can be recognized by gene expression analysis through the following technique using radioactive, fluorescent, or luminescent probes. This procedure can be carried out at the cellular level, as in FISH or by in situ hybridization with radioactive probes.
    a. Western blotting b. Southern blotting
    c. Northern blotting d. Eastern blotting

13. Which of the following techniques would be most useful to study gene expression?
    a. Northern blot
    b. Western blot
    c. Southern blot
    d. Eastern blot
14. When performing a western blot, what is the purpose of adding a secondary antibody?
    a. Separate the sample from other proteins
    b. Allow for detection of the protein sample
    c. Ensure that the primary antibody binds properly to the sample
    d. Block any interfering noise coming from the membrane
15. Control line in lateral flow immunoassay consist of what?
    a. Primary antibody
    b. Secondary antibody
    c. capture antibody
    d. None of these
16. The home bioassay for hCG is the best-known application of
    a. Enzyme linked immunoassay
    b. Lateral flow immunoassay
    c. Western blotting
    d. Radioimmunoassay
17. Arrange the following steps about ELISA (Enzyme-linked immunosorbent assay) in chronological order
    i. Incubate with antibody-enzyme complex that binds primary antibody
    ii. Coat surface with antigen, block unoccupied sites with nonspecific protein
    iii. Add substrate, formation of colored product indicates presence of specific antigen
    iv. Incubate with primary antibody against specific antigen
    a. i, iv, ii, iii
    b. i, iv, iii, ii
    c. ii, iv, iii, i
    d. ii, iv, i, iii
18. What is the role of goat anti-rabbit IgG horseradish peroxidase conjugate in the experiment?
    a. Antigen
    b. Primary antibody
    c. Secondary antibody
    d. Substrate
19. Which techniques can be used to specifically quantify transcript isoforms of a gene?
    a. Microarray
    b. RNA-Seq
    c. Northern blotting
    d. Real-time PCR
20. Yeast two-hybrid screening is used for high-throughput analysis of which of the following?
    a. DNA interaction
    b. RNA interaction
    c. Protein interaction
    d. Cell interaction
21. ChIP-Seq methods is most suitable for identifying which of the following modifications across the genome?
    a. Epigenetic modifications
    b. Genetic modifications
    c. Morphological
    d. None of these

22. Sequencing of long DNA fragments and detection nucleotide modifications by using nanopores can be achieved by which sequencing technology?
    a. Illumina sequencing
    b. Sanger sequencing
    c. PacBio sequencing
    d. Oxford Nanopore sequencing
23 Which of the following techniques can be used to perform single-cell RNA sequencing?
    a. bulk RNA-Seq
    b. Single-cell RNA-Seq (scRNA-Seq)
    c. Northern blotting
    d. Western blotting
24. The three-dimensional structure of the genome can be mapped using?
    a. ATAC-Seq
    b. ChIP-Seq
    c. Hi-C
    d. RNA-Seq
25. Which of the following methods allows the visualization of gene expression in the context of tissue morphology?
    a. RNA-Seq
    b. In situ hybridization
    c. Western blotting
    d. Flow cytometry
26. Which CRISPR system component creates cleavage at the target DNA?
    a. crRNA
    b. tracrRNA
    c. Cas9
    d. gRNA
27. Which of the following method is used for the detection and quantification of DNA methylation at single-base resolution?
    a. Bisulfite sequencing
    b. chIP-Seq
    c. RNA-Seq
    d. aTAC-Seq
28. Choose the efficient method that is used to study protein-DNA interactions at a genome-wide level
    a. Electrophoretic mobility shift assay (EMSA)
    b. Chromatin immunoprecipitation followed by sequencing (ChIP-Seq)
    c. Western blotting
    d. Co-immunoprecipitation (Co-IP)
29. What is the main advantage of using RNA-Seq over microarrays for transcriptome analysis?
    a. Lower cost
    b. Higher sensitivity and dynamic range
    c. Requires less input RNA
    d. Simpler data analysis

30. Protein-protein interactions in vivo can be identified by which of the following methods?
    a. Co-immunoprecipitation
    b. Yeast two-hybrid assay
    c. FRET (Förster resonance energy transfer)
    d. Surface plasmon resonance (SPR)
31. Alternative splicing events can be detected using?
    a. Western blotting b. Northern blotting
    c. RNA-Seq d. ELISA
32. In a given fixed cells or tissue section, which method can be applied to detect DNA or RNA sequences using fluorescently labeled nucleotides?
    a. Flow cytometry
    b. Fluorescence in situ hybridization (FISH)
    c. ELISA
    d. PCR
33. Ion Torrent Sequencing relies on release of which ion during DNA synthesis?
    a. Oxygen b. Carbon
    c. Hydrogen d. Chlorine
34. Which of the following statements best describes the versatility of the CRISPR-Cas9 system in terms of genome editing and, transcriptional regulation.?
    a. CRISPR-Cas9 is only limited to genome editing.
    b. CRISPR-Cas9 is only limited to transcriptional regulation.
    c. CRISPR-Cas9 can be implied for different applications by editing the targeted proteins or guide RNAs.
    d. CRISPR-Cas9 is mainly related for protein-protein interaction studies.
35. RNA-Seq enables the thorough examination of the transcriptome, which involves detecting new transcripts, alternative splicing occurrences, and measuring gene expression levels. What is a key benefit of RNA-Seq compared to conventional microarray methods?
    a. Known transcripts are the only ones that RNA-Seq can identify.
    b. The ability of RNA-Seq to detect gene expression has a lower dynamic range.
    c. RNA-Seq offers a more comprehensive and detailed view of the transcriptome, including novel transcripts and splice variants.
    d. Compared to microarrays, RNA-Seq requires a smaller amount of RNA input.
36. ChIP-Seq, also known as Chromatin Immunoprecipitation Sequencing, is an effective method for examining protein-DNA interactions across the entire genome. Identify the critical step in the ChIP-Seq process.
    a. Extraction of RNA from cells or tissues.
    b. Utilization of antibodies to isolate DNA-bound proteins.
    c. assessment of the absorbance of DNA-protein complexes.
    d. Execution of PCR amplification for the complete genome.

37. Hi-C is a method utilized to analyze the three-dimensional arrangement of the genome by detecting chromatin interactions.What most accurately characterizes the main objective of Hi-C?
    a. Quantifying gene expression levels.
    b. Recognizing protein-protein interactions.
    c. Mapping physical interactions among various regions of the genome.
    d. Sequencing the complete genome.
38. ATAC-Seq (Assay for Transposase-Accessible Chromatin using sequencing) is employed for the examination of chromatin accessibility. How does ATAC-Seq provide information about chromatin structure?
    a. It identifies mutations by sequencing the entire genome.
    b. Sequencing adapters are inserted into open chromatin regions using a transposase enzyme, enabling the sequencing and analysis of these regions.
    c. Gene expression levels are measured by amplifying RNA.
    d. Histone modifications are detected using antibodies.
39. What is a major benefit of using scRNA-Seq compared to bulk RNA-Seq?
    a. SCRNA-Seq gives a comprehensive insight into cell-to-cell diversity in gene expression.
    b. SCRNA-Seq enables the analysis of gene expression at the individual cell level.
    c. SCRNA-Seq is more cost-effective than bulk RNA-Seq.
    d. SCRNA-Seq is compatible with both prokaryotic and eukaryotic cells.
40. How bisulfite sequencing works can best be described by which of the following?
    a. Precipitating methylated DNA with the use of antibodies.
    b. Chemically converting unmethylated cytosines to uracil and leaving methylated cytosines unchanged, enabling subsequent sequencing to ascertain methylation status.
    c. Amplifying methylated regions of the genome through PCR.
    d. Assessing the fluorescence of methylated DNA.
41. RNA interference (RNAi) enables the specific reduction of gene expression. What accurately explains the mechanism of RNAi is:
    a. The use of antibodies in RNAi leads to the degradation of target mRNA.
    b. RNAi entails introducing double-stranded RNA (dsRNA. that gets processed into small interfering RNAs (siRNAs), which then guide the RNA-induced silencing complex (RISC. To degrade complementary mRNA.
    c. In RNAi, the target mRNA is amplified to enhance its expression.
    d. RNAi directly causes mutations in the DNA of the target gene.

42. What is the primary use of FACS, a specialized form of flow cytometry used for separating cells based on specific traits?
    a. Assessing protein-DNA interactions.
    b. Separating a mixed population of cells into distinct groups based on the presence of fluorescent markers.
    c. Analyzing the complete genome of an individual cell.
    d. Amplifying RNA for studying gene expression.

43 How would you describe the mechanism of CRISPR interference (CRISPRi)?Which option provides the best description of the mechanism of CRISPRi?
    a. CRISPRi involves using a catalytically inactive Cas9 (dCas9) protein fused to a repressor domain. It is guided by a specific gRNA to the target gene promoter, leading to the inhibition of transcription.
    b. CRISPRi involves degrading the target mRNA using siRNAs.
    c. CRISPRi involves amplifying the target gene using PCR.
    d. CRISPRi involves directly introducing mutations into the target gene.

44. What method would you employ and for what reasons in order to assess the levels of expression for a particular gene across various tissue samples?
    a. Western blotting b. Northern
    c. Real-time PCR (qPCR) d. Gel electrophoresis

45. You have completed the sequencing of a bacterial genome and have the raw sequencing reads. What's the next step in assembling the genome?
    a. Perform PCR amplification
    b. Use a genome assembly software like SPAdes or Velvet
    c. Run a gel electrophoresis
    d. Perform a Western blot

46. What technique should be used to detect protein-DNA interactions in the sample?
    a. chIP-Seq b. RNA-Seq
    c. Southern blotting d. FISH

47 In the study of how a mutation affects protein function, what method would you employ to examine protein expression and any alterations in protein size?
    a. Northern blotting b. Real-time PCR
    c. Western blotting d. Gel electrophoresis

48. What technique would offer the most extensive data for studying the global gene expression profile of a tumor sample?
    a. Microarray b. RNA-Seq
    c. qPCR d. Northern blotting

49. What technique would you employ to visualize the localization of a specific mRNA within a tissue section?
    a. Western blotting b. Flow cytometry
    c. In situ hybridization (ISH) d. RNA-Seq

50 You have found a mutation in a gene and need to ascertain its impact on the gene's transcription levels. What approach should you employ to compare the transcription levels in wild-type and mutant samples?

a. Gel electrophoresis
b. QRT-PCR (quantitative Real-Time PCR)
c. ChIP-Seq
d. Western blotting

51. Which method would you employ to ascertain if one protein interacts with another protein within living cells?

a. Western blotting
b. Co-immunoprecipitation (Co-IP)
c. Southern blotting
d. RNA-Seq

52. Which method could be used to validate the binding of a regulatory protein to the gene's promoter region in living cells?

a. RNA-Seq
b. Gel electrophoresis
c. CHIP (Chromatin Immunoprecipitation)
d. Western blotting

53. How would you isolate a specific cell type from a sample containing various cell types based on surface markers?

a. Gel electrophoresis
b. FACS (Fluorescence-Activated Cell Sorting)
c. Northern blotting
d. Western blotting

54. What technique would you utilize to ascertain the methylation status of particular DNA regions in your sample?

a. Bisulfite sequencing
b. CHIP-Seq
c. RNA-Seq
d. QRT-PCR

55. In designing an experiment to express a protein in yeast and incorporating a fluorescent tag for visualization, what characteristic should the linker possess to guarantee proper function in yeast?

a. Specific promoter for yeast
b. Signal peptide designed for secretion
c. Fluorescent tag sequence and restriction sites
d. Multiple cloning site (MCS)

56. In the process of conducting a Western blot to identify a particular protein in cell lysates, you notice a lack of signal even though you have followed the procedure. Which of the following is the least probable reason for this?

a. Use of an incorrect primary antibody
b. Inadequate transfer of protein from the gel to the membrane
c. Presence of a high concentration of blocking agent
d. Overexposure of the film

57. After effectively transferring proteins onto a membrane for a Western blot, you notice non-specific binding of your secondary antibody. What step can you improve to minimize this non-specific binding?

 a. Boost the quantity of primary antibody
 b. Lessen the duration of washing
 c. Employ an alternative blocking agent
 d. Extend the duration of gel electrophoresis running

58. During In case of failure to detect the target DNA fragment during a Southern blot, which step is crucial to ensure the successful transfer of DNA from the gel to the membrane?

 a. Using a blocking agent
 b. Ensuring proper denaturation of DNA
 c. Adding primary antibody
 d. Utilizing a secondary antibody

59. In a Northern blot to assess RNA expression levels, if you observe that the RNA has degraded after transfer, the probable cause of this issue is:

 a. Utilization of a non-denaturing gel
 b. Presence of RNase contamination
 c. Insufficient blocking of the membrane
 d. Overloading the gel

60. In a Western blot experiment, several bands at various molecular weights are observed, despite anticipating only one band for the target protein. What is the least likely explanation for this observation?

 a. The protein undergoing post-translational modifications
 b. Protein degradation occurring
 c. The antibody displaying cross-reactivity
 d. Error in diluting the primary antibody

61. In the process of setting up a Western blot to compare protein expression levels between two samples, what is the best method to guarantee equal loading of protein in each lane?

 a. Measuring the volume of each sample
 b. Utilizing a loading control antibody
 c. Visually estimating protein concentration
 d. Normalizing protein concentration using a BSA standard curve

62. During In the course of a Southern blot, instead of clear bands, you notice a blurred signal. What is the probable reason for this outcome from the options provided?

 a. DNA restriction digestion not being completed properly
 b. Excessive concentration of blocking agent
 c. Film being exposed for too long
 d. Membrane being washed inadequately

63 In order to enhance the detection sensitivity for a low-abundance protein using Western blotting, which adjustment to the protocol would be most likely beneficial?

a. Increasing the amount of blocking agent
b. Employing a more sensitive detection system
c. Decreasing the primary antibody concentration
d. Reducing the film exposure time

64. In an experiment involving Northern blotting, the goal is to differentiate between various splice variants of an mRNA. What type of probe design would be the most efficient for this purpose?

a. A probe that targets the common exon
b. A probe that targets the intronic sequence
c. A probe that targets the unique exons
d. A probe that targets the 5' untranslated region (UTR)

65. In case of high background signal while using a DIG-labeled probe for a Southern blot, the optimization of which step could help reduce this background?

a. Enhancing the concentration of the DIG-labeled probe
b. Raising the hybridization temperature
c. Lowering the stringency of the washes
d. Employing a more concentrated blocking agent

66. In troubleshooting a Western blot with high background noise and faint bands, which modification is the least likely to help resolve this issue?

a. Extending the washing time
b. Employing a more specific primary antibody
c. Reducing the concentration of the blocking agent
d. Adjusting the secondary antibody concentration

67. To successfully insert the DNA fragment with blunt ends into a plasmid vector with sticky ends, which approach would be most effective?

a. Select a different vector with blunt ends
b. attach adapters containing sticky ends to the fragment
c. Utilize a restriction enzyme to generate sticky ends on the fragment
d. Employ a ligase specific for blunt ends

68. For downstream cloning applications, if you want to add a specific sequence at the ends of your PCR products, which technique should you employ?

a. Implement restriction enzymes
b. Utilize PCR with primers that have linker sequences
c. Apply ligase directly on PCR products
d. Employ exonuclease to generate overhangs

69 In a cloning experiment, it is important to ensure that the cloned fragment is inserted in the correct orientation. Which method would be most helpful for achieving this?

a. Using blunt-end cloning

b. Using linkers with different restriction enzyme sites

c. Using a single restriction enzyme site

d. Using PCR with specific primers

70. To attach a synthetic DNA oligonucleotide to a plasmid vector, but the oligonucleotide doesn't have the required restriction sites. Which method can be utilized to incorporate these sites?

a. Employ a blunt-end ligase

b. Attach linkers with restriction sites to the oligonucleotide

c. Carry out site-directed mutagenesis

d. Utilize exonuclease to generate sticky ends

71. You have created a cDNA library and now you have to insert the cDNA fragments into a cloning vector. What is the function of adapters in this procedure?

a. They boost the effectiveness of the reverse transcription process

b. They introduce particular restriction sites to aid in cloning

c. They assist in identifying recombinant clones

d. They alter the vector to enhance its stability

72. When adding a restriction site to a DNA fragment using a linker, you observe low ligation efficiency. Which factor is the least likely cause of this problem?

a. The linker being incompletely digested

b. The linkers being at a high concentration relative to the DNA fragment

c. The use of a blunt-end ligase

d. The linker being annealed at an incorrect temperature

73. To effectively remove adapters from the ends of your DNA fragments after ligation, which method would be the most suitable?

a. Purifying the DNA fragments using gel purification

b. Amplifying the DNA fragments using PCR

c. Digesting the DNA with restriction enzymes

d. Treating the DNA fragments with exonucleases

74 In the design of a cloning vector, if you want to include a site for later addition of a tag to the expressed protein, which element should be incorporated into the vector?

a. An adapter with a restriction site

b. A linker containing a tag sequence and restriction sites

c. Multiple cloning site (MCS)

d. Strong promoter

75. Ligating multiple DNA fragments together in a specific order requires a strategy involving linkers or adapters. To achieve this, which of the following methods would be useful?
    a. Employ adapters with identical restriction sites
    b. Use linkers with unique restriction sites for each fragment
    c. Perform blunt-end ligation for all fragments
    d. Utilize PCR to amplify all fragments together
76. In the process of next-generation sequencing (NGS) library preparation, you require the attachment of sequencing adapters to your DNA fragments. What is the main purpose of these adapters?
    a. To improve the stability of the DNA fragments
    b. To insert specific restriction sites for cloning
    c. To enable easy attachment to the sequencing platform
    d. To increase the amplification efficiency
77. You are encountering poor ligation efficiency when ligating adapters to your DNA fragments during NGS library preparation. Among the following options, which one is the LEAST likely to enhance the ligation efficiency?
    a. Raising the concentration of adapters
    b. Using a higher fidelity DNA polymerase
    c. Fine-tuning the ligase enzyme concentration
    d. Confirming that the DNA fragments have compatible ends
78. When designing linkers for cloning a gene into an expression vector, it is crucial to prevent the introduction of unwanted stop codons. How can this be accomplished?
    a. Opt for blunt-end linkers
    b. Create linkers with a reading frame that aligns with the gene
    c. Employ a robust promoter
    d. Incorporate multiple cloning sites
79. You have cloned a DNA fragment with adapters into a vector and now need to confirm successful ligation. What method would be used to verify this?
    a. Verifying through PCR amplification using adapter-specific primers
    b. Using gel electrophoresis to confirm the ligation reaction
    c. Checking the vector-insert junctions by sequencing
    d. All of the above
80. What cloning strategy would you select for inserting a DNA fragment into a vector without adding extra sequences?
    a. Blunt-end cloning
    b. Linker-mediated cloning
    c. Adapter-mediated cloning
    d. TA cloning

81. You are currently planning an experiment to introduce a protein into yeast and would like to incorporate a linker to attach a fluorescent tag for visualization purposes. What characteristic should the linker possess to guarantee proper functionality in yeast?
    a. Yeast-specific promoter
    b. Signal peptide for secretion
    c. Fluorescent tag sequence and restriction sites
    d. Multiple cloning site (MCS)
82. You After conducting a Southern blot to identify a specific DNA sequence in a sample, you notice the absence of a signal after transferring the DNA to the membrane and using a labeled probe for hybridization. Which among the options provided is the least likely cause of this problem?
    a. Proper transfer of the DNA to the membrane did not occur
    b. The probe's sequence does not correspond to the target DNA
    c. The labeling of the probe was incorrect
    d. Lack of membrane washing post hybridization
83. During a Western blot experiment, observing multiple bands at varying molecular weights when investigating a single protein could be explained by any of the following:
    a. The primary antibody binding non-specifically
    b. Inadequate transfer of proteins to the membrane
    c. Degradation of the specific protein
    d. All of the above
84. When using Northern blotting to compare the expression levels of a specific mRNA across different samples, what control should be included to ensure the validity of the results?
    a. A DNA ladder
    b. A housekeeping gene mRNA
    c. An unrelated protein probe
    d. An empty lane
85. In a Western blot experiment, high background signal is seen on the membrane. What step is most likely to reduce this background?
    a. Increase the concentration of the primary antibody
    b. Reduce the blocking time
    c. Ensure the membrane is washed more thoroughly
    d. Use a higher concentration of the secondary antibody
86 In a Western blot, you are using a chemiluminescent substrate for detection. When the blot is developed, the signal appears to be very weak. What could potentially enhance the detection signal among the provided choices? Could it be
    a. Shortening the exposure time
    b. Increasing the concentration of the chemiluminescent substrate
    c. Using a more sensitive film or detector
    d. Reducing the amount of secondary antibody

87. In During a Southern blot experiment, genomic DNA was digested using a restriction enzyme before electrophoresis, leading to the observation of unexpected band patterns. What factors could account for these unexpected results?
    a. Incomplete cutting of the DNA by the restriction enzyme
    b. Hybridization of the probe to multiple genomic locations
    c. Degradation of the DNA prior to digestion
    d. All of the above

88. You have to clone a piece of DNA into a vector without adding any more sequences to it. Which method of cloning would you pick?
    a. Cone with blunt ends b. TA cloning
    c. Adapter-mediated cloning d. linker-mediated cloning

89. Finding the chromatin accessibility across the genome in your sample is what you are interested in. For this objective, which method would be most suitable?
    a. RNA-Seq b. CHIP-Seq
    c. ATAC-Seq d. FISH

90. For measuring the binding affinity of a protein-DNA interaction, the technique that would provide quantitative data is?
    a. Electrophoretic mobility shift assay (EMSA)
    b. Western blotting
    c. Surface plasmon resonance (SPR)
    d. RNA-Seq

91. For studying the genome-wide DNA methylation patterns in a sample the most efficient technique would be?
    a. ATAC-Seq b. CHIP-Seq
    c. bisulfite sequencing d. RNA-Seq

92. Technique used for mapping the three-dimensional organization of the genome in cells is?
    a. CHIP-Seq b. RNA-Seq
    c. Hi-C d. ATAC-Seq

93. Choose the technique best suited to determine the sequence of a small RNA molecule:
    a. Western b. RNA-Seq
    c. Northern d. Sanger sequencing

94. Technique used for identification of transcription factor binding sites across the genome is?
    a. RNA-Seq b. CHIP-Seq
    c. ATAC-Seq d. Northern blotting

95. Which technique can provide the most comprehensive analysis of effect of drug on the entire transcriptome of cancer cells ?
    a. Microarray b. Western blotting
    c. RNA-Seq d. QPCR

96. How you can validate the differential expression of a few candidate genes identified by RNA-Seq?
    a. Western blotting b. QRT-PCR
    c. CHIP-Seq d. FISH

97. Technique used to determine the spatial organization of specific RNA molecules within cells is?
    a. RNA-Seq b. CHIP-Seq
    c. In situ hybridization (ISH) d. Western blotting

98. What technique can be used to determine the protein expression profile of a cell line under different conditions?
    a. Northern blotting b. RNA-Seq
    c. Western blotting d. CHIP-Seq

99. You study the regulatory elements of a specific gene. What technique can you use to identify enhancer regions associated with this gene?
    a. aTAC-Seq
    b. RNA-Seq
    c. ChIP-Seq with antibodies against histone modifications associated with enhancers
    d. Sanger sequencing

100. You suspect that a specific RNA-binding protein is involved in mRNA splicing. Which technique would you use to identify the RNA targets of this protein?
    a. RNA-Seq
    b. Western blotting
    c. CLIP-Seq (Crosslinking and Immunoprecipitation Sequencing)
    d. FISH

101. To isolate a pure population of cells with a specific surface marker from a mixed cell sample, which technique is most suitable?
    a. Gel electrophoresis
    b. qRT-PCR
    c. FACS (Fluorescence-Activated Cell Sorting)
    d. Western blotting

102. To analyze the methylation status of various CpG sites within a gene promoter, which technique would you use?
    a. RNA-Seq b. CHIP-Seq
    c. Bisulfite sequencing d. ATAC-Seq

103. To understand the functional impact of a genome-wide association study (GWAS) finding, which technique links the genetic variant to a specific regulatory element?
    a. Hi-C b. ATAC-Seq
    c. CRISPR-Cas9 d. eQTL mapping

104. To identify and confirm the interaction between a long non-coding RNA (lncRNAand a specific protein, which technique should be used?

a. RNA immunoprecipitation (RIP) b. RNA-Seq

c. CHIP-Seq d. Hi-C

105. Which technique allows the measurement of mRNA association with ribosomes to determine global translational efficiency?

a. RNA-Seq b. Ribosome profiling (Ribo-Seq)

C. chIP-Seq d. qRT-PCR

106. For the highest resolution map of chromatin contacts to study chromatin organization in the nucleus, which technique is used?

a. Hi-C b. CHIA-PET

c. ATAC-Seq d. RNA-Seq

107. To determine the phosphorylation status of a specific protein under different conditions, which technique would you use?

a. Western blotting with phospho-specific antibodies

b. RNA-Seq

c. ATAC-Seq

d. QRT-PCR

108. Which technique provides single-cell resolution of chromatin accessibility to study the epigenome of immune cells?

a. Bulk ATAC-Seq

b. Single-cell ATAC-Seq (scATAC-Seq)

c. RNA-Seq

d. CHIP-Seq

109. To analyze the global distribution and abundance of post-translational modifications on proteins, which high-throughput technique is best?

a. Western blotting

b. Mass spectrometry-based proteomics

c. RNA-Seq

d. CHIP-Seq

110. Which technique is used to map N6-methyladenosine (m6a. modifications on a transcriptome-wide scale to study RNA modifications?

a. RNA-Seq

b. MeRIP-Seq (Methylated RNA Immunoprecipitation Sequencing)

c. CHIP-Seq

d. ATAC-Seq

111. To identify RNA-protein interactions for various non-coding RNAs, which technique would you use?
   a. CLIP-Seq (Crosslinking and Immunoprecipitation Sequencing)
   b. RNA-Seq
   c. Hi-C
   d. QRT-PCR

112. For identifying and characterizing the microbial community in a clinical sample suspected of containing multiple bacterial species, which sequencing technique would you use?
   a. Sanger sequencing
   b. RNA-Seq
   c. Metagenomic sequencing
   d. CHIP-Seq

113. Which sequencing technique would you use to identify DNA methylation patterns in a plant species with an unannotated genome?
   a. RNA-Seq
   b. Whole-genome bisulfite sequencing (WGBS)
   c. chIP-Seq
   d. Sanger sequencing

114. To validate a single nucleotide polymorphism (SNP) associated with a disease in a large number of samples, which sequencing technique is most accurate?
   a. RNA-Seq
   b. CHIP-Seq
   c. Targeted resequencing
   d. ATAC-Seq

115. Which sequencing technique would you use to investigate alternative splicing contributing to protein diversity in a cancer cell line?
   a. Whole-genome sequencing
   b. RNA-Seq
   c. CHIP-Seq
   d. ATAC-Seq

116 To identify transcription start sites (TSS) of a specific gene in different tissues, which technique is most suitable?
   a. Whole-genome sequencing
   b. RNA-Seq
   c. CHIP-Seq
   d. CAGE (Cap Analysis of Gene Expression)

117. Which sequencing technique would you use to identify histone modifications associated with gene regulation in differentiated cells?
   a. RNA-Seq
   b. CHIP-Seq
   c. ATAC-Seq
   d. Sanger sequencing

118. To investigate the genetic basis of a rare hereditary disease in a family, which sequencing technique provides the most comprehensive information?
   a. Whole-exome sequencing (WES)
   b. RNA-Seq
   c. chIP-Seq
   d. Targeted resequencing

119. Which sequencing technique would you use to study gene expression levels in a single cell?
   a. Whole-genome sequencing
   b. Single-cell RNA-Seq (scRNA-Seq)
   c. CHIP-Seq
   d. ATAC-Seq
120. To identify regulatory elements controlling gene expression in a specific cell type, which sequencing technique provides the best insights?
   a. RNA-Seq
   b. Whole-genome sequencing
   c. aTAC-Seq
   d. Sanger sequencing
121. Which sequencing technique would you choose to detect structural variants such as large insertions, deletions, and rearrangements in a cancer genome?
   a. RNA-Seq
   b. Whole-genome sequencing
   c. CHIP-Seq
   d. Targeted resequencing
122. To study the binding sites of a transcription factor across the entire genome in a specific cell type, which sequencing technique should you use?
   a. RNA-Seq
   b. CHIP-Seq
   c. ATAC-Seq
   d. Whole-genome sequencing
123. Which sequencing technique would provide the most detailed comparison of gene expression profiles in healthy versus diseased tissues?
   a. Whole-genome sequencing
   b. RNA-Seq
   c. CHIP-Seq
   d. Sanger sequencing
124. Which sequencing technique would you use to profile small RNA species involved in gene regulation?
   a. Whole-genome sequencing
   b. Small RNA-Seq
   c. CHIP-Seq
   d. ATAC-Seq
125. To assemble the complete genome of a bacterial strain with an unknown sequence, which sequencing technique would you use?
   a. RNA-Seq
   b. Whole-genome sequencing
   c. CHIP-Seq
   d. ATAC-Seq
126. Which sequencing technique would provide data on the three-dimensional structure of chromatin to study the effect of a genetic variant?
   a. RNA-Seq
   b. CHIP-Seq
   c. Hi-C
   d. ATAC-Seq
127. To amplify a specific DNA fragment from a complex genomic DNA mixture with the highest specificity, which PCR technique should you use?
   a. Standard PCR
   b. Nested PCR
   c. Real-time PCR (qPCR)
   d. Reverse transcription PCR (RT- PCR)

128. Which PCR method is best for quantifying the amount of a specific RNA transcript in a sample?
  a. Standard PCR
  b. Nested PCR
  c. Real-time PCR (qPCR)
  d. digital PCR (dPCR)
129. To identify and quantify different splice variants of a gene of interest, which PCR technique would be most useful?
  a. Standard PCR
  b. Nested PCR
  c. Real-time PCR (QPCR)
  d. Reverse transcription PCR (RT-PCR)
130. Which PCR method would be most suitable for detecting a low-abundance viral genome in a clinical sample with high sensitivity?
  a. Standard PCR
  b. Real-time PCR (QPCR)
  c. Digital PCR (DPCR)
  d. Nested PCR
131. To determine the presence of a specific bacterial pathogen in a food sample and obtain quantitative results, which PCR technique should you use?
  a. Standard PCR
  b. Nested PCR
  c. Real-time PCR (QPCR)
  d. Reverse transcription PCR (RT-PCR)
132. When validating the amplification efficiency of your PCR assay for quantitative analysis, which parameter would you analyze in real-time PCR (qPCR)?
  a. Melting curve analysis
  b. Threshold cycle (Ct)
  c. Gel electrophoresis
  d. Annealing temperature
133. If you are comparing the expression levels of multiple genes in different tissues, which PCR technique would be most appropriate?
  a. Standard PCR
  b. Real-time PCR (QPCR)
  c. digital PCR (DPCR)
  d. Reverse transcription PCR (RT-PCR)
134 To differentiate between specific and non-specific amplification products when suspecting contamination in your PCR reactions, which technique would be most effective?
  a. Standard PCR
  b. Gel electrophoresis
  c. Real-time PCR (qPCR) with melting curve analysis
  d. Digital PCR (dPCR)

135 For amplifying a very long DNA fragment (>10 kb. with high fidelity, which PCR technique and enzyme should you use?

a. Standard PCR with Taq polymerase
b. Long-range PCR with a high-fidelity DNA polymerase
c. Real-time PCR (qPCR)
d. Digital PCR (dPCR)

136. When designing primers for a PCR experiment, which factor is most critical to ensure specific and efficient amplification of your target sequence?

a. Primer length
b. Primer GC content
c. Annealing temperature
d. All of the above

137. To detect and quantify a single nucleotide polymorphism (SNP) in a population sample, which PCR-based technique would provide the most accurate results?

a. Standard PCR
b. Real-time PCR (qPCR) with allele-specific probes
c. Reverse transcription PCR (RT-PCR)
d. Nested PCR

138. For specifically amplifying only one member of a gene family with high sequence similarity, which primer design strategy would be most effective?

a. Use long primers to increase specificity
b. Design primers in regions of the gene with the least sequence similarity
c. Increase the annealing temperature to enhance specificity
d. All of the above

139. To determine the methylation status of specific CpG sites in a DNA sample, which PCR technique would you use?

a. Standard PCR
b. Bisulfite sequencing PCR
c. Real-time PCR (QPCR)
d. Nested PCR

140. For detecting low-frequency mutations in a mixed population of DNA molecules with high sensitivity, which PCR technique should you choose?

a. Standard PCR
b. Real-time PCR (qPCR)
c. Digital PCR (DPCR)
d. Nested PCR

141. Which PCR technique is most suitable for a rapid, point-of-care diagnostic test for a viral infection?

a. Standard PCR
b. Real-time PCR (qPCR)
c. Digital PCR (dPCR)
d. Loop-mediated isothermal amplification (LAMP)

142. For high-level protein production in E. coli after cloning a gene into an expression vector, which vector feature is most critical?

a. Origin of replication
b. Multiple cloning site (MCS)
c. Strong promoter
d. Antibiotic resistance gene

143. If a cloned gene results in an insoluble protein forming inclusion bodies in E. coli, which strategy might improve protein solubility?
   a. Use a different antibiotic resistance marker
   b. change the host strain to one optimized for protein solubility
   c. Increase the temperature of the expression culture
   d. Remove the promoter from the vector

144. To study post-translational modifications of a gene in a eukaryotic expression system, which host cell type should you choose?
   a. E. coli
   b. Saccharomyces cerevisiae (yeast)
   c. Mammalian cells
   d. bacillus subtilis

145. After cloning a gene into an expression vector and observing no protein expression, which of the following is NOT a likely reason for this issue?
   a. Incorrect orientation of the inserted gene
   b. Mutation in the antibiotic resistance gene
   c. Weak promoter driving the gene
   d. Toxicity of the protein to the host cells

146 To facilitate the purification process of a recombinant protein expressed in E. coli, which tag should you use?
   a. His-tag
   b. Flag-tag
   c. GST-tag
   d. Any of the above

147. If an inducible expression vector in E. coli shows no detectable protein expression upon induction, what is the most likely cause?
   a. Incorrect antibiotic selection
   b. Mutation in the cloned gene
   c. Insufficient inducer concentration
   d. Strong promoter

148 To ensure proper glycosylation of a protein produced in a mammalian expression system, which vector feature is essential?
   a. Strong bacterial promoter
   b. Signal peptide sequence
   c. His-tag for purification
   d. Ampicillin resistance gene

149. To express a toxic protein in E. coli while minimizing its detrimental effects on the host cells, which strategy would be most effective?
   a. Use a strong constitutive promoter
   b. Use an inducible expression system
   c. Increase the antibiotic concentration
   d. Remove the tag from the protein

150. Which of the following techniques is primarily used to study protein-DNA interactions within chromatin?
   a. Western Blotting
   b. Polymerase Chain Reaction (PCR)
   c. Chromatin Immunoprecipitation (ChIP)
   d. Enzyme-Linked Immunosorbent Assay (ELISA)

Answer Key

1	c	2	b	3	a	4	b	5	b	6	c	7	c
8	c	9	c	10	d	11	c	12	c	13	b	14	b
15	b	16	b	17	d	18	c	19	b	20	c	21	a
22	d	23	b	24	c	25	b	26	c	27	a	28	b
29	b	30	a	31	c	32	b	33	c	34	c	35	c
36	b	37	c	38	b	39	b	40	b	41	b	42	b
43	a	44	c	45	b	46	a	47	c	48	b	49	c
50	b	51	b	52	c	53	b	54	a	55	c	56	d
57	c	58	b	59	b	60	d	61	b	62	a	63	b
64	c	65	b	66	c	67	b	68	b	69	b	70	b
71	b	72	c	73	c	74	b	75	b	76	c	77	b
78	b	79	d	80	a	81	c	82	d	83	d	84	b
85	c	86	c	87	d	88	a	89	c	90	c	91	c
92	c	93	d	94	b	95	c	96	b	97	c	98	c
99	c	100	c	101	c	102	c	103	d	104	a	105	b
106	b	107	a	108	b	109	b	110	b	111	a	112	c
113	b	114	c	115	b	116	d	117	b	118	a	119	b
120	c	121	b	122	b	123	b	124	b	125	b	126	c
127	b	128	c	129	d	130	c	131	c	132	b	133	b
134	c	135	b	136	d	137	b	138	d	139	b	140	c
141	d	142	c	143	b	144	c	145	b	146	d	147	d
148	b	149	b	150	c								

22

Cell Culture and Techniques

Nayanmoni Konwar[1] and Gunda Sai Rakesh[2]

[1]*Department of Veterinary Microbiology, Institute of Veterinary Science and Animal Husbandry, Siksha 'O' Anusandhan, Deemed to be University, Campus-4, Bhubaneswar, Odisha-751030*

[2]*Department of Veterinary Microbiology, College of Veterinary Sciences and Animal Husbandry, Central Agricultural University, Selesih, Aizawl-796014*

Introduction

Cell culture is a technique that involves the isolation and in vitro maintenance of cells isolated from tissues or whole organs derived from animals, microbes or plants. This technique has immeasurable role in the field of biology. The scientific progress in biology, microbiology and biotechnology in recent years can be credited on the development of cell culture technology. With the development of cell culture the isolation of viruses has become less cumbersome, the assessment of the efficacy and toxicity of new drugs has been easier, new vaccines are being developed and there has been development in biotechnology assisted reproductive technology.

In general, animal cells have more complex nutritional requirements and usually need more stringent conditions for growth and maintenance. For the growth of the cell in vitro specific mediums are required by the cells. Previously natural mediums like plasma ,serums were used but with the advent of synthetic media the specific needs of different cell types can be catered with. Cell culture is governed by a provided set of protocols requiring a sterile pure culture of cells, various nutrients for its growth, sterile cell culture hood, appropriate aseptic techniques and the utilisation of suitable conditions for optimal viable growth of cells.

The first instance of in vitro cultivation of animal tissue was performed in 1882 when Sydney Ringer developed Ringer's solution, a balanced salt solution of a composition that is close to that of bodily fluids, and successfully kept frog hearts beating after dissection and removal from the body. After the success of Ringer's solution, many researchers tried to maintain cells but it was Ross G. Harrison who could maintain a outgrowth of nerve fibres of a frog in lymph fluid in the year 1907. In 1912, Carrel demonstrated that the long-term cultivation of the cells that have been obtained from the connective tissues of chick fetuses is possible (for several months) with a periodic exchange of the medium. It was observed that somatic cells stopped growing after a certain number of cell divisions. In 1940, Wilton R. Earle and his co-workers used carcinogens to successfully create immortal mouse fibroblasts (L cells), revealing that proliferation from a single cell is possible. In 1951, George O. Gey and his co-workers created an infinitely proliferating human cell line from the tissue of a patient with uterine cervical cancer (HeLa cells). Due to the development of these established cell lines, the procedure of cell culture became very feasible and it enabled researchers worldwide to perform assays by using the same homogenous population of cells. This state of affairs made it easier to examine and to precisely quantify the subtle differences in the of culture media on cells.

With the advent of Cell culture scientist has been able to study the genetic abnormalities which can be determined by chromosomal analysis of cells derived, for example, from expectant mothers. Similarly, viral isolations could be done easily and the viral titre could be estimated both qualitatively and quantitatively on isolated cells in culture. In industry, cultured cells are used routinely to test both the pharmacological and toxicological effects of pharmaceutical compounds. This technology offered a user-friendly system to the scientist as it is relatively cheap to run and the exploitation of which avoids the legal, moral and ethical questions which are generally associated with animal experimentation. Cell culture techniques have also been beneficial for the production of cell culture adapted vaccines against various viral disease of both human and veterinary importance. Polio vaccine was the first vaccine which utilized this technique for development of the vaccine. Until now many cell culture adapted vaccines has been development which has proven to be efficacious. Furthermore, successful development of culture techniques for stem cells will provide a much needed cell-based strategy for treating diseases where organ transplant is currently the only available option. Thus we can say that cell culture technique is one of the most beneficial technologies developed by scientist for the betterment of both human and animal health.

1. Trypsin is used for dissociating the tissue into single cells.
   a. True b. False
2. In the secondary culture, cells are obtained from ____________________
   a. Primary culture b. The organism
   c. Organ culture d. Phenotypic culture
3. EDTA binds the ____________ ions.
   a. Magnesium b. Iron
   c. Carbon d. Calcium
4. The foundation for the development of cell culture technique was laid by
   a. Roux b. Arnold
   c. Ross d. Harrison
5. Who is regarded as the father of tissue culture
   a. Harrison b. Arnold
   c. Ross d. Roux
6. Use of trypsin to free cells from tissue matrix for cell culture was described by
   a. Jolly and Koch b. Beebe and Ewing
   c. Sims and Stillman d. Gottieb Maberland
7. Cell culture technique became simpler only after advent of
   a. Antibiotics b. Trypsin
   c. Cell culture media d. All of the following

8. Which of the following is true regarding animal cell culture technique
   a. Lactic acid is source of carbon
   b. Cells have high requirement of L-glutamine
   c. Cholin is necessary for cell adhesion and cytoskeleton
   d. All of the following
9. Which of the following is the structural fibre in cell culture system
   a. Collagen b. Elastin
   c. Fibronectin d. Both a and b
10. Optimum pH required for the growth of mammalian cells is
   a. 5.3-7.0 b. 6.5-7.0
   c. 7.2-7.4 d. 8.1-8.9
11. The optimum temperature of any cell or organ is called
   a. Critical temperature b. Threshold temperature
   c. Ceiling temperature d. None of the above
12. For culture of avian cells the optimum temperature requirement is
   a. 37°℃ b. 40°℃
   c. 42°℃ d. 35°℃
13. Which of the following is the oldest cell line
   a. Hela cell line b. Vero cell line
   c. CHO cell line d. BHK cell line
14. The ratio of CO2 : O2 used in cell culture system should be
   a. 1:5 b. 1:13
   c. 1:19 d. 1:25
15. Which of the following is easy and rapid method to interpret viability of cells in culture system
   a. Trypan blue dye exclusion b. Neutral red assay
   c. Fluorescein dye assay d. All of the following
16. Vero cell line is obtained from Kidney cells of
   a. African green monkey b. Chinese hamster
   c. Calf d. Swine
17. Advantages of cell culture techniques over other techniques is due to
   a. Reproducibility b. Convenience over animal model
   c. Potential for large scale production d. All of the above
18. Cell culture techniques was first developed by
   a. Harrison b. Koch
   c. Pasteur d. Fischer
19. Chicken embryo kidney cell culture is an example of
   a. Primary cell culture b. Cell line
   c. Secondary cell culture d. None

20. Foetal bovine serum is sterilized by

a. Hot air oven | b. Autoclaving
c. Filtering | d. UV radiation

21. Most tissue culture reagents can be stored at what temperature

a. −20◦ C | b. -40° C
c. 37°C | d. 4°C

22. Cryopreservation of cells are done at what temperature

a. -70°C | b. -196°C
c. -40°C | d. -110°C

23. Organisms which can cause contamination in cell culture system

a. Bacteria | b. Mycoplasma
c. Fungi | d. All of the above

24. Swabing of working surfaces should be done with

a. 80% alcohol | b. 70% alcohol
c. 10% alcohol | d. 100% alcohol

25. Flaming is not advisable laminar flow because

a. It disrupts the laminar flow
b. Can damage the HEPA filter
c. Omelt some of the plastic interior fittings.
d. All of the above

26. Normal fibroblast cell lines perform best at what pH

a. pH 7.4 to pH 7.7 | b. pH 7.2 to pH 7.4
c. pH 7 to pH 7.4 | d. pH 7to pH 7.2

27. Which class of biosafety cabinet is mist commonly preferred for cell culture works

a. Class I | b. Class II
c. Class III | d. None

28. What is the purpose of CO_2 incubator in cell culture laboratory

a. To maintain physiological pH | b. To provide CO_2
c. To kill bacteria | d. To grow viruses

29. What is the alternate method of buffering the cell culture system without CO2 incubator

a. Ddition of bicarbonate | b. Addition of HEPES
c. Addition of seum | d. Addition of aminoacids

30. What is used in order to avoid contamination in cell culture

a. Antibiotics | b. Anticoagulants
c. Antiseptics | d. Alcohol

31. Percentage of CO_2 required for cell culture system is

a. 10% | b. 2.5%
c. 5% | d. 8%

32. ________________ is used for observing cells in cell culture lab
   a. Inverted phase contrast microscopes   b. Phase contrast microscope
   c. Confocal microscope   d. Dark field microscope

33. The common contaminant in cell culture is mycoplasma which is a
   a. Fungi   b. Bacteria
   c. Virus   d. Mould

34. In case of bacterial contamination in cell culture the changes that we can observe is
   a. The cells will be overgrowth
   b. The media becomes turbid and acidic
   c. The pH becomes alkaline
   d. All of the above

35. Fungal contamination can be detected in cell culture by
   a. Presence of moving organism   b. Presence of hyphae
   c. Presence of dead cell   d. None of the above

36. The cells which are derived directly from tissues following enzymatic dissociationare known as
   a. Cell lines   b. Secondary cell culture
   c. Primary cell culture   d. All of the above

37. The process by which cells are harvested, diluted in fresh growth medium and replaced in a new culture flask to promote further growth
   a. Trypsinization   b. Filtration
   c. Subculturing   d. Incubation

38. Trypsin is commonly used in combination with EDTA because
   a. Chelates the Ca ions   b. Helps in buffering
   c Cell structure preservation   d. None

39. Cryoprotectent used for cryopreservation of cell lines is
   a. Isopropyl alcohol   b. DMSO
   c. EDTA   d. Foetal bovine serum

40. The degree of viability is most commonly determined by differentiating living from dead cells using
   a. The dye exclusion method   b. Wright staining method
   c. Geimsa staining   d All of the above

41. What is the full form of HEPA
   a. High efficiency processed air
   b. High efficiency particulate air
   c. Highly effective particulate air
   d. High efficiency particulate atmosphere

42. The first immortalise cell line was named as
   a. CEK cell lines   b. BHK cell lines
   c. HeLa cell lines   d. MDCK cell lines

43. HeLa cell are the cells which are derived from
    a. Cervical cancer cells
    b. Mammary cancer cells
    c. Uterine cancer cells
    d. None of the above
44. The viral oncogenes which are used for development of cell lines are
    a. T antigen from SV40 virus
    b. E6 and E7 oncogenes from human papilloma virus
    c. Both a and b
    d. None
45. Due to certain limitations of oncogenes to transform cell line Cell culture experts in the recent time they use a gene called
    a. Human telomerase reverse transcriptase (hTERT)
    b. Reverse transcriptase
    c. Telomerase
    d. T antigen
46. When was the first human cell lines established
    a. 1960s
    b. 1920s
    c. 1990s
    d. 1950s
47. The pioneer in cell culture techniques was
    a. Roux
    b. Harrision
    c. Grey
    d. Kohler and Milestein
48. The first person to develop cell culture technique in vitro was
    a. Ross Granville Harrison
    b. Wilhelm Roux
    c. Leo Loeb
    d. Robert Koch
49. The scientist who first developed the idea of continous cell culture system was
    a. Harrision
    b. Roux
    c. Gey
    d. Burrows and Carrel
50. In January, 1912, Carrel and his coworkers developed the first "cell line" derived from the fragments of
    a. Chicken embryo fibroblast
    b. Chicken embryo liver
    c. Chicken embryo heart
    d. Chicken embryo kidney
51. Use of incubators for cell cultures was recommended by
    a. Carrel and Burrows
    b. Herrell and coworkers
    c. Pannett and Compton
    d. None of them
52. The classification of Synthetic media. several groups based on the type of supplements added are
    a. Serum-containing media
    b. Serum-free media
    c. Protein-free media
    d. All of the Above
53. The medium used for human zygote cultures for the first time was
    a. Ham's F-10, supplemented with serum
    b. RPMI 1640
    c. DMEM
    d. M199

54. Which of the following was the first widely used chemically defined medium

a. Eagle'sBasal medium
b. DMEM medium
c. MEM medium
d. M199 medium

55. __________developed plague assay technique for quantitation of animal viruses

a. George Gey
b. Renato Dulbecco
c. Gregor Mendel
d. Harrision

56. Which of the following materials are required for counting cells before seeding in flask

a. Haemocytometer
b. Microscope
c. Trypan blue
d. All of them

57. What is the commonly used indicator in cell culture media

a. Methyl red
b. Phenolpthalein
c. Bromothymol blue
d. Phenol red

58. What is the common viral contaminant in Foetal bovine serum used for cell culture

a. Bovine viral diarrhoea virus
b. Bovine spongiform encephelopathy
c. Rinderpest virus
d. Foot and mouth disease virus

59. The first virus to be isolated in cell culture was

a. Rabies virus
b. FMD virus
c. Polio virus
d. Rota virus

60. The origin of Vero cell line is

a. African green monkey kidney
b. Rhesus monkey Kidney
c. Bovine kidney
d. None

61. What is the first recombinant influenza vaccine licensed in US

a. Optaflu
b. FluBlock
c. NASOVAC-S4
d. FLUARIX

62. The COVAXIN vaccine is prepared by culturing the SARS-CoV-2 sample in which cell line

a. BHK-21 cell line
b. HeLa cell line
c. Vero cell line
d. Macrophage culture

63. Trypsin used for cell culture is derived from

a. The pancreas of pigs
b. Liver of pigs
c. Pancreas of cattle
d. Stomach of pigs

64. Caustic alkaline detergents render the surface of the glass unsuitable for cell attachment and require subsequent neutralization with

a. 1M HCL
b. 0.5M H_2SO_4
c. 0.1 M HCl or H_2SO_4
d. 2M HCL

65. Syncythia formation is observed in cells infected by which virus
    a. New Castle disese virus
    b. Infectious Bursal disease virus
    c. avian adenovirus
    d. All of them
66. For chicken embryo fibroblast culture the embryos should be of what age
    a. 10-15 days
    b. 13-15 days
    c. 9-11days
    d. 5-6 days
67. For preparation of chicken embryo liver cell culture the embryos should be the age of
    a. 12-15 days
    b. 13-15 days
    c. 16-18 days
    d. 0 day post hatch
68. DF-1 cell line is derived from which primary cell culture
    a. Chicken embryo fibroblast culture
    b. Duck embryo fibroblast culture
    c. Mouse embryo fibroblast
    d. None of the above
69. BHK-21 cell line is derived from which animal
    a. Mice
    b. Rat
    c. Pig
    d. Hamster
70. MDCK cell line is derived from which animal
    a. Monkey
    b. Mouse
    c. Dog
    d. Cat
71. MDBK cell line is derived from which animal
    a. Bovine
    b. Ovine
    c. caprine
    d. Swine
72. Rabies cell culture based vaccine is prepared in
    a. Human diploid cell culture
    b. Purified chick embryo cell culture (PCEC)
    c. Vero cell
    d. All of the above
73. The cells which provide physical support to help the cell cultures adhere and grow are
    a. Feeder cells
    b. Adherent cells
    c. Suspension cells
    d. Stem cells
74. The cells which grow and remain suspended in the culture medium is known as
    a. Feeder cells
    b. Adherent cells
    c Suspension cells
    d. Stem cells
75. Which cell line is used for propagation of foot and mouth disease virus
    a. Vero cell line
    b. BHK-21 cell line
    c. MDCK cell line
    d. QT-35 cell line

76. Cell line used for Lumpy skin disease propagation is
   a. BHK-21
   b. Vero cell line
   c. MDCK cell line
   d. MDBK cell line
77. Which of the following is NOT a primary cell culture?
   a. Fibroblasts from a mouse embryo
   b. HeLa cells
   c. Hepatocytes from a rat liver
   d. Neural cells from a chick embryo
78. What is the main advantage of using continuous cell lines over primary cultures?
   a. Higher genetic similarity to the tissue of origin
   b. More representative of in vivo conditions
   c. Unlimited growth potential
   d. Lower risk of contamination
79. Which of the following cell lines is derived from human cervical cancer?
   a. Vero cells
   b. HEK293 cells
   c. HeLa cells
   d. cHO cells
80. What is the purpose of trypsinization in cell culture?
   a. To provide nutrients to the cells
   b. To detach adherent cells from the culture vessel
   c. To sterilize the culture medium
   d. To freeze cells for storage
81. Which of the following statements about the CO2 incubator is true?
   a. It is used to maintain a hypoxic environment.
   b. It regulates temperature and humidity but not CO2 levels.
   c. It maintains the pH of the culture medium by controlling CO2 levels.
   d. It is only used for bacterial cultures.
82. Which component is essential in serum for promoting cell growth?
   a. Antibiotics
   b. Growth factors
   c. pH buffers
   d. Sodium chloride
83. What is the main function of fetal bovine serum (FBS) in cell culture?
   a. To act as an antibiotic
   b. To provide essential growth factors and hormones
   c. To solidify the culture medium
   d. To decrease the pH of the culture medium
84. Which cell line is commonly used for producing recombinant proteins?
   a. HeLa cells
   b. CHO (Chinese Hamster Ovary) cells
   c. Jurkat cells
   d. COS-7 cells
85. Which of the following is NOT a characteristic of a transformed cell line?
   a. Contact inhibition
   b. Anchorage-independent growth
   c. Immortalization
   d. Altered morphology

86. Which technique is used to assess cell viability?
    a. Western blotting b. MTT assay
    c. PCR d. Flow cytometry
87. Which cell line is derived from African green monkey kidney cells?
    a. HeLa cells b. Vero cells
    c. HEK293 cells d. CHO cells
88. What is the purpose of cryopreservation in cell culture?
    a. To sterilize cells
    b. To detach cells from the culture surface
    c. To store cells at very low temperatures for long-term use
    d. To measure cell proliferation
89. Which of the following is a common method for cell transfection?
    a. Southern blotting b. Electroporation
    c. Northern blotting d. Affinity chromatography
90. Which cell line is frequently used in vaccine production?
    a. HeLa cells b. Vero cells
    c. HEK293 cells d. Jurkat cells
91. Which of the following techniques is commonly used to confirm the identity of a cell line?
    a. ELISA b. Western blot
    c. STR (Short Tandem Repeat) profiling d. Flow cytometry
92. Which of the following is a sign of bacterial contamination in cell culture?
    a. Increase in pH b. Cloudy medium
    c. Decrease in cell growth rate d. All of the above
93. Which of the following cell lines is derived from human embryonic kidney cells?
    a. HeLa cells b. Vero cells
    c. HEK293 cells d. CHO cells
94. Which of the following is NOT a commonly used cell viability assay?
    a. MTT assay b. Trypan blue exclusion test
    c. FAT d. Flow cytometry
95. Which of the following components can be used to enhance cell attachment in culture?
    a. Gelatin b. Poly-L-lysine
    c. Collagen d. All of the above
96. Which cell line is commonly used for the production of monoclonal antibodies?
    a. HeLa cells b. SP2/0 cells
    c. CHO cells d. COS-7 cells

97. Assertion (A): Cell lines can be subcultured indefinitely.

Reason (R): Cell lines are derived from primary cells which have undergone transformation to become immortal.

a. Both A and R are true, and R is the correct explanation of A.
b. Both A and R are true, but R is not the correct explanation of A.
c. A is true, but R is false.
d. A is false, but R is true.

98. Assertion (A): Serum-free media can be used for cell culture.

Reason (R): Serum-free media reduce the risk of contamination and variability in cell culture.

a. Both A and R are true, and R is the correct explanation of A.
b. Both A and R are true, but R is not the correct explanation of A.
c. A is true, but R is false.
d. A is false, but R is true.

99. Assertion (A): Cell lines are less representative of in vivo conditions than primary cells.

Reason (R): Cell lines often undergo genetic and phenotypic changes that differ from primary cells.

a. Both A and R are true, and R is the correct explanation of A.
b. Both A and R are true, but R is not the correct explanation of A.
c. A is true, but R is false.
d. A is false, but R is true.

100. Assertion (A): Cell culture media must be supplemented with antibiotics.

Reason (R): Antibiotics prevent contamination from bacteria and fungi in cell culture.

a. Both A and R are true, and R is the correct explanation of A.
b. Both A and R are true, but R is not the correct explanation of A.
c. A is true, but R is false.
d. A is false, but R is true.

101. Assertion (A): Mycoplasma contamination is a major issue in cell culture.

Reason (R): Mycoplasma contamination is often undetectable by visual inspection but affects cell physiology.

a. Both A and R are true, and R is the correct explanation of a.
b. Both A and R are true, but R is not the correct explanation of a.
c. A is true, but R is false.
d. A is false, but R is true.

102. Giemsa stain when it is used for staining cell culture it takes the following colour

a. Nucleus pink or magenta, the nucleoli dark blue, cytoplasm pale gray-blue
b. Nucleus dark blue,nucleoli pink,cytoplasm pale blue
c. Nucleus blue and cytoplasm pink
d. None of the above

103. Crystal violet is a monochromatic stain and stains the cells
   a. Nucleus dark blue and the cytoplasm light blue
   b. Nucleus pink and the cytoplasm light blue
   c. Nucleus red and cytoplasm blue
   d. None of the above

104. Stem cells in the basal layer of the epidermis is
   a. Multipotent stem cell   b. Unipotent stem cell
   c. Pluripotent stem cell   d. Totipotent stem cell

105. A diminished rate of cell proliferation, reduced saturation density and agglutination during growth in suspension is a sign of
   a. Fungal contamination   b. bacterial contamination
   c. Old media   d. Mycoplasmal contamination

106. What is the sensitive test for detection of mycoplasmal contamination in cell culture
   a. ELISA   b. FAT
   c. PCR   d. IPT

107. What are the antibiotics which are used in cell culture
   a. Penicillin   b. Streptomycin
   c. Gentamicin   d. All of the above

108. Name one anti fungal agent which is added to medium to inhibit fungal growth in cell culture
   a. Amphothericin B   b. Fluconazole
   c. Ketoconazole   d. All of the above

109. What is the best cryoprotectant for preserving cell lines
   a. Glycerol   b. Polyethylene glycoL
   c. DMSO   d. Serum

110. Most cultured cells survive best if they are cooled at
   a. 1°C/min   b. 2°C/min
   c. 5°C/min   d. 10°C/min

111. Viability of animal cell culture can be determined by 1.bradford's assay,2. Trypan blue assay, 3. Comet assay, 4.MTT assay
   a. 2 only   b. 1 and 2 only
   c. 2 and 4 only   d. 1 and 3 only

112. Which of the following is an anchorage independent cell line
   a. MCF_7 b. MDA MB 231
   c. K562   d. PC-3

113. Heat inactivation of foetal bovine serum is done at
   a. 56°C for 30 min   b. 56°C for 20 min
   c. 70°C for 10 min   d. 37°C for 15 min

114. Which of the following statements is not correct for propagation and maintenance of mammalian cells in vitro
   a. HEPES is added to maintain pH of the culture cells
   b. Transformed cells donot need an external serum supply
   c. The primary cells are obtained directly from the orhanism
   d. Trypsin is added in cell culture media toprovide nutrients
115. For developing transgenic mice embryonic stem cells are engineered to express transgene.The cells are selected by
   a. Novobiocin b. Neomycin
   c. Tetracycline d. Penicillin
116. Test performed for detection of virus that does not produce any cytopathic changes in cell culture
   a. Immuno peroxidase test b. ELISA
   c. VNT d. CFT
117. Test performed to study the quantity of virus titre in cell culture
   a. $TCID_{50}$ assay b. $TCTD_{50}$ assay
   c. VNT d. MTT assay
118. Mitogens ussed in MTT assay are
   a. Concanavalin A b. Phytohemagglutinin
   c. Lipopolysaccharide d. All of the above
119. The growth of animal cells in vitro in a suitable culture medium is called___________
   a. Gene expression b. Transgenesis
   c. Plant tissue culture d. Animal cell culture
120. Name the organism on which first cell line was observed?
   a. E.coli b. Sheep
   c. Mouse d. Drosophila
121. Which of the following is the characteristics of a normal cell?
   a. Anchorage independent b. Continuous cell lines
   c. Dependent on external growth factor d. No contact inhibition
122. Name the cell line of the human embryonic lung?
   a. HeLa b. WISH
   c. L d. MRC-5
123. Which of the following is NOT the part of growth medium for animal culture?
   a. Starch b. Serum
   c. Carbon source d. Inorganic salts
124. Which of the following is NOT the major function of the serum?
   a. Promotion of tuber and bulb formation b. Stimulate cell growth
   c. Enhance cell attachment d. Provide transport proteins

125. Which of the following culture is used for the production of primary and secondary metabolites?
   a. Cell suspension culture b. Callus culture
   c. Protoplast d. Somatic hybrid
126. Hybridoma cells have an application to produce:
   a. Antigens b. Antibodies
   c. Cancer cells d. Cell lines
127. What does HBSS stands for in cell culture
   a. Hanks Balanced Salt solution b. Hanks Basal Salt solution
   c. Both 1 and 2 d. Only 1
128. Animal cell cultures are used widely for the production of
   a. Insulin b. Somatostatin
   c. Mabs d. Thyroxine
129. The first vaccine developed from animal cell culture was
   a. Hepatitis B vaccine b. Influenza vaccine
   c. Small pox vaccine d. Polio vaccine
130. The cell line used for the production of polio vaccine was
   a. Primate kidney cell line b. CHO cell line
   c. Dog kidney cell line d. Mouse fibroblast cell line
131. The virus commonly used to infect cell cultures for the production of interferon is
   a. Corona virus b. Sendai virus
   c. Polio virus d. Small pox virus
132. What is the full form of RPMI-1640 media
   a. Roswell Park Memorial Institute b. Phenol red medium
   c. Roswell phenol red medium d. None
133. Hybrid antibodies are
   a. Antibodies produced in cell cultures
   b. Antibodies designed using rDNA technology produced in cell cultures
   c. Antibodies produced in invivo
   d. Both a and b
134. What can be observed by naked eye in a virus culture?
   a. Viroid b. Virions
   c. Viral plaques d. Virus capsid
135. What is used to suppress mycoplasma contamination in virus cultures?
   a. Abacavir b. Kanamycin
   c. Peramivir d. Zanamivir
136. Which culture media is used to grow HeLa cells?
   a. DMEM b. Agar media
   c. MS media d. LS media

137. All established cell lines have equal susceptibility to viruses.
   a. True b. False
138. The cells should be subcultured at which growth phase
   a. Lag phase b. Log phase
   c. Stationary d. Decline phase
139. Pyruvate is included in the formulation of some media, as an alternative source of
   a. Vitamins b. Amino acids
   c. Energy d. Protein
140. What is the reisistance of water that is suitable for preparation of cell culture medium
   a. 16-18MΩ b. 20 MΩ
   c. 25 MΩ d. 50 MΩ
141. For virus titration which type of cell culture plate is recommended
   a. 48 well cell culture plate b. 96 well cell culture plate
   c. 12 well cell culture plate d. 6 cell cell culture plate
142. For sterilizing media and serum what process is mostly used
   a. Autoclaving b. Irradition
   c. Filtering d. Hot air oven
143. What is the percentage of FBS in growth medium
   a. 10% b. 8%
   c. 5% d. 2.4%
144. What is the percentage of serum in maintenance medium
   a. 4% b. 2%
   c. 10% d. 5%
145. What concentration of antibiotic-antimycotic 100x strength is used in cell cultre
   a. 10X b. 2X
   c. 1X d. 5X
146. What should be the temperature of the water for thawing cryopreserved cells
   a. 42°C b. 37°C
   c. 25°C d. 4°C
147. 1. Cytopathic effect produced by all viruses are same
   2. The degree of cytopathic changes increases with passage of virus
   a. Only 1 is true b. Only 2 is true
   c. Both 1 and 2 are true d. Both are false
148. Cell culture adapted vaccines are prepared for the following which virus
   a. Polio virus b. Rotavirus
   c. Hepatitis virus d. All of the above
149. CHO cell lines is derived from
   a. Chinese hamster kidney cells b. Chines Hamster ovary cells
   c. Chicken heart cells d. Chicken embryonic kidney cells

150. Which of the following are commonly produced in animal cell cultures
   a. Interferon   b. Mab
   c. Vaccines   d. All of the above

Answer Key

1	a	2	a	3	d	4	a	5	a	6	c	7	d
8	d	9	d	10	c	11	c	12	b	13	a	14	c
15	a	16	a	17	d	18	a	19	a	20	c	21	a
22	b	23	d	24	b	25	d	26	a	27	b	28	a
29	b	30	a	31	c	32	a	33	b	34	b	35	b
36	c	37	c	38	a	39	b	40	a	41	b	42	c
43	a	44	c	45	a	46	d	47	a	48	a	49	d
50	c	51	a	52	d	53	a	54	a	55	b	56	d
57	d	58	a	59	c	60	a	61	b	62	c	63	a
64	c	65	a	66	c	67	b	68	a	69	d	70	c
71	a	72	d	73	a	74	c	75	b	76	d	77	b
78	c	79	c	80	b	81	c	82	b	83	b	84	b
85	a	86	b	87	b	88	c	89	b	90	b	91	c
92	c	93	c	94	c	95	d	96	b	97	a	98	a
99	a	100	b	101	a	102	a	103	a	104	b	105	d
106	c	107	d	108	a	109	c	110	a	111	c	112	c
113	a	114	d	115	a	116	a	117	a	118	d	119	d
120	c	121	c	122	d	123	a	124	a	125	a	126	b
127	d	128	c	129	d	130	a	131	b	132	a	133	b
134	a	135	b	136	a	137	b	138	b	139	c	140	a
141	b	142	c	143	d	144	c	145	b	146	b	147	d
148	d	149	b	150	d								

23

Biotechnology in Reproduction

T. Sarath[1], S. Manokaran[2], R. Rajkumar[1] and A. Thangamani[2]

[1]*Vetrinary Clinical Complex*

[2]*Department of Veterinary Gynaecology and Obstetrics, Veterinary College and Research Institute, Salem - 636 112*

Biotechnology is being harnessed in various aspects of the livestock industry to hasten breed development for improved animal health and welfare, enhanced reproduction, and improved nutritional quality and safety of animal-derived foods. Various biotechnology methods are used in improving the breeding stock of animals. These include artificial insemination (AI), embryo transfer (ET), in-vitro fertilization (IVF), sexing of semen and embryos, micromanipulation of oocytes/ embryos, transgenesis, somatic cell nuclear transfer and the emerging technology on genomics and marker-assisted selection (MAS).

Artificial Insemination: One of the earliest perfected technology is artificial insemination (AI) where new breeds of animals are produced through the introduction of the male sperm from one superior male to the female reproductive tract without mating. AI reduces transmission of venereal disease, lessens the need of farms to maintain breeding males, facilitates more accurate recording of pedigrees, and minimizes the cost of introducing improved genetics. Various technologies have evolved that led to the efficient use of AI in developing desired livestock, including the methods of freezing semen or cryopreservation and sperm sexing.

Embryo Transfer: Embryo transfer (ET) from one mother to a surrogate mother makes it possible to produce several livestock progenies from a superior female. Selected females are induced to superovulate hormonally and inseminated at an appropriate time relative to ovulation depending on the species and breed. Week-old embryos are flushed out of the donor's uterus, isolated, examined microscopically for number and quality, and inserted into the lining of the uterus of surrogate mothers.

ET increases reproductive rate of selected females, reduces disease transfer, and facilitates the development of rare and economically important genetic stocks as well as the production of several closely related and genetically similar individuals that are important in livestock breeding research.

***In vitro* Fertilization:** In case other artificial reproductive techniques fail due to difficulties such as blocked reproductive systems, non-responsive ovaries in the females, marginal semen quality and quantity in the male, and presence of disease, in vitro fertilization (IVF) is used. The fertilization of the sperm and the egg is conducted in vitro (outside the animal's body) at specific environmental and biochemical conditions. To date, successful IVFs have been conducted in various animal species due to advances in embryo production and cryopreservation of reproductive cells. Since the birth of the first rabbit conceived through IVF in 1959, IVF offsprings have been born in mice, rats, hamsters, cats, guinea pig, squirrels, pigs, cows, monkeys, and humans.

Semen sexing: Semen sexing is a biotechnology-based technique that uses flow cytometry or cell sorters to separate sperm into X-sperm, Y-sperm, and unsexable sperm. This process is used to breed animals like cattle, sheep, and pigs, and may also be used for companion animals like cats, dogs, and horses.

Embryo sexing: This technique involves collecting embryos and then biopsying or aspirating them to determine their sex. Some of the techniques employed commercially for the embryo sexing are chromosomal analysis of demi-embryos, immunological detection of embryonic H- Y antigen, use of Y-specific probes, Fluorescence in situ hybridization, rapid sexing method for preimplantation embryos of bovine using loop-mediated isothermal amplification (LAMP) reaction and ultrasonic examination of fetal structures.

Micromanipulation of oocytes / embryos: Micromanipulation is a technology which is used to physically interact with a sample (gametes or embryos) under a microscope, where a level of precision of movement is necessary that cannot be achieved by the unaided human hand. It includes Zona thinning, Partial Zona drilling or dissection (PZD), Zona drilling (ZD), Subzonal sperm injection (SUZI) and Intra Cytoplasmic Sperm Injection (ICSI).

Transgenesis: Transgenesis is a biotechnology technique that involves introducing a foreign gene into an animal's genome, which can then be passed on to its offspring. This process is used to create genetically modified animals (GMAs) or genetically engineered animals. There are different methods of transgenesis such as DNA microinjection, DNA transfer into gametes and DNA Electroporation. Transgenic farm animals can be used both in breeding and biomedicine.

Somatic Cell Nuclear Transfer: Somatic cell nuclear transfer (NF) is a technique in which the nucleus (DNA. of a somatic cell is transferred into a female egg cell or oocyte in which the nucleus has been removed to generate a new individual, genetically identical to the somatic cell donor. This technique was used to generate Dolly from a differentiated adult mammary epithelial cell which demonstrated that genes that are already inactivated in differentiated tissues can be completely reactivated. NF technology creates possibility of generating clones from superior genotype and can be used to efficiently evaluate effects of genotype x environment interactions and testing or dissemination of transgenics. Problems on high rate of pregnancy loss, survival of newborn and increased incidence of abnormal development due to incorrect reprogramming of nuclear DNA (epigenetic inference) and unusual conditions during in-vitro processes make this a pre-commercial technology.

Genomics and Marker-Assisted Selection (MAS) Applications

The discovery and identification of DNA sequences or molecular markers associated with important animal traits has various applications that include trait improvement, heritability determination, and product traceability.

Molecular marker-assisted introgression (MAI): Markers are used to guide livestock breeders in selecting individuals expressing the introgressed gene. A series of backcrossing to the recipient parent is usually done in conventional breeding. With the use of molecular markers, the time and number of backcrossing cycles incurred in selection and identification of the desired individual are reduced. Today, molecular markers are being used in various livestock trait improvement activities such as growth, meat quality, wool quality, milk production and quality, and disease resistance.

1. First successful embryo transfer technology was reported in which of the following animal
   a. Dog
   b. Rabbit
   c. Cat
   d. Sow
2. Which among the following is the most successful method of gene transfer?
   a. Retroviruses
   b. Liposomes
   c. Pronuclear microinjection
   d. Biolistics
3. The embryo transfer in Horse was reported by
   a. Oguri and Tsutsumi
   b. Nicholas
   c. Fekete and Little
   d. Heape
4. The pregnancy rate from transfer of fresh embryos in cows ranges from
   a. 30-40%
   b. 40-50%
   b. 65-80%
   d. >80%
5. In embryo transfer program in cows, carbachol has been used to
   a. Reduce uterine contractions
   b. Dilate cervix
   c. Reduce the frothiness of the flush
   d. Two of the options are correct
6. The most popular method of embryo freezing is
   a. Slow freezing
   b. Rapid freezing
   c. Vitrification
   d. Two of the options are correct
7. What are the reasons for using embryo transfer in pigs
   a. Establish new herds from herds with pseudorabies
   b. Obtain boars for closed commercial herd
   c. Obtain more offspring from superior gilts and sows
   d. All the above
8. What are the major limiting factors identified at an early stage in Embryo transfer programmes in goats
   a. Variability of response to superovulatory treatments
   b. Premature regression of corpus luteum
   c. All of the above
   d. None of the above
9. The number of cattle embryos that are ideally transferred into a recipient is
   a. 1
   b. 2
   c. 3
   d. 4
10. Approaches to cryopreservation of pig embryos are
    a. Vitrificatoion
    b. Removing cytoplasmic lipids from early embryos
    c. Conventional method of freezing
    d. All of the above

11. Zona layer removal by which species involves rhythmic expansions and contractions of the blastocyst aided by production of zona lysin from the estrogen sensitized uterine epithelium.
    a. Pig
    b. Mouse
    c. Rabbit
    d. None of the above
12. Which of the following is the advantage of assisted fertilization and blastocyst hatching.
    a. Normal rate of congenital malformation
    b. No risk of conjoint turning
    c. High success with standard transfer techniques
    d. More labor intensive
13. What is the primary goal of micromanipulation techniques in IVF?
    a. To increase the number of embryos available for transfer
    b. To improve embryo implantation rates
    c. To ensure the genetic diversity of embryos
    d. None of the above
14. What is the role of phenol red in embryo culture media?
    a. To act as an energy source for embryo metabolism.
    b. To serve as a pH indicator in the media.
    c. To provide an osmolality adjustment to the media.
    d. To enhance the motility of sperm used in fertilization.
15. What does the immunobead test detect on the sperm surface?
    a. Acrosome reaction
    b. Sperm motility defects
    c. Antisperm antibodies
    d. Zona penetration
16. What is the primary advantage of ultrafiltration over distilled or bottled water?
    a. Less expensive
    b. Requires frequent cleaning
    c. Leaches organic compounds
    d. Higher contaminant carryover
17. Which pattern of sperm motility is important for binding to and penetrating the zona pellucida of the egg?
    a. Curvilinear velocity (VCL)
    b. Hyperactivation
    c. Straight line velocity (VSL)
    d. Average path velocity (VAP)
18. Which of the following involves the injection of immotile live sperm directly into the vitellus?
    a. SUZI
    b. ZIFT
    c. ICSI
    d. PZD
19. How long is the fertilizable life of oocytes in humans?
    a. 4 hours
    b. 10 hours
    c. 24 hours
    d. 48 hours

20. When is secondary insemination performed?
    a. Only in cases of fertilized oocytes
    b. When fertilization occurs after the first insemination
    c. When oocytes are unfertilized and immature during the first insemination
    d. To improve the polyspermic rate
21. What is the primary method for separating X and Y chromosome-bearing spermatozoa in farm animals?
    a. Flow cytometry
    b. Gradient centrifugation
    c. Electrophoresis
    d. Microscopy
22. Which of the following is a benefit of sexing spermatozoa in farm animals?
    a. Increased fertility
    b. Improved sperm motility
    c. Reduced sperm abnormalities
    d. Ability to predetermine offspring sex
23. What is the name of the fluorescent dye used to stain X and Y chromosome-bearing spermatozoa for flow cytometric sorting?
    a. Hoechst 33342
    b. DAPI
    c. PI
    d. FITC
24. Which farm animal species has the largest difference in DNA content between X and Y chromosome-bearing spermatozoa?
    a. Cattle
    b. Pigs
    c. Sheep
    d. Horses
25. What is the typical purity of sorted X or Y chromosome-bearing spermatozoa using flow cytometry?
    a. 80-90%
    b. 90-95%
    c. 95-98%
    d. 98-99%
26. Which of the following is a limitation of flow cytometric sorting of X and Y chromosome-bearing spermatozoa?
    a. Low throughput
    b. High cost
    c. Damage to spermatozoa
    d. All of the above
27. What is the purpose of using a sheath fluid in flow cytometric sorting of X and Y chromosome-bearing spermatozoa?
    a. To maintain sperm viability
    b. To improve sorting efficiency
    c. To reduce sperm agglutination
    d. To enhance fluorescence signal
28. Which of the following is a potential application of sexed spermatozoa in farm animals?
    a. Artificial insemination
    b. In vitro fertilization
    c. Embryo transfer
    d. All of the above

29. What is the name of the technology used to sort X and Y chromosome-bearing spermatozoa based on their DNA content?
    a. Beltsville Sperm Sexing Technology
    b. Flow Cytometric Sperm Sexing
    c. Microfluidic Sperm Sexing
    d. Magnetic Activated Cell Sorting
30. Which of the following is a benefit of using sexed spermatozoa in farm animals?
    a. Increased reproductive efficiency
    b. Improved genetic selection
    c. Reduced reproductive costs
    d. All of the above
31. Which one of the following is not a G- protein coupled receptor in poultry?
    a. GPR3
    b. GPR9
    c. GPR12
    d. GPR6
32. GPR-12 receptor expression was upregulated by?
    a. Progesterone
    b. Estrogen
    c. Acetylcholine
    d. Calcium
33. GWAS stands for
    a. Genome Wide Association Study
    b. Genetic Wife Authorized Study
    c. Genetic World Authorized Study
    d. Genome World Association Study
34. What is the primary purpose of Artificial Insemination in poultry?
    a. To increase the number of eggs laid
    b. To control the sex ratio of offspring
    c. To enhance genetic quality and diversity
    d. To reduce the cost of feed
35. Embryo transfer in poultry involves:
    a. Transferring sperm between males
    b. Transferring fertilized eggs to a new host hen
    c. cloning of embryos
    d. Freezing embryos for future use
36. CRISPR technology in poultry biotechnology is primarily used for
    a. Sexing embryos
    b. Freezing sperm
    c. Genetic modification
    d. Transferring eggs
37. In poultry breeding, what is a primary benefit of using genetic engineering techniques?
    a. Increasing the feed conversion ratio
    b. Enhancing disease resistance
    c. Reducing the need for artificial insemination
    d. Improving egg shell quality
38. Which technique involves replicating individuals with desirable traits?
    a. Genetic modification
    b. Cloning
    c. Embryo transfer
    d. Artificial insemination

39. ________ is a method used to improve genetic diversity and quality by selecting and breeding individuals with desirable traits.

a. Gene cloning
b. Genetic engineering
c. In breeding
d. Embryo transfer

40. The use of __________ technology allows precise modification of genes to achieve specific traits in poultry

a. Cryopreservation
b. Sexing
c. CRISPR
d. Embryo transfer

41. The first successful embryo transfer buffalo calf was born in _________

a. Japan, 1988
b. Australia, 1880
c. France, 1920
d. USA, 1983

42. The conception rate of buffalo by artificial insemination using frozen semen is _________

a. 25 – 45 %
b. 55 - 75 %
c. 85 - 95 %
d. 5 15 %

43. Majority of buffaloes in tropical climate fails to express estrus signs during ________ season.

a. Winter
b. Summer
c. Autumn
d. Rainy

44. The concentration of progesterone hormone in buffalo blood during estrus is _______

a. 0.01 ng/ml
b. 0.20 ng/ml
c. 0.8 ng/ml
d. 1.6 ng/ml

45. SCNT stands for

a. Sperm Cell Nuclear Treatment
b. Stromal cell Nuclear Transplant
c. Stem Cell Nuclear Therapy
d. Somatic Cell Nuclear Transfer

46. In ________ species, the corpus luteum have no yellow colour at any stage of development.

a. Buffalo
b. Sheep
c. Horse
d. Pig

47. Staining of Cumulus oocyte complex using brilliant cresyl blue, that can be used as a marker for determining the oocyte quality for biotechnological techniques like cloning is based on

a. Intracellular activity of Aromatase
b. Intracellular activity of Glucose-6-Phosphate dehydrogenase
c. Intracellular activity of Pyruvate dehydrogenase
d. Intracellular activity of DNA Polymerase

48. The optimal duration of In Vitro Maturation (IVM) for bubaline oocytes is ____ hours.

a. 24
b. 48
c. 72
d. 96

49. FITC – PSA and Chlortetracycline fluorescence assay is used to evaluate the __________ status of sperm, so that it can aid to evaluate the capacitation of sperm.

    a. Mitochondrial   b. Acrosomal
    c. Tail   d. Nuclear

50. The chromosomal number in swamp and riverine buffalo is

    a. 50, 48   b. 60, 64
    c. 48, 50   d. 50, 60

51. If frozen semen is used, sperm motility can be enhanced. (hypermotility) by:

    a. Caffeine   b. Theophylline
    c. Lactic acid   d. Percoll density gradient

52. In cattle, sperm capacitation is typically achieved using:

    a. Heparin   b. Caffeine
    c. Theophylline   c. None of the above

53. For in vitro culture (IV c. of sheep embryos, the oviductal epithelial cells are often used as a:

    a. Culture medium   b. Energy source
    c. Hormonal supplement   d. Co-culture system

54. The optimal temperature for in vitro culture of embryos is typically:

    a. 37°C   b. 39°C
    c. 41°C   d. 43°C

55. Carbon dioxide (CO□) is often added to the atmosphere of in vitro culture chambers to:

    a. Maintain pH   b. Increase oxygen levels
    c. Reduce temperature   d. Stimulate cell division

56. What stages can pig embryos develop to when cultured in mouse excised oviducts?

    a. Morula and blastocyst stage   b. 1-cell to 4-cell stage
    c. 8-cell to 16-cell stage   d. 16-cell to 32-cell stages

57. What is the purpose of adding heat-treated serum or bovine serum albumin to in vitro fertilization media?

    a. To provide an energy source   b. To support spermatozoal motility
    c. To enhance the acrosome reaction   d. To maintain pH balance

58. Which of the following is NOT a criterion for evidence of fertilization?

    a. Penetration of sperm into the ooplasm
    b. Swelling of the sperm head and pronuclear formation
    c. Morphologically normal cleavage
    d. Presence of a second polar body

59. What is the optimal pH range for embryo culture media?

    a. 6.5-7.0   b. 7.0-7.4
    c. 7.2-7.6   d. 7.5-8.0

60. What is the typical osmolality range used for embryo culture media?
   a. 250-270 mOsm/kg
   b. 270-300 mOsm/kg
   c. 300-330 mOsm/kg
   d. 330-360 mOsm/kg

61. The birth of Piglets from embryo transfer was discovered by ______
   a. Heape
   b. Kvansnickii
   c. Willadsen
   d. Marden& chang

62. The birth of calf after IVF was discovered in which year _____
   a. 1951
   b. 1890
   c. 1982
   d. 1996

63. In which species the birth of an offspring boss from embryo transfer was discovered ____
   a. Rat
   b. Rabbit
   c. Both a & b
   d. None of the above

64. Birth of buffalo calf from embryo transfer was discovered by
   a. Nicholas
   b. Warwick& berry
   c. Willadsen
   d. drost et al

65. First commercial embryo transfer company formed for farm animals was discovered by____
   a. Alberta livestock transplants Ltd
   b. Oguri & Tsutsumi
   c. Brackett *et al*
   d. Prather *et al*

66. The protocols for superovulation of sheep and goat based on_____and multiple injections of porcine FSH
   a. Progesterone pessary
   b. Gonadotropins
   c. LH
   d. ECG

67. In which species, the LH hormone used for superovulation______
   a. Cattle
   b. Goat
   c. Pig
   d. sheep

68. At what level, the gonadotropin (pFSH) is injected in the superovulation protocol in cattle and buffalo_______
   a. 20-30 mg
   b. 1500 IU
   c. 80 mg
   d. 60 mg

69. In which species, the PGF is not used in superovulation protocol____
   a. Cattle
   b. Sheep
   c. Pig
   d. Goat

70. In which species, Feed altrenogest is given as pretreatment in superovulation protocol_____
   a. Cattle
   b. Buffalo
   c. Sheep
   d. Goat

71. The first began at the Animal Research Station in Cambridge using donor nuclei from early embryos in Nuclear transfer is
   a. Yanagimachi
   b. Roslin
   c. Willadsen
   d. Houdebine
72. Steen Willadsen in the mid-1980s in Cambridge was to demonstrate the possibility of producing sheep clones by fusing a
   a. Nucleated blastomere donor with an Enucleated recipient
   b. Enucleated blastomere donor with an Nucleated recipient
   c. a. & b. are correct
   d. a. are incorrect
73. The cloned embryos contain fewer cells than normal embryos are cattle, rabbit
   a. 9% & 43%
   b. 10% & 15%
   c. 19% & 45%
   d. 3% & 35%
74. According to Yanagimachi , high cloning success rate in
   a. Elite cattle
   b. Japanese black cattle
   c. Guernsey
   d. brown Swiss
75. The cloned foal, named 'Prometea' was derived from a cell taken in a skin biopsy from the mare mother
   a. Recipient
   b. Donor
   c. a. & b are correct
   d. None of the above
76. SCNT has been reported in the pig the viability of embryos with an extremely rate of cloned piglet production.
   a. High
   b. Medium
   c. Low
   d. Very low
77. Nuclear transfer procedures currently used to produce cloned animals.
   a. Enucleated recipient oocyte fusing the donor and recipient cells with electrical pulses
   b. The donor nucleus is injected into enucleated oocytes by piezo-actuated microinjection
   c. Whole-cell injection into the oocyte
   d. All are correct
78. Bhojwani (2003) used the 'zona-free' method of SCNT as described by Vajta and reported the first birth of a calf by cloning technology, this success followed the transfer of blastocysts to recipients, of which only one gave birth.
   a. 18 & 18
   b. 13 & 15
   c. 16 & !8
   d. 17 & 17
79. In Japan, Atabay (2004) used vitrified bovine oocytes as recipient cytoplasts for somatic-cell nuclear transfer (SCNT)
   a. Sheep
   b. Buffalo
   c. Bovine
   d. Pig

80. The successful cloning of sheep from an adult somatic cell and the birth to play an important role in the development of new procedures for genetic engineering in farm animals is

a. Dolly b. lurcy
c. Bonnie d. Rosie

81. For identification of interesting new models, genetic screening, and characterization of remains a long and arduous task.

a. Positional effect b. Thance mutation
c. Insertional mutagenesis d. Transgenic line

82. In gene transfer, animals receiving new genes are referred to as transgenic, a term first coined by an d. in 1981

a. Gordon and Ruddle b. Ruddle and Brinsten
c. brinsten and Gordon d. Yanagimachhi and brinsten

83. A is a direct familial lineage derived from one or more transgenic founders, characterized by the passing of the transgene(s) to successive generations as a stable genetic element.

a. Transgenic line b. non transgenic line
c. Both a and b. d. None of the above

84. DNA microinjection is usually accomplished in ova at the stage.

a. one cell stage b. 2 cell stage
c. 4 cell stage d. 16 cell stage

85. Retroviruses effectively transduce only cells.

a. Mitotically active cells b. Germ cells
c. somatic cells d. Dormant cells

86. Cells are derived from early pre implantation embryos and maintained in culture for a sufficient period for one to perform various in vitro manipulations.

a. Pluripotent ES cells b. Germ cells
c. Somatic cells d. none of the above

87. Efforts to genetically alter growth rates and patterns have included production of transgenic swine and cattle expressing a. foreign,

a. Foreign c-ski oncogene b. GDF-8 (myostatin) gene,
c. Both aand b. D. none of the above

88. Advantages offered by swine over other domestic species include a favourable response to

a. Hormonal superovulation protocols b. breeding capacity
c. both a and b. d. None of the above

89. Have been used as intermediate hosts to maintain ova at various stages of development, for the most part using a ligated oviduct as the storage depot.

a. Rabbit b. Cattle
c. Sheep d. None of the above

90. Is the most useful as it can indicate transgene copy number, length of a given target sequence, and possible sequence mutation.
   a. Southern blotting b. Northern blotting
   c. Western blotting d. None of the above
91. Advanced reproductive biotechnologies, ________is increasingly being conducted in small ruminants.
   a. Cloning by somatic cell nuclear transfer (SCNT)
   b. Multiple ovulation embryo transfer technology (MOET)
   c. Artificial insemination (AI)
   d. In-vitro produced embryos (IVP)
92. ________is the only reproductive technology used on any scale in countries where sheep and goats are important in farming.
   a. Embryo transfer b. Invitro fertilization
   c. Artificial insemination d. In Vitro-produced Embryos
93. As with cattle, the cost of a lamb or kid born after Embryo Transfer is likely to be ________times greater than one born after Artificial insemination.
   a. 10 b. 30
   c. 50 d. 80
94. Immunizing goats against________by way of a commercially available vaccine (Vaxtrate) which suppresses gonadotrophin secretion, steroidogenesis, sperm production, the production of male odour and agonistic behaviour between males.
   a. FSH b. LH
   c. GnRH d. Testosterone
95. Companies currently working on transgenic protein production for sheep is________
   a. GTC (Framingham, Massachusetts, USA)
   b. Pharming (Leiden, The Netherlands)
   c. Pharming BioProtein Technology (Paris, France)
   d. GTC PPL Therapeutics (Edinburgh, UK)
96. Measurement of the crown–rump length enables the gestational age of the embryo to be accurately estimated up to day------, using a linear regression equation.
   a. 30 b. 35
   c. 40 d. 45
97. The intravaginal sponge treatment is likely to be longer in goats than in sheep, due to________________________
   a. Longer estrus cycle in goat compared to sheep
   b. Longer estrus cycle in sheep compared to goat
   c. Short estrus cycle in goat compared to sheep
   d. Short estrus cycle in sheep compared to goat

98. Embryos are usually collected ______days after breeding by laparotomy or laparoscopy.

a. 6-8 b. 7-8

c. 8-9 d. 9-10

99. Artificial insemination is done on the understanding that it permits higher selection intensities for males and allows the monitoring of bucks for the selection for major genes, such as the ________

a. Alpha-sl-casein gene b. DNAH1 gene

b. Amelogenin gene d. SRY chromosome

100. In males, -----------------is considered as a most promising non-invasive and non-contact imaging technique to study scrotal thermoregulation and infertility problems associated with testicular pathologies and thermal stress.

a. Thermometry

b. Infrared thermography

c. Passive Integrated Transponder

d. Implantable and skin surface radio transmitters

101. From the following methods which is used for increasing the chances of successful Invitro Fertilization in exotic animals

a. Invitro Maturation (IVM) b. Ovum Pick-Up (OPU)

c. Cloning d. Both a and b

102. In exotic animals genetic engineering can increase the

a. Disease resistance b. Disease susceptibility

c. Adaptability d. Genetic potentia

103. Which of the following methods helps to overcome the breeding challenges and increase the genetic diversity

a. Embryo Transfer b. Cloning

c. Cryopreservation d. Artificial Insemination

104. For the conservation of Giant Panda and Amur Leopard the two methods which contributed more are_________

a. Genetic Engineering and Cloning

b. Embryo Transfer and Artificial Insemination

c. Cryopreservation and Cloning

d. Embryo Transfer and Cloning

105. The hormone responsible for the superovulation in Sumatran Rhinos is

a. Follicle Stimulating Hormone b. Luteinizing Hormone

c. Gonadotrophic Releasing Hormone d. Progesterone

106. The application of reproductive biotechnology in ferrets is

a. Biomedical Research b. Pet Breeding

c. Conservation efforts d. All the above

107. What is the primary goal of reproductive biotechnology in exotic animals
  a. To increase the population numbers
  b. To reduce extinction risk
  c. To enhance genetic diversity
  d. All the above
108. What are some ethical considerations surrounding reproductive biotechnology in exotic animals
  a. Animal welfare, genetic integrity, and ecosystem impact
  b. Cost efficiency and convenience
  c. Public opinion and political support
  d. Scientific curiosity and research experts
109. What is superovulation and how it is induced in exotic animals
  a. Superovulation is the release of multiple egg, induced by hormones
  b. Superovulation is the release of single egg , induced by mating
  c. Superovulation is release of multiple sperms, induced by hormones
  d. Superovulation is the release of single egg , induced by hormones
110. What role does embryo transfer play in reproductive biotechnology of exotic animals
  a. To transfer the embryo from one female to another
  b. To transfer sperm from one male to another
  c. To transfer eggs from one female to another
  d. To transfer genetic material from one female to another
111. Which biotechnological method is commonly used for conservation of endangered wild animal species?
  a. In Vitro Fertilization (IVF)
  b. Gene Editing
  c. Artificial Insemination (AI)
  d. Cloning
112. What is the primary advantage of using artificial insemination in wildlife conservation?
  a. Increased genetic diversity
  b. Higher birth rate
  c. Reduced need for natural mating
  d. Easier transportation of gametes over long distances
113. Which reproductive technology involves the transfer of fertilized embryos from one individual to a surrogate mother?
  a. Embryo Transfer
  b. Cloning
  c. Somatic Cell Nuclear Transfer
  d. In Vitro Fertilization (IVF)
114. What is a key challenge in applying Assisted Reproductive Technologies (ART) in wild animals?
  a. Cost of the procedure
  b. Ethical concerns
  c. Limited knowledge of species-specific reproductive biology
  d. Unavailability of advanced technology

115. Cryopreservation of sperm and embryos in wildlife species is primarily used for what purpose?
   a. Genetic modification
   b. Long-term storage for breeding programs
   c. Cloning
   d. Increasing reproductive rates in captivity
116. Which technique is used to manipulate genes directly in wildlife for conservation purposes?
   a. Gene therapy
   b. CRISPR-Cas9
   c. Somatic Cell Nuclear Transfer
   d. Artificial Insemination
117. What is the role of cloning in wild animal conservation?
   a. To increase genetic diversity
   b. To replicate endangered animals
   c. To alter animal genetics for disease resistance
   d. To artificially enhance reproduction rates
118. Which hormone is most commonly used to induce ovulation in wild animals during assisted reproduction?
   a. Estrogen
   b. Progesterone
   c. Follicle Stimulating Hormone (FSH)
   d. Testosterone
119. In vitro fertilization (IVF) in wild animals is most useful for which of the following reasons?
   a. It guarantees successful pregnancies
   b. It allows fertilization in a controlled environment
   c. It avoids genetic disorders
   d. It increases the population size faster
120. Which reproductive biotechnological technique has the greatest potential to restore extinct species?
   a. In Vitro Fertilization
   b. Artificial Insemination
   c. Gene Editing
   d. Cloning
121. Which of the following molecule is produced by Endometrial epithelial cells that inhibit T cell proliferation
   a. Cytokine TGF β
   b. Prostaglandin E2
   c. Both a & b
   d. None of the above
122. Which of the following molecule is produced by stromal cells that inhibit T cell proliferation
   a. Cytokine TGF β
   b. Prostaglandin E2
   c. Both a & b
   d. None of the above
123. What was the major opsonin in uterine fluid of mares
   a. IgA
   b. IgG
   c. C3b
   d. Fibronectin

124. What is the primary mechanism by which the placenta protects the fetus from immune rejection?
   a. Acting as a physical barrier
   b. Producing immunosuppressive molecules
   c. Altering its own antigenicity
   d. All of the above

125. What is the likely cause of the decrease in maternal lymphocytes in the uterus during early pregnancy?
   a. Interferon-gamma secreted by the conceptus
   b. Immunosuppressive molecules produced by the placenta
   c. Hormonal changes associated with pregnancy
   d. Unknown

126. What is the primary reason for the survival of the fetal allograft?
   a. The placenta is less antigenic than other foreign tissues
   b. Lymphocyte activation is inhibited at the maternal-fetal interface
   c. Both a and b
   d. Neither a nor b

127. In the sheep, progesterone appears to inhibit lymphocyte function by inducing the secretion of which protein from the uterine endometrium
   a. Ovine uterine serpin
   b. IL-4
   c. IFN-τ
   d. None of the above

128. What are the major lymph nodes filtering lymph derived from the reproductive tract?
   a. Medial iliac lymph nodes
   b. lumbo aortic lymph nodes
   c. Both a and b
   d. Neither a nor b

129. What is the effect of ovariectomy on the development of uterine infections in mares?
   a. Increased susceptibility to infection
   b. decreased susceptibility to infection
   c. No effect on susceptibility to infection
   d. Increased susceptibility to infection initially, followed by decreased susceptibility

130. What are the specific proteins secreted by the reproductive tract that help limit bacterial growth?
   a. Lysozyme and lactoferrin
   b. Opsonin and complement
   c. Cytokines and chemokines
   d. Immunoglobulins and complement

131. What is the primary function of immunization against Luteinising Hormone Releasing Hormone (LHRH) in animals?
   a. Stimulate ovulation
   b. Suppress pituitary secretion of LH and FSH
   c. Increase reproductive activity
   d. Enhance testosterone production
132. What is the effect of immunization against follicle stimulating hormone (FSH) in male animals?
   a. Increases spermatogenesis
   b. Decreases testosterone production
   c. Disrupts spermatogenesis
   d. Increases LH secretion
133. Immunization against which hormone can lead to a delay in puberty in female animals
   a. Oxytocin
   b. Prostaglandin F2α
   c. Luteinising hormone releasing hormone (LHRH)
   d. Gonadotrophin
134. Which of the following antigens has been targeted for immunization to create a contraceptive vaccine in animals
   a. Zona pellucida antigens
   b. Progesterone
   c. Luteinising hormone
   d. Testosterone
135. Immunization against which hormone is suggested for blocking implantation in female animals
   a. Prolactin
   b. Oestrogen
   c. Progesterone
   d. Oxytocin
136. Immunization against which hormone could prevent premature luteolysis in postpartum cows?
   a. Prolactin
   b. Oxytocin
   c. Progesterone
   d. Prostaglandin F2α
137. Which antigen is essential for sperm-egg interaction and has been used in immunization studies
   a. PH-20
   b. FA-1
   c. SP-10
   d. LDH-C4
138. What is the effect of immunization against LHRH in sexually mature animals?
   a. It enhances reproductive function.
   b. It causes gonadal quiescence and reverses animals to a prepubertal state.
   c. It increases testosterone levels.
   d. It improves fertility rates in farm animals

139. Immunization against which hormone can cause multiple ovulations in farm animals?

a. Testosterone
b. Oxytocin
c. Inhibin
d. Progesterone

140. What was the primary outcome of immunizing ewes against estradiol-17β?

a. An increase in fertility
b. Induced anovulation and anoestrus
c. No effect on reproductive cycles
d. Enhanced ovarian function

141. What is the main advantage of embryo cryopreservation over sperm or oocyte preservation in terms of genetic integrity?

a. It contains the complete genetic quota.
b. It avoids any risk of mutation during storage.
c. It simplifies the thawing process.
d. It reduces the risk of contamination during storage.

142. Cryopreservation helps maintain genetic diversity in animal breeding programs. What is one significant way this technology aids in advanced animal genetics research?

a. It allows rapid genetic modification of inbred strains.
b. It ensures that embryos remain in constant development in vitro.
c. It preserves mutations and special genetic combinations for future studies.
d. It eliminates the risk of disease transmission between species.

143. Which biophysical factor primarily influences the variability in cryopreservation success across different mammalian species?

a. The availability of liquid nitrogen.
b. The stage of embryonic development.
c. The duration of storage in cryogenic tanks.
d. The genetic background of the species.

144. When considering freezing techniques, what is the main disadvantage of fast freezing in embryo cryopreservation?

a. Increased formation of large ice crystals.
b. Higher risk of solution effects.
c. Loss of genetic material during freezing.
d. Formation of multiple embryos from a single zygote.

145. Cryoprotectants such as glycerol or dimethyl sulfoxide (DMSO) are used in cryopreservation to:

a. Accelerate the freezing process.
b. Lower the freezing temperature and reduce cellular dehydration.
c. Increase the formation of ice crystals.
d. Prevent contamination during storage.

146. Why is liquid nitrogen at -196°C commonly used for long-term embryo cryopreservation?
   a. It allows gradual thawing and rehydration of embryos.
   b. It prevents any biologic activity in the preserved embryos.
   c. It increases metabolic activity during the storage period.
   d. It simplifies the embryo classification process before freezing.
147. Which of the following is a key consideration when handling embryos prior to cryopreservation?
   a. Ensuring embryos remain at 0°C before freezing.
   b. Using sterile techniques and transferring embryos into fresh culture medium every 2 hrs
   c. Storing embryos in small test tubes without medium.
   d. Manipulating embryos at room temperature to reduce bacterial contamination.
148. What is a major advantage of using programmable freezers for cryopreserving embryos?
   a. They reduce the need for cryoprotectants.
   b. They ensure precise control of the cooling rate.
   c. They allow embryos to be stored without cryogenic materials.
   d. They prevent any risk of genetic drift during freezing.
149. During the thawing process of cryopreserved embryos, which factor is crucial to limit ice crystal growth and ensure embryo viability?
   a. Slow thawing and gradual rehydration.
   b. Rapid warming and careful dilution of cryoprotectant.
   c. Reducing the thawing temperature below -100°C.
   d. Prolonged exposure to room temperature before thawing.
150. Which method is most effective for assessing the survival of cryopreserved embryos post-thawing?
   a. Morphologic evaluation immediately after thawing.
   b. Testing embryo development in culture to the blastocyst stage.
   c. Transferring embryos to an oviduct of a different species.
   d. Measuring the rate of metabolic activity immediately after thawing.

Answer Key

1	b	2	c	3	a	4	c	5	b	6	c	7	d
8	c	9	b	10	d	11	b	12	a	13	b	14	b
15	b	16	a	17	b	18	c	19	d	20	c	21	a
22	d	23	a	24	a	25	c	26	d	27	a	28	d
29	a	30	d	31	b	32	a	33	a	34	c	35	b
36	c	37	b	38	b	39	b	40	d	41	d	42	a
43	b	44	c	45	d	46	a	47	b	48	a	49	b
50	c	51	c	52	a	53	a	54	b	55	a	56	a
57	c	58	d	59	c	60	d	61	c	62	c	63	c
64	d	65	a	66	a	67	a	68	a	69	c	70	d
71	c	72	a	73	a	74	b	75	a	76	c	77	d
78	a	79	b	80	a	81	a	82	b	83	a	84	a
85	a	86	a	87	c	88	c	89	a	90	a	91	a
92	c	93	a	94	c	95	d	96	c	97	a	98	a
99	a	100	b	101	d	102	d	103	a	104	a	105	a
106	d	107	d	108	a	109	a	110	a	111	c	112	d
113	a	114	c	115	b	116	b	117	b	118	c	119	b
120	d	121	a	122	b	123	b	124	d	125	a	126	c
127	a	128	c	129	a	130	a	131	b	132	c	133	c
134	a	135	c	136	d	137	a	138	b	139	c	140	b
141	a	142	c	143	b	144	a	145	b	146	b	147	b
148	b	149	b	150	b								

24

Clinical Biochemistry

Ravi Shankar Kumar Mandal[1], Sonam Bhatt[1], Vivek Joshi[2] and Anil Kumar[1]

[1]Department of Veterinary Medicine, Bihar Veterinary College, Patna- 800014

[2]ICAR-Indian Veterinary Research Institute, Izatnagar- 243122

Introduction

Water is the most abundant compound in the body, and most of life's essential processes take place in this aqueous environment. Although there is substantial variation, the total body water (TBW) of most domestic animals is approximately 60% of body weight (0.60 l/kg).Electrolytes are substances that exist as positive or negative charged particles in aqueous solution. The positively charged particles are "cations," and the negatively charged particles are "anions". The osmotic properties of a solute in solution are related to the number of particles in solution and not to its weight or its charge. One osmole of a non-dissociable substance is equal to its molecular weight in grams. One osmole of any substance that dissociates in solution into two or more particles is equal to the molecular weight in grams divided by the number of particles into which each molecule dissociates. Osmolarity is defined as the number of osmoles per l of final solution, whereas osmolality is the number of osmoles per kilogram of water. Although the expressions are similar, osmolality more correctly describes the osmotic properties as measured in the clinical laboratory.

The biochemical mechanism by which the chemical energy contained in foodstuffs are made available to the animal are collectively described as metabolism. The digestion of carbohydrate in the animal begins with the initial contact of the carbohydrate in their foodstuffs with the enzymes of salivary juice. Salivary α-amylase splits the α1,4-glucosidic bonds of various polysaccharides. Salivary amylase is similar in major respects to pancreatic α amylase.

A variety of stimuli can initiate gastric secretion. The sight or smell of food or the presence of food within the mouth causes gastric secretion by a reflex mechanism involving the vagus nerve. In the dog, gastric juice is produced in the resting state at a rate of approximately 5 ml/h. Pepsinogen is the zymogen, or inactive precursor, of pepsin, the principal proteolytic enzyme of gastric juice. Pepsin is capable of hydrolyzing peptide bonds of most proteins, mucin being one important exception. Rennin is another proteolytic enzyme produced by the gastric mucosa and has characteristics that are similar to those of pepsin. The oxyntic cells produce HCl. When the normal mucosa is stimulated, both Cl _ and H _ are secreted together, but current evidence suggests that H _ and Cl – are secreted by separate, closely coupled mechanisms.

The hepatocytes continuously secrete bile into the bile canaliculi; it is transported through a system of ducts to the gallbladder, where it is modified, concentrated, and storedduring digestion, bile is discharged into the lumen of the duodenum, where it aids in emulsification, hydrolysis, and solubilization of dietary lipids.

Clinical biochemistry in nephrology is mainly used to diagnose and monitor renal dysfunction or damage. The mammalian kidney consists of tens of thousands to millions of nephrons that function as parallel units. The larger the species, the greater the number of nephrons per kidney. The number of nephrons progressively increases during fetal development and is complete at birth (e.g., in sheep or humans) or during the few days following birth (e.g., in rat). Blood is supplied to the kidneys by the renal arteries. Depending on the location of the glomeruli, blood is then supplied to a network perfusing the cortical tubules or to the vasa recta vessels, which penetrate deep into the medulla in " hairpins " parallel to the loops of Henle. As a result of glomerular filtration, all small hydrosoluble plasma molecules, including water and ions, are freely filtered but high molecular weight proteins are not.

Skeletal muscle comprises approximately 50% of the body's mass. It is largely composed of long multinucleated spindle shaped skeletal muscle cells (myofibers) that are highly specialized by virtue of a structured array of muscle-specific contractile proteins and conductile membranes containing ion channels and pumps. Muscles in the body differ in their constituent myofiber populations and vascular and nerve supply, which affects the speed and force developed during muscle contraction as well as the neuromuscular disorders with which they are afflicted.

The detection of proteins in serum by their catalytic activity as a reporter of tissue damage is a cornerstone of medical laboratory analyses. Alanine aminotransferase (ALT), formerly known as glutamic pyruvate transaminase, catalyzes the reversible transamination of L-alanine and 2-oxoglutarate to pyruvate and L-glutamate. Aspartate aminotransferase (formerly glutamic oxaloacetic transaminase; GOT) catalyzes the transamination of L-aspartate and 2-oxoglutatarate to oxaloacetate and glutamate.

Minerals have a variety of functions in the body. They activate enzymatically catalyzed reactions, provide skeletal support, aid in nerve transmission and muscle contractions, serve as components of certain transport proteins and hormones, and function in maintaining water and electrolyte balance. Vitamins are organic molecules that are needed in minute amounts to function as essential enzymes, enzyme precursors, or coenzymes in many of the body's metabolic processes. With a few exceptions, most vitamins cannot be synthesized by the body and must be sup lied in the food. Vitamin A is necessary for support of growth, health, and life of higher animals.

1. The number of osmoles per liter of final solution is

   a. Osmolarity b. Osmolality

   c. Molarity d. Molality

2. The number of osmoles per kilogram of water

   a. Osmolarity b. Osmolality

   c. Molarity d. Molality

3. Which ion is primary determinant of plasma osmolality
   a. Potassium b. Chloride
   c. Sodium d. Hydrogen
4. Release of anti-diuretic hormone is closely related to
   a. Potassium b. Chloride
   c. Sodium d. Hydrogen
5. Renin is released in response to reduced renal perfusion produced by hypotension, volume depletion, or increased sympathetic activity by the
   a. Hepatocyte b. Gastric mucosa
   c. Lung d. Juxtaglomerular cells
6. Atrial natriuretic factor (ANF), also known as atrial natriuretic peptide (ANP), exists as a group of diverse peptide hormones produced in the
   a. Hepatocyte b. Heart
   c. Lung d. Juxtaglomerular cells
7. Metabolic acidosis is characterized by a
   a. Addition of hydrogen ions b. Loss of bicarbonate ions
   c. Dccreasc in pII d. All of thc abovc
8. The intracellular movement of hydrogen in exchange for potassium helps to prevent an excessive increase of the ECF hydrogen ion concentration in the face of an acid load. This exchange is called
   a. Chloride shift b. Cation shift
   c. Hydrogen shift d. Potassium shift
9. Lingual lipase is secreted by ....
   a. Von Ebner's gland b. Parotid glands
   c. Mandibular gland d. Submaxillary gland
10. Salivary amylase enzymatic activity is absent in the saliva of
   a. Dog b. Horse
   c. Cattle d. All
11. The only hormone known to stimulate HCl is
   a. Gastrin b. Secretin
   c. Glucagon d. Insulin
12. Amylase is ....containing metalloenzyme, catalyzes the specific hydrolysis of' α -1,4-glucosidic bonds, which are present in starch and glycogen.
   a. Calcium b. Zinc
   c. Magnesium d. Iron
13. Pancreatic amylase has an optimal pH for activity of 6.7 to 7.2 and is activated by
   a. Calcium b. Chloride
   c. Bicarbonate d. Phosphate

14. Choose the correct statement
    a. The pancreatic peptidases are secreted as the inactive proenzymes.
    b. The pancreatic peptidases are secreted as the active enzymes.
    c. At acidic pH, trypsinogen can be converted autocatalytically to trypsin.
    d. All
15. The secretin-stimulated pancreatic juice has a
    a. Large volume b. High HCO3-
    c. Low enzymatic activity d. All of the above
16. Source of secretin is
    a. D cells of pancreas b. S cells of duodenum
    c. G cells of pyloric antrum d. L cells of small intestine
17. The major precursor for carbohydrate synthesis in mature ruminants is
    a. Acetic acid b. Propionic acid
    c. Butyric acid d. Lactic acid
18. Starch and glycogen are composed of long chains of glucose molecules linked together by repeating
    a. α -1,4-glucosidic bonds b. β -1,4-glucosidic bonds
    c. α -1,6-glucosidic bonds d. β -1,6-glucosidic bonds
19. Cellulose is composed of long chains of glucose molecules linked together by repeating
    a. α -1,4-glucosidic bonds b. β -1,4-glucosidic bonds
    c. α -1,6-glucosidic bonds d. β -1,6-glucosidic bonds
20. At acidic pH, affinity of cobalamin is higher for
    a. Haptocorrin b. Intrinsic factor
    c. Both d. None
21. At neutral pH, affinity of cobalamin is higher for
    a. Haptocorrin b. Intrinsic factor
    c. Both d. None
22. Which is the most important non-erythroid source of bilirubin
    a. Myoglobin b. Cytochromes
    c. Peroxidase d. catalase
23. Conjugation of bilirubin with glucuronic acid is catalyzed by
    a. Uridine-diphosphate glucuronosyltransferas
    b. Serum glutamic-pyruvic transaminase
    c. Serum glutamic-oxaloacetate transaminase
    d. Gamma-glutamyl transferase
24. Bilirubin is carried in plasma by
    a. Albumin b. α-1 globulin
    c. Both a and b d. Transferrin

25. Conjugated bilirubin is also known as
    a. Indirect reacting bilirubin
    b. Water insoluble bilirubin
    c. Water soluble bilirubin
    d. Free bilirubin
26. Conjugated bilirubin is carried to small intestine by biliary system and intestinal bacterial flora reduce bilirubin to compounds of similar structure, which are collectively called as
    a. Biliverdin
    b. Bilirubin
    c. Urobilinogen
    d. Urobilin
27. Fecal urobilinogen is oxidized to ...., which is an orange substance and is excreted in feces
    a. Biliverdin
    b. Bilirubin
    c. Urobilinogen
    d. Urobilin
28. For calculation of Icterus index, yellow colour of serum or plasma is compared with standard solution of
    a. Potassium permanganate
    b. Potassium dichromate
    c. Ehrlich's diazo reagent
    d. Concentrated hydrochloric acid
29. Ehrlich's diazo reagent is used in estimation of
    a. Van den Bergh's tets
    b. Icterus index
    c. Rothera's test
    d. BSP excretion test
30. Major source of serum glutamic oxaloacetic transaminase is
    a. Muscle
    b. Liver
    c. Kidney
    d. Pancreas
31. Alkaline phosphatase is a microsomal enzyme, with its principal activity being intracellular, except in the case of___________, where it acts mainly in an extracellular location
    a. Hepatocytes
    b. Osteoblast
    c. Myocytes
    d. Renal cells
32. The major source of blood NH3 is
    a. Liver
    b. Gastrointestinal tract
    c. Kidney
    d. Lung
33. The following disaccharide is orally administered to manage hepatic encephalopathy
    a. Sucrose
    b. Mannose
    c. Lactulose
    d. Lactose
34. ___________ is a mitochondrial enzyme with a key role in the detoxification of ammonia (ammonia scavenger)?
    a. Glutamate dehydrogenase
    b. Ornithine carbamoyltransferase
    c. Arginase
    d. γ–Glutamyltranspeptidase
35. Conjugated bilirubin, which is water soluble, reacts ....with diazotized sulfanilic acid in aqueous solution
    a. Promptly
    b. Slowly
    c. Both
    d. None

36. After addition of accelerator to the aqueous solution the diazo reaction with unconjugated bilirubin can be complete d. The accelerators used are
    a. Methanol
    b. Ethanol
    c. Botha and b
    d. Ammonia
37. Clay coloured feces is observed in
    a. Pre-hepatic jaundice
    b. Hepatic jaundice
    c. Extrahepatic bile duct obstruction
    d. Intrahepatic cholestasis
38. The bile acid is
    a. Cholic acids
    b. Chenodeoxycholic acid
    c. Hyocholic acid
    d. All of the above
39. Conversion of cholesterol to 7 α -hydroxycholesterol is the initial, rate-limiting step in the synthesis of cholic acid, which is catalyzed by
    a. Cholesterol 7 α –hydroxylase
    b. Sterol 27-hydroxylase
    c. Cholesterol 25-hydroxylase
    d. Cholesterol 24-hydroxylase
40. The secondary bile acids are formed in the
    a. Live
    b. Small intestine
    c. Large intestine
    d. all of the above
41. The driving force of filtration through glomerulus is
    a. Plasma colloi dal (oncotic. pressure
    b. Hydrostatic pressure of cardiac origin
    c. Urine hydrostatic pressure within the Bowman's capsule
    d. All
42. The albumin concentration in primitive urine is
    a. 20-30 mg/L
    b. 40-50 mg/L
    c. 60-70 mg/L
    d. 90-100 mg/L
43. Preservatives used for preservation of urine
    a. Boric acid
    b. Thymol
    c. Toluene
    d. All
44. Urinary enzymes are
    a. N-acetyl- β –glucosaminidase
    b. Gamma-glutamyl transferase
    c. Glutathione-S-transferase
    d. All
45. Protein estimation in urine is done by
    A. Benedict's test
    b. Ross test
    c. Robert's test
    d. All of the above
46. Foam test is used in urine to detect
    a. Ketone
    b. Bile
    c. Glucose
    d. Calcium
47. Gmelintets is used in urine for detection of
    a. Ketone
    b. Bile
    c. Glucose
    d. Calcium

48. Fanconi-like syndromes are observed in some breeds of dogs, mainly basenjis, characterized by multiple defects in the reabsorption of glucose, sodium, potassium, calcium, phosphate, amino acids, and water by the tubule, developed due to

a. Gentamicin toxicity | b. Calcitriol deficiency
c. Maleic acid | d. All of the above

49. Unregulated or wide spread activation of endothelial cells can have drastic consequences, as observed with

a. Disseminated intravascular coagulation
b. atherosclerosis
c. Vascular disease
d. All of the above

50. The normal circulating life span of mammalian platelets is in the range of

a. 20-30 days | b. 30-50 days
c. 3-10 days | d. 120 days

51. Open-canalicular system (OCS) is absent in the platelets of

a. Cattle | b. Horse
c. Asian elephant | d. All of the above

52. The phenomenon of glucose molecules irreversibly binding to proteins is widespread in biological system, and the products are known as glycated proteins. When the protein of the complex is albumin or total serum protein, the product is called

a. HbA1c | b. Fructosamine
c. Both | d. None

53. The measurement of HbA1c in canines reflect the average blood glucose level over the previous

a. 6 weeks | b. 10 weeks
c. 12 weeks | d. 16 weeks

54. The measurement of fructosamine in canines reflect the average blood glucose level over the previous

a. 2 weeks | b. 4 weeks
c. 6 weeks | d. 8 weeks

55. Normal blood glucose level in cow is in range of

a. 45-75 mg/dl | b. 75-115 mg/dl
c. 85-150 mg/dl | d. 85-130 mg/dl

56. The chief synthetic and catabolic organ for cholesterol is the

a. Muscle | b. Intestine
c. Liver | d. Heart

57. Ketosis which occurs when a dairy cow receives insufficient calories to meet lactational demands plus body maintenance is

a. Underfeeding ketosis | b. Alimentary ketosis
c. Spontaneous ketosis | d. Nervous ketosis

58. Manganese absorption is increased under following condition
    a. Mn deficiency b. Fe deficiency
    c. Both of the above d. None
59. Hydroxylation process of Cholecalciferol to 25-hydroxycholecalciferol occurs in
    a. Kidney b. Intestine
    c. Bone d. Liver
60. The conversion of 25-hydroxycholecalciferol to calcitriol in the kidneys occurs in response to elevated level of
    a. Thyroxine b. Calcitonine
    c. Epinephrine d. Parathyroid hormone
61. Parakeratosis develops due to deficiency of
    a. Cu b. Ca
    c. Zn d. Mg
62. Lethal acrodermatitis, an autosomal recessive disorder in bull terriers is due to congenital deficiency of
    a. Cu b. Ca
    c. Zn d. Mg
63. For optimal maintenance, dose of Vitamin A recommended as
    a. 20-50 IU/Kg b. wt. b. 50-75 IU/Kg b. wt.
    c. 100-200 IU/Kg b. wt. d. 400-500 IU/Kg b. wt
64. In some animals deficiency of following enzyme results in need of a dietary source of vitamin C
    a. L- Gulonolactone hydroxylase b. L- Gulonolactone oxidase
    c. D- Gulonolactone monooxygenase d. D- Gulonolactone hydroxylase
65. Of the mammals, that do not produce ascorbic acid is
    a. Primates b. Guinea pig
    c. Both a and b d. None
66. Impaired collagen synthesis is principal feature of deficiency of
    a. Ascorbic acid b. Niacin
    c. Riboflavin d. Biotin
67. "Diseases of four D's- dermatitis, diarrhea, dementia and death" is due to deficiency of
    a. Ascorbic acid b. Niacin
    c. Riboflavin d. Biotin
68. Black tongue in dogs is due to deficiency of
    a. Ascorbic acid b. Niacin
    c. Riboflavin d. Biotin
69. Curled toe syndrome in birds is due to deficiency of
    a. Manganese b. Niacin
    c. Riboflavin d. Thiamin

70. Fox fed uncooked fish products and in cats given both fresh fish and canned cat food that has suffered excessive processing losses, results in deficiency of

a. Ascorbic acid b. Niacin
c. Riboflavin d. Thiamin

71. Sodium metabisulfite as preservative in food can degrade

a. Pantothenic acid b. Thiamin
c. Riboflavin d. Niacin

72. Biotin functions in enzymatic carboxylation as a co-factor for enzyme

a. Acetyl Co A carboxylase b. Propionyl CoA carboxylase
c. Pyruvate carboxylase d. All of the above

73. Choline is particularly noteworthy because it plays a key role in

a. Methyl group metabolism b. Carcinogenesis
c. Lipid transport d. All of the above

74. The primary sign of choline deficiency is

a. Cardiomegaly b. Encephalopathy
d. Fatty liver d. Renal failure

75. Oxidation of fatty acids requires their transportation from the cytosol into the mitochondrial matrix where they undergo β-oxidation. Following compound is necessary for transportation process of fatty acids

a. Taurine b. Carnitine
c. Coenzyme Q d. Inositol

76. Globulin level in cerebrospinal fluid (CSF) is estimated by

a. Foam test b. Sulfosalicylic acid test
c. Pandy's test d. Schales mercuric nitrate method

77. Specific gravity of normal CSF is

a. 1.003 to 1.008 b. 1.008 to 1.013
c. 1.013 to 1.018 d. 1.018 to 1.023

78. Increased cell count in CSF is interpreted as

a. Leucocytosis b. Pleocytosis
c. Erythrocytosis d. Thrombocytosis

79. Test for platelet dysfunction is

a. Clot retraction method b. PF-3 test
c. Platelet adhesiveness d. All of the above

80. A leukocyte that has ruptured and in which the cell nucleus appears as a pale staining smear without prescribed form or shape is called

a. Basket cell b. Dohle bodies
c. Mast cell d. Tart cell

81. Intraerythrocytic mass of denatured globin, irregular in shape and appearing as a refractile granule when slightly out of focus, is

a. Howell-Jolly bodies b. Heinz bodies
c. Acanthocyte d. Target cell

82. Erythrocyte with a central rounded area of pigmented material, surrounded by a clear zone without pigment and a dense ring of cytoplasm about the periphery of the erythrocyte, is

a. Howell-Jolly bodies b. Heinz bodies
c. Acanthocyte d. Target cell

83. Mean corpuscular hemoglobin concentration (MCH c. is expressed as

a. Concentration of hemoglobin in the average erythrocyte
b. Amount of hemoglobin by weight in the average erythrocyte
c. Average volume of individual erythrocyte
d. All of the above

84. Regenerative anemia s seen in case of

a. Acute hemorrhage b. Blood parasites
c. Equine infectious anemia d. All of the above

85. Positive Coomb's test is indication for

a. Systemic lupus erythematous
b. Autoimmune hemolytic anemia
c. Collagen vascular disease associated with antinuclear antibodies
d. All of the above

86. Bence-Jones proteinuria is a condition where a type of protein called Bence-Jones protein is found in the urine, present in

a. Canine distemper b. Multiple myeloma
c. Leptospirosis d. Aflatoxicosis

87. Wallace – Diamond or Watson method is confirmatory test for

a. Protein b. Glucose
c. Urobilinogen d. Blood

88. Mucous secreting glands are present in the renal pelvis and in ureter close to the kidney and presence of large amount of homogenous mucus is normal in the urine of following species

a. Equine b. Canine
c. Bovine d. Swine

89. Alkaline urine with high plasma bicarbonate concentration is seen in

a. Metabolic acidosis b. Respiratory acidosis
c. Metabolic alkalosis d. Respiratory alkalosis

90. Alkaline urine with low plasma bicarbonate concentration is seen in

a. Metabolic acidosis b. Respiratory acidosis
c. Metabolic alkalosis d. Respiratory alkalosis

91. Acidic urine with low plasma bicarbonate concentration is seen in

a. Metabolic acidosis b. Respiratory acidosis
c. Metabolic alkalosis d. Respiratory alkalosis

92. Acidic urine with high plasma bicarbonate concentration is seen in
    a. Metabolic acidosis b. Respiratory acidosis
    c. Metabolic alkalosis d. Respiratory alkalosis

93. Normal blood glucose level in dog is
    a. 35-70 mg/dl b. 65-118 mg/dl
    c. 120-140 mg/dl d. 140-180 mg/dl

94. Free thyroxine (FT_4) level in blood of dog is
    a. 0.05- 0.5 ng/dl b. 0.5-2.7 ng/dl
    c. 2.7-4.5 ng/dl d. 4.5-6.5 ng/dl

95. Normal blood calcium level in cattle is
    a. 4.5-8.5 mg/dl b. 9.7-12.4 mg/dl
    c. 12.4-15.0 mg/dl d. 15-20 mg/dl

96. Normal blood cholesterol level in cat is
    a. 95-130 mg/dl b. 135-270 mg/dl
    c. 5.1-54.2 mg/dl d. 50-80 mg/dl

97. Normal blood magnesium level of cow is
    a. 1.8-2.3 mg/dl b. 2.5-5 mg/dl
    c. 5-7.5 mg/dl d. 7.5-9.0 mg/dl

98. Normal blood Hemoglobin A1c (HbA1cconcentration in dog is
    a. 2.3-6.4 % b. 6.4-7.8 %
    c. 10.2-15.8 % d. 15.8-20.2 %

99. Normal blood aspartate aminotransferase (AST) level in horse is
    a. 78-132 U/L b. 226-366 U/L
    c. 32-84 U/L d. 1-30 U/L

100. Normal blood alanine amino transferase (ALT) level in dog is
    a. 21-102 U/L b. 120-204 U/L
    c. 220-400 U/L d. 400-500 U/L

Answer Key

1	a	2	b	3	c	4	c	5	d	6	b	7	d
8	b	9	a	10	d	11	a	12	a	13	b	14	a
15	d	16	b	17	b	18	a	19	b	20	a	21	b
22	b	23	a	24	c	25	c	26	c	27	d	28	b
29	a	30	a	31	b	32	b	33	c	34	a	35	a
36	c	37	c	38	d	39	a	40	c	41	b	42	a
43	d	44	d	45	c	46	b	47	b	48	d	49	d
50	c	51	d	52	d	53	a	54	a	55	a	56	c
57	a	58	b	59	d	60	d	61	c	62	c	63	c
64	b	65	c	66	a	67	b	68	b	69	c	70	d
71	b	72	d	73	d	74	c	75	b	76	c	77	a
78	b	79	d	80	a	81	b	82	d	83	a	84	d
85	d	86	b	87	c	88	a	89	c	90	a	91	a
92	b	93	b	94	b	95	b	96	a	97	a	98	a
99	b	100	a										

25

Biochemistry of Hormones

Sasmita Barik[1] and Shiv Kumar Yadav[2]

Department of Veterinary Physiology and Biochemistry, College of Veterinary Sciences and Animal Husbandry, Guru Angad Dev Animal and Veterinary Sciences University, Ludhiana, Punjab

[2]KVK, Shahjahanpur, Uttar Pradesh

Introduction

Most glands of the body deliver their secretions by means of ducts. These are called exocrine glands. There are few glands that produce chemical substance that they directly secrete into the blood stream for transmission to various target tissues. These are ductless or endocrine glands. The secretions of endocrine glands are called as hormones. Therefore, it is a chemical substance which is produced in one part of the body, enters the circulation and is carried to distant target organs and tissues to modify their structures and functions. Hormones are stimulating substances and act as body catalysts. The hormones catalyze and control diverse metabolic processes. Despite their varying actions and different specificity's depending on the target organ, the hormones have several characteristics in common with enzymes. They act as body catalysts resembling enzymes in some aspect. They are required only in small quantities. They are not used up during the reaction. They differ from enzymes because they are produced in an organ other than that in which they ultimately perform their action. The major hormone secreting glands are as follows— Pituitary, Thyroid, Parathyroid, Adrenal, Pancreas, Ovaries and Testes. The hormones are classified into following main classes according to the chemical structures:

1. Peptides and protein: All hypothalamic releasing and inhibiting hormone, Oxytocin; ADH Insulin, glucagon, somatostatin, pancreatic polypeptide Calcitonin Hormones regulating digestion (Gastrin, secretin cholecystokinin) Erythropoietin
2. Biogenic amines: T3, T4 (Thyroid hormones) Epinephrine and Norepinephrine Histamine Serotonin Melatonin
3. Steroids: Aldosterone, cortisol Androgens (Male sex hormone) Calcitrol Testosterone Estrogens, Progesterone (Female sex hormones)

The few important properties of hormones are as follows:

1. Action in low concentration Hormones act in a very low conc.
2. Hormones are not ordinarily stored, except in the gland of origin.
3. They do not have any cumulative action, because they are destroyed and excreted as soon as their functions are over.

4. Some hormones work quickly and are destroyed quickly e.g. epinephrine, other perform their work slowly and are also disposed of slowly e.g. Thyroxine.
5. 3'-5' c-AMP plays a unique role in the action of many protein hormones.
6. The action of most protein hormones is inhibited in absence of calcium even though ability to increase or decrease c-AMP is comparatively unimpaired.

Hormone secretion is strictly under control of several mechanisms. like:

1. Neuroendocrinal Control mechanism
2. Feedback Control Mechanism

Hormones of Anterior pituitary gland

1. Growth hormone
2. Thyroid stimulating hormone
3. Follicle stimulating hormone
4. Prolactin
5. Melanocyte stimulating hormone

Growth hormone from all mammalian species consist of a single polypeptide with a molecular weight of about 21500. It consists of 191 amino acids. There are two disulfide bridges between the adjacent cysteine residues (53-165 and 182-189). Growth hormone brings about positive nitrogen balance by retaining nitrogen. It stimulates overall protein synthesis. Growth hormone is a diabetogenic hormone, antagonizes the effect of insulin. Hypersecretion of GH can result in hyperglycemia, Hyposecretion causes stunted stature due to premature cessation of growth of the epiphyseal cartilages and consequently of long bones.

Thyroid Stimulating Hormone (TSH) is produced by basophil cells of anterior pituitary and is glycoprotein in nature. Its molecular weight is approximately 30,000. This consists of a α and β subunits. The α-subunit of TSH, LH, HCG and FSH are nearly identical. The biological specificity of thyrotropin must therefore be in β-subunit. The TSH stimulates the synthesis thyroid hormones at all stages such as iodine uptake, organification and coupling. It enhances the release of stored thyroid hormones.

Adrenocorticotropic Hormone (ACTH) or Corticotropin is a single polypeptide containing 39 amino acids.Two forms have been isolated, α-corticotropin and β-corticotropin. ACTH increases the synthesis of corticosteroids by the adrenal cortex and also stimulates their release from the gland. Profound changes in the adrenal structure, chemical composition and enzymatic activity are observed as a response to ACTH.

Follicle stimulating hormone (FSH) and leutenizing Hormone (LH) are pituitary gonadotrophins that influence the function and maturation of the testes and ovary. Both of them are glycoproteins with sialic acid, hexose and hexosamine as the carbohydrate moiety (16%). Molecular weight of FSH is 25000 and that of LH is 40000. LH causes final maturation of graffian follicle and stimulates ovulation. It also stimulates secretion of estrogen by the theca and granulosa cells. It helps in the formation and development of corpus luteum for leutinization of cells. FSH promotes follicular growth and prepares the graffian follicle for the action of LH and enhances the release of estrogen induced by LH. In males it stimulates seminal tubule and testicular growth, and plays an important role in maturation of spermatozoa.

Prolactin is a simple monomeric protein with 199 amino acids with three -S-S linkages. It stimulates mammary growth and secretion of milk. By acting through specific glycoprotein receptors on plasma membrane of mammary gland cells.The hormones secreted by intermediate lobe or middle lobe of pituitary gland are called melanocyte-stimulating hormones or MSH. MSH darkens the skin and is involved in skin pigmentation by deposition of melanin by melanocytes.

The hormones of posterior pituitary gland are Vasopressin (ADH) and Oxytocin These are small peptides containing nine amino acids. Oxytocin differs from Vasopressin with respect to 3rd and 8th amino acid residues. Their biological activities depend on C-terminal glycinamide, the side chain amide groups of glutamine and asparagine, the hydroxy phenyl group of tyrosine, and the intra-chain – S – S – linkage between cysteine 1st and 6th amino acidaDH reabsorbs water from the kidneys by distal tubules and collecting ducts. Contraction of smooth muscle is the primary function of oxytocin.

The principal hormones secreted by the follicular cells of thyroid are: (1) Thyroxine (T4) (2) Tri-iodo thyronine (T3) and (3) 'Reverse' T3. The hormones T4, T3 and "reverse" T3 are iodinated amino acid tyrosine. The iodine in thyroxine accounts for 80% of the organically bound iodine in thyroid venous blood. Small amounts of 'reverse' tri-iodo thyronine, Monoiodotyrosine (MIT) and another compound are also liberated. The hormones of thyroid gland play an active role in the metabolism. Their main affects are on protein and carbohydrate metabolism.

The hormones of parathyroid glands are (1) Parathormone (PTH) (2) Calcitonin. Parathormone is a linear polypeptide consisting of 84 amino acids. N-terminal amino acid is alanine and C-terminal is glutamine. Bovine PTH has molecular wt of 9500. Parathormone from different species differ only slightly in structure. The parathyroid gland is the principal target organ for bone and kidneys. It increases the rate of bone reabsorption with consequent mobilization of calcium and phosphate. An early effect on osteocytes leads to release of calcium from crystals of mature bone into blood, occurs within 15-30 minutes and does not initially depend upon the synthesis of RNA by osteocytes. It directly increases renal tubular reabsorption of calcium and direct renal excretion of phosphate. Calcitonin is a calcium regulating hormone.

The adrenal gland is composed of an outer cortex and inner medulla. The cortex is responsible for secretion of steroid hormones. The medulla is responsible for secretion of epinephrine. The adrenal cortex hormones are of two types: Glucocorticoids and Mineralocorticoids. Glucocorticoids primarily affect metabolism of carbohydrates, proteins and lipids and relatively have minor effects on electrolytes and water metabolism, e.g. cortisol, cortisone and corticosterone. Mineralo-corticoids are those which primarily affect the reabsorption of Na^+ and excretion K^+ (Mineral metabolism) and distribution of water in tissues, e.g. Aldosterone. Two biologically active compounds have been isolated from the adrenal medulla and synthesized. They are: Epinephrine and Norepinephrine (Nor adrenaline). The naturally occuring forms are laevorotatory, the synthetic are racemic, the former being almost twice as active as the latter. The above two hormones are called catecholamines and are closely related to tyrosine and synthesized in body from tyrosine.

The sex hormones or gonadal hormones are secreted by the testes, ovary, corpus luteum and to a small extent from placenta and adrenal cortex. They are all steroid compounds related to cholesterol. Sex hormones are of 3 types: Androgens, oestrogens and gestrogens. Androgens are hormones capable of producing certain characteristic musculinizing effects, i.e. they maintain the normal structure and function of the prostate and seminal vesicles and influence the development of secondary male sex characteristics, such as hair distribution and voice. The naturally occuring androgens in man are- Testosterone Epiandrosterone(3β - androsterone) Androsterone Dehydro epiandrosterone (DHEA). Two main types of female hormones are secreted by the ovary: The follicular or Estrogenic hormones The Pro gestational hormone. Estrogens are hormones capable of producing certain biological effects, the most characteristic of which are the changes which occur in mammals of estrus. They include growth of female genital organs and the appearance of female secondary sex characteristics. The growth of the mammary duct system and numerous other phenomena which vary somewhat in different species. The naturally occurring estrogens in humans are: β–Estradiol Estrone Estriol. Progesterone is the hormone of the corpus luteum, the structure of which develops in the ovary from the ruptured Graffian follicle. It is also formed by the placenta, which secretes progesterone, during the later part of pregnancy. Progesterone is also formed in the adrenal cortex, as a precursor of both C19 and C21 corticosteroids. It is also formed in the testes. Relaxin is a hormone concerned with the relaxation of pelvic tissues and cavity operating in conjunction with other factors. Relaxin is produced, during pregnancy, in tissues of the reproductive system, e.g., principally by corpus luteum and also by placenta. Its production is stimulated by progesterone, pregnenotone and related adrenocortical steroids, e.g. deoxy corticosterone. Pregnancy activates the placental hormones. The implanted blastocyst forms the trophoblast which is subsequently organized into the placenta. The placenta provides the nutritional connection between the embryo and the maternal circulation. Human placenta produces and secretes two peptide hormones and two steroid hormones. Human chorionic gonadotropin hormone (hcG) Chorionic somatomammotropin (CS) Progestins Estrogens.

1. Hormones are
   a. Peptides b. Steroids
   c. Cholesterol d. All
2. The only correct statement about hormone receptors is
   a. Receptors for protein hormones are present in cytosol
   b. Receptors for steroid hormones are membrane bound
   c. Hormone-receptor binding is irreversible
   d. Receptors can undergo down regulation and up regulation
3. Hormone receptors possess all the following properties except
   a. All of them are proteins
   b. They possess a recognition domain
   c. They bind hormones with a high degree of specificity
   d. Number of receptors in a target cell is constant
4. All the following hormones use cAMP asa second messenger except
   a. Estrogen b. FSH
   c. Luteinizing d. Glucagon
5. Hormone that binds to intracellular receptor is
   a. Adrenocorticotropic hormone b. Thyroxine
   c. Follicle stimulating hormone d. Glucagon

6. Hormone that acts through second messenger camp is
   a. Insulin b. Glucagon
   c. Calcitriol d. ADH
7. Hormone secreted from anterior pituitary is
   a. GH b. ADH
   c. FSH d. LH
8. Vasopressin is also known as
   a. Antidiabetogenic hormone b. Antidiuretic hormone
   c. Somatotropic hormone d. Pitoxin
9. Which of the following is used for inducing labour
   a. Prostaglandins b. Prostacyclins
   c. Vasopressin d. Thromboxanes
10. Which of the following does not have disulphide bond?
   a. Oxytocin b. Vasopressin
   c. Insulin d. Glucagon
11. A hormone secreted from posterior pituitary is
   a. Vasopressin b. Thyrotropic hormone
   c. Prolactin d. A drenocorticotropic hormone
12. Total number of amino acids in growth hormone is
   a. 91 b. 191
   c. 151 d. 291
13. Growth hormone causes
   a. Decreased peripheral utilization of glucose
   b. Decreased hepatic production via gluconeogenesis
   c. Increased glycolysis in muscle
   d. Decreased lipolysis
14. Epinephrin promotes the glycogenolysis in
   a. Muscle b. Liver
   c. Heart d. None of these
15. Prostacyclins is
   a. Inhibition of platelet aggregation b. Contraction of uterus
   c. Decrease of gastric secretion d. Relieving asthma
16. Acromegaly results due to excessive release of
   a. Thyroxine b. Insulin
   c. Growth hormone d. Glucagon
17. Thyrotropin releasing hormone is a
   a. Dipeptide b. Tripeptide
   c. Octapeptide d. Decapeptide

18. The number of amino acids in prolactin is
    a. 134
    b. 172
    c. 146
    d. 199
19. Adrenocorticotropic hormone (ACTH) is a single polypeptide containing
    a. 72 amino acid
    b. 49 amino acid
    c. 40 amino acid
    d. 58 amino acid
20. The sequence of amino acids in human growth hormone and the synthesis were done by
    a. Sanger
    b. Krebs
    c. Chah Holi
    d. Molisch
21. Proopiomelanocortin is the precussor of
    a. ACTH
    b. β-tropin
    c. Endorphins
    d. All of these
22. Biological activity of ACTH requires
    a. 10-N-terminal amino acid
    b. 24-N-terminal amino acid
    c. 24-C-terminal amino acid
    d. 15-C-terminal amino acid
23. ACTH stimulates the secretion of
    a. Glucocorticoids
    b. Thyroxine
    c. Epinephrine
    d. Luteinizing hormone
24. Adrenalin is synthesized from
    a. Adenine
    b. Adenosine
    c. Tyrosine
    d. Tryptophan
25. Corticotropin releasing hormone controls the direct release of
    a. Pro-opiomelanocortin
    b. α MSH
    c. β MSH
    d. Endorphins
26. Excessive secretion of ACTH causes
    a. Cushing's syndrome
    b. Addison's disease
    c. Myxoedema
    d. Thyrotoxicosis
27. Insulin increases the permeability of glucose across the plasma membrane of muscle cells by
    a. Acting on adenylate cycle
    b. By loosening the integrity of the membrane
    c. Through Ca2+ ions
    d. By hexose carries of intracellular organelles
28. The immediate parent of α, β endorphins is
    a. Pro-opiomelanocortin
    b. β-lipotropin
    c. ATCH
    d. Lipoprotein
29. ACTH induces rise in
    a. Cyclic AMP
    b. Calcium
    c. Cyclic GMP
    d. Magnesium

30. Glucocorticoids causes hyperglycemia due to
    a. Inactivation of protein phosphatase
    b. Inactivation of fructose 1,6-biphosphatase
    c. Stimulation of synthesis of pyruvate carboxylase
    d. Stimulation of synthesis of eltroxykinase
31. Catecholamine hormones are synthesized in the
    a. Chromaffin cells of adrenal medulla
    b. Zona glomerulosa of adrenal cortex
    c. Zona fasciculate of adrenal cortex
    d. Zona reticularis of adrenal cortex
32. The predominant glucocorticoid is
    a. Cortisol b. Aldosterone
    c. Dehydroephiandrosterone d. Androstenedione
33. A specific cortisol binding protein, transcortin is a
    a. Albumin b. α2-Globulin
    c. α1-Globulin d. β-Globulin
34. Cortisol is synthesized in
    a. Zona fasiculata b. Zona glomerulosa
    c. Zona reticularis d. chromaffin cells
35. All mammalian steroid hormones are formed from
    a. Purine b. cholesterol
    c. Pyrimidine d. Pyrrole
36. Aldosterone synthesis occurs in
    a. Zona reticularis b. Zona fasciculata
    c. Zona glomerulosa d. chromaffian cells
37. The most important effect of aldosterone is to
    a. Increase the rate of tubular reabsorption of sodium
    b. Decrease the rate of tubular reabsorption of potassium
    c. Decrease the reabsorption of chloride
    d. Decrease the renal reabsorption of sodium
38. One of the potent stimulators of aldosterone secretion is
    a. Increased sodium concentration
    b. Decreased potassium concentration
    c. Increased potassium concentration
    d. Increased ECF volume
39 In the rennin-angiotensin system the primary hormone is
    a. Angiotensinogen b. Angiotensin I
    c. Angiotensin II d. Angiotensin III

40. Steroid hormones are synthesized from
    a. adenine b. Vitamin
    c. Protein d. Cholesterol
41. The hormone required for uterine muscle contraction ais
    a. Progesterone b. Oxytocin
    c. Estrogen d. Vasopressin
42. Melanogenesis is stimulated by
    a. MSH c. LH
    b. FSH d. HCG
43. The number of amino acids in antidiuretic hormone is
    a. 9 b. 27
    c. 18 d. 36
44. ADH
    a. Reabsorbs water from renal tubules
    b. Excretes water from renal tubules
    c. Excretes hypotonic urine
    d. Causes low specific gravity of urine
45. The number of amino acids in the hormone oxytocin is
    a. 7 b. 14
    c. 9 d. 18
46. Epinephrine is rapidly metabolized by
    a. Monoamine oxidase b. Deaminase
    c. Transminase d. Decarboxylase
47. Insulin regulates fatty acid synthesis by
    a. Dephosphorylating of acetyl CoA carboxylase
    b. Activating phosphorylase
    c. Inhibiting malonyl CoA formation
    d. Controlling Carnitine-Acyl CoA transferase activity
48. Increased reabsorption of water from the kidney is the major consequence of the secretion of the hormone?
    a. Cortisol b. Vasopressin
    c. Insulin d. aldosterone
49. TSH hormone biochemically is a
    a. Protein b. Glycoprotein
    c. Fat d. carbohydrate
50. An increase in the osmolality of extracellular compartment will
    a. Inhibit ADH secretion
    b. Stimulate ADH secretion
    c. Cause no change in ADH secretion
    d. Stimulate the volume and osmoreceptor

51. All the following hormones use cAMP as a second messenger except
    a. Estrogen   b. Luteinizing
    c. FSH   d. Glucagon
52. All the following hormones promote hyperglycemia except
    a. Epinephrine   b. Insulin
    c. Norepinephrine   d. Glucagon
53. The secondary sexual characters in females is effected by
    a. Estrogens.   b. MIS
    c. Gluco corticoids   d. None of these
54. Gastric Secretion is regulated by the hormone:
    a. Glucagon   b. Epinephrin
    c. Gastrin   d. ACTH
55. Which of the following hormones is not involved in carbohydrate metabolism?
    a. ACTH   b. Vasopressin
    c. Glucagon   d. Growth hormone
56. Which one is required for converting glucose to glycogen in liver is
    a. Latic acid   b. UTP
    c. GTP   d. Pyruvic acid
57. For Catecholamine biosynthesis the rate limiting enzyme is
    a. DOPA decarboxylase   b. DOPAMINE β-hydroxylase
    c. Tyrosine hydroxylase   d. Phenylalanine hydroxylase
58. The biosynthesis of both Catecholamine and serotonin require
    a. Tyrosine hydroxylase   b. N-methyl transferase
    c. Aromatic amino acid decarboxylase   d. Tryptophan pyrrolase
59. Epinephrine stimulates glycogenolysis in
    a. Liver   b. Muscle
    c. Liver and muscle   d. Kidney
60. Epinephrine is derived from norepinephrine by
    a. Decarboxylation   b. Hydroxylation
    c. Oxidation   d. N-methylation
61. Glucagon hormone is called
    a. Hypoglycemic factor   b. Hyper glycemic factor
    c. Antidiauritic factor   d. Thyrotropin-releasing factor
62. Which of the following statements is correct?
    a. Thyroxine inhibits utilization of glucose
    b. Insulin increases utilization of glucose
    c. Glucagon promotes muscle glycogenolysis
    d. Insulin inhibits lipogenesis from carbohydrates

63. This pancreatic hormone promotes glycogenesis
    a. Insulin b. Stomato station
    c. Glucagon d. Pancreozymine
64. Epinephrine causes in muscle:
    a. Gluconeogenesis b. Glycogenesis
    c. Glycolysis d. Glycogenolysis
65. Aldosteronism alteration causes pathology of
    a. addison's b. Grave's
    c. cushing's d. Hartnup's
66. Insulin like growth hormones are produced by
    a. Hypophysis b. Pancreas
    c. Liver d. Thyroid
67. Somatostatin is produced by
    a. Hypothalamus b. Pancreas
    c. Hypothalamus and pancreas d. Hypothalamus and Adrenals
68. Prolactin release inhibiting hormone is believed to be
    a. Serotonin b. Dopanine
    c. Norepinephrine d. Acetyl choline
69. Which of the following organ prefers fructose to glucose
    a. Liver b. Testes
    c. Pancreas d. Heart
70. Which of the following hormone is not under the control of ACTH?
    a. Adosterone b. Cortisol
    c. Corticosterone d. Deoxycorticosterone
71. Excess secretion of thyroid hormones causes
    a. Hyperthyroidism b. Myxoedema
    c. Cretinism d. Cushing syndrome
72. Which one of the following is not liberated by the adenohypophysis
    a. Growth hormone b. TSH
    c. ACTH d. Gonadotropin
73. Insufficient free T3 and T4 results in
    a. Grave's disease b. Myxoedema
    c. Cushing syndrome d. Gigantism
74. Epinephrin promotes the glycogenolysis in
    a. Muscle b. Liver
    c. Both d. None
75. Which of one of the following is released by hypothalamus
    a. Somatostatin b. Somatotropic hormone
    c. Somato medin C d. Luteinising hormone

76. In primary hypothyroidism the useful estimation is of
   a. T3
   b. T4
   c. TBG
   d. Autoantibodies
77. Prostaglandins are
   a. c2 unsaturated acids
   b. c2 saturated alcohols
   c. c20 saturated acids
   d. c27 saturated alcohols
78. The blood sugar raising action of the hormone of suprarenal cortex is due to
   a. Glyconeogenesis
   b. Glycogenolysis
   c. Glucagon like activity
   d. Due to inhibition of glomerular filtration of glucose
79. Thyroperoxidase enzyme contains
   a. Heme
   b. Copper
   c. Zinc
   d. Magnesium
80. This hormone has disulphide group:
   a. Glucagon
   b. T4
   c. Insulin
   d. Epinephrine
81. Which of the following hormones are synthesized as prehormones
   a. Vasopressin and oxytocin
   b. Growth hormone and insulin
   c. Insulin and parathyroid hormone
   d. Insulin and Glucagon
82. Thyroproxidase requires hydrogen peroxide as oxidizing agent. The H2O2 is produced by
   a. FADH2 dependent enzyme
   b. NADH dependent enzyme
   c. NADP dependent enzyme
   d. NADPH dependent enzyme
83. TSH stimulates the synthesis delete
   a. Thyroxine
   b. Adrenocorticoids
   c. Epinephrine
   d. Insulin
84. Which of one of the following is not GUT hormone
   a. Motiline
   b. Gastrin
   c. Secretion
   d. Calcitonin
85. The tyrosine residues per molecule of thyroglobulin is
   a. 85
   b. 95
   c. 115
   d. 135
86. Which of one ring in the structure of the following is aromatic?
   a. Androgens
   b. Cholesterol
   c. Estrogens
   d. bile acids
87. The number of amino acids in parathormone is
   a. 65
   b. 84
   c. 115
   d. 122

88. Which one of the following statements is incorrect?
    a. Insulin increases glucose phosphorylation
    b. Insulin increases glycolysis
    c. Insulin augments HMP shunt
    d. Insulin promotes gluconeogenesis
89. Thyroid hormones are synthesized by the iodination of the amino acid:
    a. Glycine b. Phenylalanine
    c. Alanine d. Tyrosine
90. Parathormone causes
    a. Reduces the renal clearance or excretion of cblcium
    b. Increases renal phosphate clearance
    c. Increases the renal clearance of calcium
    d. Decreases the renal phosphate clearance
91. Whcih of the following hormone does not activate adenylate cyclase?
    a. Epinephrine b. Glucagon
    c. Parathyroid hormone d. Insulin
92. The number of amino acids in the peptide hormone calcitonin is
    a. 16 b. 24
    c. 32 d. 40
93. Pheochromacytoma is a tumor of
    a. Adrenal medulla b. Bone
    c. Head of Pancreas d. Pituitary
94. The characteristic of hyperparathyroidism is
    a. Low serum calcium
    b. High serum phosphorous
    c. Low serum calcium and high serum phosphorous
    d. High serum calcium and low serum phosphate
95. Target tissue of insulin is
    a. Red blood cells b. Renal tubular cells
    c. GI tract epithelial cells d. Liver
96. The number of amino acids in the A and B chain of insulin respectively is
    a. 19 and 28 b. 21 and 30
    c. 25 and 35 d. 29 and 38
97. Which of the following hormone is a peptide of less than ten amino acids?
    a. Insulin b. Oxytocin
    c. Growth hormone d. Parathyroid hormone
98. Calcitonin causes
    a. Calcinuria and phosphaturia b. Decrease in urinary calcium
    c. Decrease in urinary phosphorous d. Increase in blood calcium level

99. T3 is
  a. Thyroxine
  b. Triodo thyronine
  c. Triodo tyrosine
  d. Reverse tri iodo thyronine

100. In A chain of the insulin molecule the Nterminal amino acid is
  a. Glycine
  b. Valine
  c. Serine
  d. Phenylalanine

101. Parathyroid hormone
  a. Is released when serum Ca++ is too high
  b. Inactivates vitamin D
  c. Is secreted when Ca++ is too low
  d. depends on vitamin K for adequate activity

102. This pancreatic hormone increases the blood-sugar level:
  a. Insulin
  b. Glucagon
  c. Pancreozymin
  d. Pancreatic polypeptide

103. One of the following is not used as a second messenger by hormones:
  a. MRNA
  b. CAMP
  c. Calcium ions
  d. Myoinisotol

104. Insulin resistance is encountered in
  a. Addison's disease
  b. Hypothyroidism
  c. Hypopituctarism
  d. Acromegaly

105. Which one of the following statements is fully correct?
  a. Hormones are needed in the diet
  b. Hormones can be elaborated only by endocrine glands
  c. All the hormones enter the cells and perform their function
  d. Hormones are substance synthesized in the body in small quantities and control and regulate metabolic events

106. Richest source of prostaglandins in a human male is
  a. Blood
  b. Semen
  c. Urine
  d. C.S.F.

107. In the A chain of insulin molecule the Cterminal amino acid is
  a. Asparagine
  b. Threonine
  c. Valine
  d. Tyrosine

108. In hyperparathyroidism there is
  a. Hypocalcemia
  b. Hypokalemia
  c. Hypophophatemia
  d. Hyperkalemia

109. There is polyuria without glycosuria in this disorder
  a. Diabetes insipidus
  b. Diabetes millitus
  c. Bronze diabetes
  d. Juvenile diabetes

110. In the B chain of insulin molecule, the N terminal amino acid is
   a. Proline b. Threonine
   c. Phenylalanine d. Lysine
111. In hypophysectonized animals, fasting produces
   a. Severe hyperglycemia b. Hypoglycemia
   c. No change in blood sugar d. Mild hyper glycemia
112. In the insulin molecule, the number of interchain disulphide brides is
   a. 1 b. 2
   c. 3 d. 4
113. In the B chain of insulin molecule, the C-terminal amino acid
   a. Threonine b. Tyrosine
   c. Glutamate d. Valine
114. Insulin stimulates
   a. Hepatic glycogenolysis b. Hepatic glycogenesis
   c. Lipolysis d. Gluconeogenesis
115. Vasoconstrictor effect of ADH is mediated by
   a. CAMP b. CGMP
   c. Protein kinase C d. Angiotensin II
116. Calcitomica is antagonist to
   a. Serotonin c. Thyroxine
   c. Tri iodo thyronine d. Para thyroid hormone
117. Biological activity of gastrin is present in the
   a. Four N-terminal amino acids b. Four C-terminal amino acids
   c. Five N-terminal amino acids d. Five C-terminal amino acids
118. Gastrin is a polypeptide made up of
   a. Five amino acids b. Twelve amino acids
   c. Seventeen amino acids d. Twenty amino acids
119. The number of intrachain disulphide bridges in insulin is
   a. 1 b. 2
   c. 3 d. 4
120. Insulin exists in polymeric forms, for polymerization it requires
   a. Calcium b. Magnesium
   c. Manganese d. Zinc
121. The number of amino acids in pre-pro insulin is
   a. 51 b. 86
   c. 109 d. 132
122. Proinsulin has
   a. 74 amino acids b. 86 amino acids
   c. 105 amino acids d. 109 amino acids

123. Retention of sodium in the body leads to a retention of
   a. Potassium
   b. Water
   c. Potassium and water
   d. Neither potassium nor water

124. Progesterone is transported in blood by
   a. Transcortin
   b. Sex hormone binding globulin
   c. Albumin
   d. Testosterone estrogen binding globulin

125. Placenta secretes all of the following except
   a. FSH
   b. Progesterone
   c. Estrogen
   d. Chorionic gonadotropin

126. Secretion of androgens is increased by
   a. LH
   b. ACTH
   c. FSH
   d. Growth hormone

127. Action of insulin on lipid metabolism is
   a. It increases lipolysis and increases triglyceride synthesis
   b. It decreases lipolysis and increases triglyceride synthesis
   c. It decreases lipolysis and decreases triglyceride synthesis
   d. It increases synthesis of triglyceride and increased ketogenesis

128. Insulin increases the activity of
   a. Pyruvate kinase
   b. Phosphorylase
   c. Triacylglycerol kinase
   d. Fructose 2, 6-bisphosphatase

129. Insulin decreases the activity of
   a. CAMP dependent protein kinase
   b. HMG CoA-reductas
   c. Phosphodiesterase
   d. Acetyl CoA-carboxylase

130. Testosterone is transported in blood by
   a. Transcortin
   b. Testosterone binding globulin
   c. Testosterone estrogen binding globulin
   d. Albumin

131. The most potent hormone concerned with the retention of sodium in the body is
   a. Cortisone
   b. Corticosterone
   c. Aldosterone
   d. Cortisol

132. Aspirin blocks the synthesis of
   a. Prostaglandins only
   b. Prostacyclins only
   c. Thromboxanes only
   d. All of these

133. Administration of TSH increases serum T3 and T4 in
   a. Hyperthyroidism of pituitary origin
   b. Hyperthyroidism of thyroid origin
   c. Hypothyroidism of pituitary origin
   d. Hypothyroidism of thyroid origin

134. High level of T3 and T4 and low TSH in serum indicates
   a. Hyperthyroidism of pituitary or igin
   b. Hypothyroidism of pituitary origin
   c. Hyperthyroidism of thyroid origin
   d. Hypothyroidism of thyroid origin
135. The α-cells of pancreas islets produce
   a. Insulin b. Glucagon
   c. Somatostatin d. Pancreatic polypeptide
136. The number of amino acids in single chain polypeptide glucagons is
   a. 21 b. 31
   c. 29 d. 39
137. Total number of amino acids in human chorionic gonadotropin is
   a. 53 b. 145
   c. 92 d. 237
138. Glucagon enhances
   a. Hepatic glycogenolysis b. Muscle glycogenolysis
   c. Hepatic glycogenesis d. Lipogenesis
139. The production of progesterone by corpus luteum cell is stimulated by
   a. LH b. ACTH
   c. TSH d. MSH
140. In the biosynthesis of testosterone the rate limiting step is conversion of
   a. Cholesterol to pregnenolone
   b. Pregnenolone to progesterone
   c. Progesterone to 17 α-hydroxy progesterone
   d. 17 α-Hydroxy progesterone to androstenedione
141. Glucagon
   a. Increases protein synthesis b. Inhibits lipolysis in adipocytes
   c. Increases gluconeogenesis in liver d. Stimulates muscle glycogenolysis
142. Proteoglycans are made up of proteins and
   a. Glucosamine b. Sialic acid
   c. Mannosamine d. Mucopolysaccharides
143. The precursor of testosterone is
   a. Aldosterone b. Estrone
   c. Methyl testosterone d. Pregnenolone
144. A hormone produced by corpus luteum and placenta, concerned with relaxation of pelvis tissue is
   a. HCG b. Chorionic somatommotropin
   c. Relaxin d. Progestins

145. Synthetic progesterone used in oral contraceptive is
   a. Norethindrone b. Pregnenolone
   c. Androstenodione d. Stilbestrol
146. Androgens are synthesised in
   a. Leydig cells in testes b. Sertoli cells in testes
   c. Seminiferous tubules d. Prostate gland
147. In Addison's disease, there is excessive retention of
   a. Potassium b. Chloride
   c. Sodium d. Water
148. Secretion of mineralcorticoids is increased by
   a. ACTH b. Hypokalaemia
   c. Angiotensin d. Hypernatraemia
149. Mineralocorticoids increase the tubular secretion of
   a. Sodium b. Chloride
   c. Potassium d. Bicarbonate
150. The leyding cell activity is controlled by
   a. Intestitial cell stimulating hormone
   b. Adernocortex stimulating hormone
   c. Thyroid stimulating hormone
   d. Melanocyte stimulating harmone

Answer Key

1	d	2	d	3	d	4	a	5	b	6	d	7	a
8	b	9	a	10	a	11	a	12	c	13	a	14	c
15	a	16	b	17	b	18	d	19	b	20	a	21	d
22	b	23	a	24	a	25	c	26	a	27	d	28	a
29	a	30	c	31	a	32	a	33	c	34	a	35	b
36	c	37	a	38	c	39	c	40	d	41	b	42	a
43	a	44	a	45	c	46	a	47	b	48	c	49	b
50	b	51	d	52	b	53	a	54	b	55	b	56	b
57	c	58	b	59	c	60	d	61	d	62	a	63	a
64	d	65	a	66	a	67	b	68	c	69	b	70	a
71	a	72	a	73	b	74	b	75	b	76	d	77	c
78	a	79	a	80	b	81	c	82	d	83	a	84	d
85	c	86	b	87	b	88	d	89	d	90	a	91	d
92	c	93	a	94	d	95	d	96	b	97	b	98	a
99	b	100	a	101	c	102	b	103	c	104	a	105	d
106	c	107	a	108	b	109	a	110	c	111	b	112	b
113	a	114	b	115	c	116	d	117	b	118	c	119	a

120	d	121	c	122	b	123	b	124	a	125	a	126	a
127	b	128	a	129	a	130	c	131	b	132	d	133	c
134	c	135	b	136	c	137	d	138	a	139	a	140	d
141	c	142	a	143	d	144	c	145	a	146	a	147	a
148	b	149	c	150	a								

26

Diagnostic Biochemistry

***Lalhmangaihzuali*[1] *and Mohammed Hasif Ganimattoullah*[2]**

[1]*Division of Biochemistry, ICAR-IVRI, Uttar Pradesh*

[2]*Institute of Veterinary Science and Animal Husbandry, Siksha O Anusandhan University, Bhubneshwar, Orissa*

Introduction

Diagnostic biochemistry, is a branch of laboratory medicine that focuses on the analysis of bodily fluids to diagnose and monitor diseases. This field plays a crucial role in understanding the biochemical mechanisms underlying various conditions, enabling accurate diagnosis, prognosis, and management. The biological samples for diagnosis include blood, urine, cerebrospinal fluid, pleural fluid and tissues.

Factors Affecting Serum Enzyme Activity or Protein Level

1. **Organ Mass and Enzyme Tissue Concentration:**
    - Higher enzyme concentrations in organs can lead to greater increases in serum enzyme activity during disease. For instance, the liver's large mass contributes to potential increases in serum ALT activity.
2. **Cell Location**
    - The proximity of cellular enzymes to the blood, urine, or other fluids determines the fluid in which an enzyme's activity will increase upon cell injury. For example, renal tubular gamma-glutamyltransferase (GGT) is released into urine, not blood, following injury.
3. **Release Mechanisms of Cytoplasmic Enzymes**
    - Alterations in the cell membrane are essential for cytoplasmic enzymes to access the blood. When cell necrosis occurs, perforations and tears in the cell membrane enable the release of cytosolic contents. Membrane blebs also allow the release of cytoplasmic enzymes, either directly into the blood or into the interstitial space, from where they can be transported by the lymphatic system to the bloodstream.
4. **Blood Clearance Rates of Enzymes**
    - Serum enzyme activity depends on the clearance rate from the blooddiseases can affect enzyme clearance, complicating diagnostic test interpretations. For example, pancreatic amylase increases in renal failure due to decreased clearance.

5. **Enzyme Induction**

   - Increased serum enzyme activity can result from increased production, not just cell injury. This induction can be due to hormonal changes, diseases like cholestasis, or drug effects.

Different organ/tissue function tests

Liver function test

- **Alanine Aminotransferase (ALT)**: Also known as serum glutamic-pyruvic transaminase (SGPT). An enzyme found primarily in the liver. Elevated levels indicate liver cell damage or inflammation. Elevated serum ALT activity is specific for detecting liver injury in dogs and cats, but not in horses and cattle.
- **Aspartate Aminotransferase (AST)**: Formerly known as serum glutamic oxaloacetic transaminase (SGOT). AST activity is relatively high in the liver, skeletal muscle, and cardiac muscle, with variations across different species. Elevated serum AST levels are seen in both reversible and irreversible hepatocyte injuries, including hepatocellular injury and cholestasis. All domestic animals have high AST activity in livers, making serum AST a common marker for assessing liver cell damage. However, since AST activity is also high in the kidneys, heart, and skeletal muscles, increased serum AST levels are considered less specific for liver disease compared to elevated serum ALT levels.
- **Alkaline Phosphatase (ALP)**: An enzyme found in the liver, bone, and other tissues. Elevated levels can indicate cholestasis (bile flow obstruction), liver disease, or bone disorders. Commonly elevated in young growing animals due to bone growth.
- **Gamma-Glutamyl Transferase (GGT)**: GGT activity is primarily associated with biliary epithelial cells in animals. Elevated serum GGT levels are frequently seen with cholestasis (bile duct obstructions) and conditions that lead to biliary hyperplasia in all species. Serum GGT activity is especially useful as a clinical indicator of cholestasis in horses and cattle, owing to their higher liver GGT activity compared to dogs and cats.
- **Arginase**: In mammals, there are two isoforms of arginase: arginase type I and type II. Arginase type I is a cytosolic enzyme primarily expressed in the liver, where it plays a crucial role in urea synthesis. In contrast, arginase type II is a mitochondrial enzyme found in many tissues, including the kidney. Due to the higher arginase activity in the liver compared to other organs, increased serum arginase activity is considered specific to liver function.
- **Ornithine carbamoyltransferase (OCT):** OCT is considered as a liver-specific in domestic animals and is used to detect hepatocellular necrosis.
- **Bilirubin**: A byproduct of the breakdown of red blood cells, processed by the liver. Total Bilirubin is the sum of unconjugated and conjugated bilirubin levels in the blooddirect Bilirubin reflects the level of conjugated bilirubin. Indirect Bilirubin can be calculated by subtracting direct bilirubin from total bilirubin. Elevated Unconjugated Bilirubin can indicate hemolytic anemia or ineffective erythropoiesis, where there is increased breakdown of red blood cells. Elevated

Conjugated Bilirubin often suggests liver dysfunction, such as hepatitis or biliary obstruction, where the ability to excrete bilirubin by liver is impaired.

- **Bile Acids**: Produced by the liver and involved in fat digestion. Elevated bile acid is indicative of liver dysfunction, particularly when there is impaired hepatic uptake, conjugation, or excretion of bile acids. This can occur in conditions such as cholestasis, hepatitis, cirrhosis, or hepatic insufficiency. Elevated postprandial bile acid levels can indicate liver dysfunction or portosystemic shunts.

Neuromuscular function test

- **Creatine Kinase (CK):** Creatine kinase is the most commonly utilized serum enzyme test for diagnosing neuromuscular diseases in domestic animals.
- **Aspartate Aminotransferase (AST)**: Increases in AST activity is common in various muscle disorders characterized by the necrosis of muscle fibers.
- **Lactate Dehydrogenase (LDH):** LDH molecules are tetrameric, composed of M (muscle) and H (heart) subunits, forming five isoenzymes distinguishable by electrophoresis. LDH5 (M4) is predominantly found in skeletal muscle, while LDH1 (H4) is prevalent in heart muscle. Elevated LDH levels are observed in muscle disorders with myonecrosis and various hepatic disorders, but without isoenzyme analysis, LDH measurements lack organ specificity.
- **Myoglobin:** Increased levels of myoglobin are detected in human muscle disorders. Due to its specificity to skeletal and cardiac muscles and its rapid clearance from plasma, myoglobin levels are considered specific for muscle necrosis.
- **Others:** Troponin I assay are employed to detect myocardial degeneration across various species. Serum carbonic anhydrase III has been suggested as a marker for rhabdomyolysis.

Kidney Function Test

- **Creatinine**: Creatinine is the test most often used to diagnose and monitor kidney disease in human and animal clinical pathology. Elevated plasma creatinine levels can indicate impaired kidney function, while low levels may be associated with low muscle mass
- **Urea**: Urea the primary form of nitrogen elimination in mammals, is freely filtered by the kidney glomeruli and reabsorbed in the collecting tubule. Its passive reabsorption increases when urine flow is reduced, leading to elevated plasma urea in dehydrated or hemorrhagic patients, and decreased P-Urea in overhydrated patients.
- **Cystatin C**: The plasma concentration of cystatin C rises in cases of renal failure. It is the most sensitive marker for detecting renal failure in humans

Thyroid Function Tests

- **Total Thyroxine (T4)**: Measures the total amount of thyroxine in the blood. Low levels suggest hypothyroidism, while high levels indicate hyperthyroidism.
- **Free Thyroxine (fT4)**: Measures the free (unbound. thyroxine in the blood. Free T4 is less affected by non-thyroidal illnesses and is more specific for diagnosing thyroid dysfunction.

- **Thyroid-Stimulating Hormone (TSH)**: Measures the level of TSH in the bloo d. High levels indicate hypothyroidism in dogs. Low levels of TSH have no specific clinical significance in cats due to their naturally low TSH levels.
- **Triiodothyronine (T3) and Free T3 (fT3)**: Measures total and free triiodothyronine. These tests are less commonly used due to variability and less diagnostic value compared to T4 and fT4.
- **Thyroid Autoantibodies**: Detects the presence of antibodies against thyroid tissue, which can indicate autoimmune thyroiditis, a common cause of hypothyroidism in dogs.

Lipid profile test

- **Total Cholesterol**: Measures the overall level of cholesterol in the blood. Elevated levels can indicate hypercholesterolemia.
- **High-Density Lipoprotein (HDL) Cholesterol**: Often referred to as "good" cholesterol. Higher levels are generally protective against cardiovascular disease.
- **Low-Density Lipoprotein (LDL) Cholesterol**: Known as "bad" cholesterol. Elevated levels are associated with an increased risk of atherosclerosis and heart disease.
- **Very Low-Density Lipoprotein (VLDL) Cholesterol**: Transports triglycerides in the blood. Elevated VLDL is often seen in hypertriglyceridemia.
- **Triglycerides**: Measures the level of triglycerides in the blood. High levels indicate hypertriglyceridemia, which is a risk factor for pancreatitis and cardiovascular disease.

1. What is diagnostic biochemistry also known as?
   a. Molecular biology b. Clinical biochemistry
   c. Immunology d. Genetics
3. Which of the following is NOT a factor affecting serum enzyme activity or protein level?
   a. Organ mass b. Enzyme tissue concentration
   c. Cell location d. Blood pH
4. What can higher enzyme concentrations in organs lead to?
   a. Lower serum enzyme activity
   b. Greater increases in serum enzyme activity during disease
   c. No change in serum enzyme activity
   d. Decreased enzyme production
5. Where would renal tubular gamma-glutamyltransferase (GGT) be released following renal tubular epithelial cell injury?
   a. Blood b. Urine
   c. Cerebrospinal fluid d. Interstitial fluid
6. What is necessary for cytoplasmic enzymes to access the blood?
   a. Increased enzyme production b. Cell membrane alterations
   c. Enzyme inhibitors d. pH changes

7. What can perforations and tears in the cell membrane cause during cell necrosis?
   a. Enzyme activation
   b. Release of cytosolic contents
   c. Cell regeneration
   d. Enzyme inhibition
8. What is the main cause of increased serum enzyme activity during enzyme induction?
   a. Cell injury
   b. Increased enzyme production
   c. Decreased enzyme clearance
   d. Enzyme inhibition
9. Which enzyme is used as a specific marker for liver injury in dogs and cats?
   a. Alanine Aminotransferase (ALT)
   b. Aspartate Aminotransferase (AST)
   c. Akaline Phosphatase (ALP)
   d. Gamma-Glutamyl Transferase (GGT)
10. In which species is serum ALT activity NOT specific for liver injury?
   a. Dogs
   b. Cats
   c. Horses
   d. Humans
11. What does elevated serum AST activity indicate?
   a. Liver cell damage only
   b. Muscle damage only
   c. Both liver and muscle damage
   d. Bone disorders
12. What condition is commonly indicated by elevated ALP levels in young growing animals?
   a. Liver disease
   b. Bone growth
   c. Muscle necrosis
   d. Kidney failure
13. In which species is serum GGT activity especially useful as an indicator of cholestasis?
   a. Dogs and cats
   b. Horses and cattle
   c. Birds and reptiles
   d. Humans
14. Which isoform of arginase is primarily expressed in the liver?
   a. Arginase type I
   b. Arginase type II
   c. Both type I and type II
   d. Neither type I nor type II
15. What is the function of ornithine carbamoyltransferase (OCT) in domestic animals?
   a. Detects hepatocellular necrosis
   b. Indicates kidney function
   c. Measures muscle damage
   d. Assesses bone growth
16. Which type of bilirubin is a byproduct of red blood cell breakdown?
   a. Conjugated bilirubin
   b. Unconjugated bilirubin
   c. Both conjugated and unconjugated bilirubin
   d. Direct bilirubin
17. What does elevated unconjugated bilirubin typically indicate?
   a. Liver dysfunction
   b. Hemolytic anemia
   c. bone disorders
   d. Muscle necrosis

18. What condition is suggested by elevated conjugated bilirubin levels?
    a. Hepatitis
    b. Muscle injury
    c. Bone growth
    d. Dehydration
19. What can elevated postprandial bile acid levels indicate?
    a. Normal liver function
    b. Liver dysfunction or portosystemic shunts
    c. Kidney disease
    d. Bone disorders
20. Which enzyme is most commonly utilized for diagnosing neuromuscular diseases in domestic animals?
    a. Creatine Kinase (CK)
    b. Alanine Aminotransferase (ALT)
    c. Lactate Dehydrogenase (LDH)
    d. Myoglobin
21. What does an increase in AST activity commonly indicate in muscle disorders?
    a. Necrosis of muscle fibers
    b. Muscle regeneration
    c. Normal muscle function
    d. Decreased enzyme production
22. Which LDH isoenzyme is predominantly found in skeletal muscle?
    a. LDH1 (H4)
    b. LDH2 (H3M)
    c. LDH3 (H2M2)
    d. LDH5 (M4)
23. What does elevated LDH levels in muscle disorders indicate?
    a. Myonecrosis
    b. Bone growth
    c. Liver regeneration
    d. Kidney dysfunction
24. Which biomarker is considered specific for muscle necrosis?
    a. Myoglobin
    b. Bilirubin
    c. Alkaline Phosphatase (ALP)
    d. Gamma-Glutamyl Transferase (GGT)
25. What is the most sensitive marker for detecting renal failure in humans?
    a. Creatinine
    b. Urea
    c. Cystatin C
    d. Bilirubin
26. What condition is suggested by elevated plasma creatinine levels?
    a. Impaired kidney function
    b. Bone disorders
    c. Normal kidney function
    d. Muscle regeneration
27. What does low plasma creatinine levels typically indicate?
    a. High muscle mass
    b. Low muscle mass
    c. Kidney dysfunction
    d. Liver disease
28. What happens to plasma urea levels in dehydrated patients?
    a. Decrease
    b. Increase
    c. Stay the same
    d. Fluctuate randomly

29. Which test measures the total amount of thyroxine in the blood?
    a. Free Thyroxine (fT4)
    b. Total Thyroxine (T4)
    c. Triiodothyronine (T3)
    d. Free Triiodothyronine (fT3)
30. What does low Total Thyroxine (T4) levels suggest?
    a. Hyperthyroidism
    b. Hypothyroidism
    c. Normal thyroid function
    d. Liver dysfunction
31. What does high Free Thyroxine (fT4) levels indicate?
    a. Hypothyroidism
    b. Hyperthyroidism
    c. Kidney dysfunction
    d. Muscle necrosis
32. High levels of hypothyroidism in dogs indicate
    a. Thyroid-Stimulating Hormone (TSH)
    b. Triiodothyronine (T3)
    c. Free Thyroxine (fT4)
    d. Total Thyroxine (T4)
33. What do high levels of LDL cholesterol indicate?
    a. Lower risk of atherosclerosis
    b. Increased risk of atherosclerosis
    c. Normal cardiovascular health
    d. bone growth
34. What is the role of High-Density Lipoprotein (HDL) cholesterol?
    a. Transports triglycerides
    b. Indicates liver dysfunction
    c. Protects against cardiovascular disease
    d. Measures muscle damage
35. Which type of cholesterol is known as "bad" cholesterol?
    a. High-Density Lipoprotein (HDL)
    b. Low-Density Lipoprotein (LDL)
    c. Very Low-Density Lipoprotein (VLDL)
    d. Total Cholesterol
36. Which cholesterol type is often elevated in hypertriglyceridemia?
    a. High-Density Lipoprotein (HDL)
    b. Low-Density Lipoprotein (LDL)
    c. Very Low-Density Lipoprotein (VLDL)
    d. Total Cholesterol
37. What do high triglyceride levels indicate?
    a. Hypercholesterolemia
    b. Hypertriglyceridemia
    c. Normal cardiovascular health
    d. Bone disorders
38. What are total cholesterol levels used to measure?
    a. Overall cholesterol in the blood
    b. Only HDL cholesterol
    c. Only LDL cholesterol
    d. Only VLDL cholesterol
39. What can elevated serum GGT levels indicate?
    a. Muscle necrosis
    b. Liver disease
    c. Kidney disease
    d. Heart disease

40. In which organ is Aspartate Aminotransferase (AST) activity relatively high, aside from the liver?
    a. Kidneys
    b. Brain
    c. Skeletal muscle
    d. Lungs
41. Elevated levels of which enzyme can indicate cholestasis or bile duct obstruction?
    a. Alanine Aminotransferase (ALT)
    b. Aspartate Aminotransferase (AST)
    c. Alkaline Phosphatase (ALP)
    d. Ornithine Carbamoyltransferase (OCT)
42. Which enzyme's activity is especially useful for indicating cholestasis in horses and cattle?
    a. Alanine Aminotransferase (ALT)
    b. Gamma-Glutamyl Transferase (GGT)
    c. Aspartate Aminotransferase (AST)
    d. Arginase
43. Which isoform of arginase is primarily expressed in the liver?
    a. Arginase type I
    b. Arginase type II
    c. Arginase type III
    d Arginase type IV
44. What is the primary clinical significance of increased serum ornithine carbamoyltransferase (OCT) activity?
    a. Detecting bone disorders
    b. Detecting hepatocellular necrosis
    c. Diagnosing renal failure
    d. Diagnosing thyroid dysfunction
45. What condition is indicated by elevated unconjugated bilirubin levels?
    a. Cholestasis
    b. Hemolytic anemia
    c. Biliary obstruction
    d. Hepatitis
46. Elevated conjugated bilirubin levels often suggest dysfunction in which organ?
    a. Kidney
    b. Heart
    c. Liver
    d. Pancreas
47. Which enzyme is most commonly utilized to diagnose neuromuscular diseases in domestic animals?
    a. Lactate Dehydrogenase (LDH)
    b. Myoglobin
    c. creatine Kinase (CK)
    d. Aspartate Aminotransferase (AST)
48. Which isoenzymes are distinguishable by electrophoresis and are found in both muscle and heart tissues?
    a. Creatine Kinase (CK)
    b. Lactate Dehydrogenase (LDH)
    c. Myoglobin
    d. Troponin I
49. Increased levels of which molecule are detected in muscle disorders and are specific for muscle necrosis?
    a. Lactate Dehydrogenase (LDH)
    b. Creatine Kinase (CK)
    c. Myoglobin
    d. Troponin I

50. Which biomarker is the most sensitive for detecting renal failure in humans?
 a. Creatinine b. Urea
 c. Cystatin C d. Total Thyroxine (T4)

51. Elevated levels of which molecule in the blood can indicate impaired kidney function?
 a. Thyroxine (T4) b. Urea
 c. Cystatin C d. Creatinine

52. In cases of dehydration, which nitrogenous waste product is likely to be elevated due to increased passive reabsorption in the kidney?
 a. Creatinine b. Urea
 c. Uric acid d. Ammonia

53. Low levels of which thyroid hormone suggest hypothyroidism?
 a. Total Thyroxine (T4) b. Free Thyroxine (fT4)
 c. Thyroid-Stimulating Hormone (TSH) d. Triiodothyronine (T3)

54. Which elevated levels indicate hypothyroidism in dogs?
 a. Total Thyroxine (T4) b. Free Thyroxine (fT4)
 c. Thyroid-Stimulating Hormone (TSH) d. Triiodothyronine (T3)

55. Which thyroid test is less affected by non-thyroidal illnesses and is more specific for diagnosing thyroid dysfunction?
 a. Total Thyroxine (T4) b. Free Thyroxine (fT4)
 c. Thyroid-Stimulating Hormone (TSH) d. Triiodothyronine (T3)

56. Which component of a lipid profile is often referred to as “good” cholesterol?
 a. Total Cholesterol
 b. High-Density Lipoprotein (HDL) Cholesterol
 c. Low-Density Lipoprotein (LDL) Cholesterol
 d. Very Low-Density Lipoprotein (VLDL) Cholesterol

57. Which lipid profile component is associated with an increased risk of atherosclerosis and heart disease when elevated?
 a. Total Cholesterol
 b. High-Density Lipoprotein (HDL) Cholesterol
 c. Low-Density Lipoprotein (LDL) Cholesterol
 d. Triglycerides

58. Which lipid profile component is elevated in hypertriglyceridemia and is a risk factor for pancreatitis?
 a. Total Cholesterol
 b. High-Density Lipoprotein (HDL) Cholesterol
 c. Low-Density Lipoprotein (LDL) Cholesterol
 d. Triglycerides

59. What is the primary form of nitrogen elimination in mammals, which is freely filtered by the kidney glomeruli?

  a. Creatinine b. Urea

  c. Ammonia d. Uric acid

60. Which liver enzyme is specific for detecting liver injury in dogs and cats, but not in horses and cattle?

  a. Alanine Aminotransferase (ALT)

  b. Aspartate Aminotransferase (AST)

  c. Alkaline Phosphatase (ALP)

  d. Gamma-Glutamyl Transferase (GGT)

61. Which enzyme activity is commonly elevated in young growing animals due to bone growth?

  a. Alanine Aminotransferase (ALT)

  b Aspartate Aminotransferase (AST)

  c. Alkaline Phosphatase (ALP)

  d. Gamma-Glutamyl Transferase (GGT)

62. Which enzyme is primarily associated with biliary epithelial cells in animals?

  a. Alanine Aminotransferase (ALT)

  b. Gamma-Glutamyl Transferase (GGT)

  c. Aspartate Aminotransferase (AST)

  d. Arginase

63. What condition can be indicated by elevated postprandial bile acid levels?

  a. Hyperthyroidism

  b. Liver dysfunction or portosystemic shunts

  c. Hypercholesterolemia

  d. Hypothyroidism

64. Which test is most often used to diagnose and monitor kidney disease in human and animal clinical pathology?

  a. Cystatin C b. Urea

  c. Creatinine d. Total Thyroxine (T4)

65. What is the primary role of arginase type I in the liver?

  a. Protein synthesis b. Urea synthesis

  c. Lipid metabolism d. Glucose metabolism

66. Which enzyme is considered specific for muscle necrosis due to its rapid clearance from plasma?

  a Creatine Kinase (CK) b. Lactate Dehydrogenase (LDH)

  c. Myoglobin d. Troponin I

67. Elevated serum GGT levels are frequently seen with which condition?

  a. Hyperthyroidism b. Cholestasis (bile duct obstructions)

  c. Hypercholesterolemia d. Rhabdomyolysis

68. Which test is used to diagnose Cushing's disease in dogs?
    a. Blood Glucose Test
    b. Cortisol Levels Test
    c. Thyroid Function Test
    d. Urinalysis
69. Which electrolyte is crucial for assessing hydration status in animals?
    a. Sodium
    b. Potassium
    c. Chloride
    d. Calcium
70. What is the significance of measuring fructosamine in diabetic animals?
    a. To monitor short-term glucose levels
    b. To monitor long-term glucose levels
    c. To assess liver function
    d. To evaluate kidney function
71. What is the significance of measuring fructosamine in diabetic animals?
    a. To monitor short-term glucose levels
    b. To monitor long-term glucose levels
    c. To assess liver function
    d. To evaluate kidney function
72. Which test is used to diagnose thyroid disorders in cats?
    a. Blood Glucose Test
    b. T4 (Thyroxine) Test
    c. Cortisol Levels Test
    d. Urinalysis
73. Which technique separates molecules based on size and charge?
    a. Spectrophotometry
    b. Chromatography
    c. Electrophoresis
    d. Mass Spectrometry
73. What is the primary purpose of an immunoassay in veterinary biochemistry?
    a. To measure enzyme activity
    b. To detect and quantify specific proteins and hormones
    c. To analyze chemical composition
    d. To separate complex mixtures
74. What does POCT stand for in veterinary diagnostics?
    a. Point-of-Care Testing
    b. Post-Operative Clinical Test
    c. Primary Outpatient Chemical Test
    d. Patient-Oriented Care Test
75. Which enzyme level is measured to diagnose pancreatitis in animals?
    a. ALT
    b. Lipase
    c. AST
    d. ALP
76. What does an elevated cortisol level indicate in dogs?
    a. Diabetes
    b. Cushing's disease
    c. Liver disease
    d. Hypothyroidism
77. Which test detects early signs of kidney damage in animals?
    a. Urinalysis
    b. Blood Glucose Test
    c. Urine Protein/Creatinine Ratio
    d. Serum Biochemistry Panel

78. Which electrolyte is critical for muscle function in animals?
    a. Sodium
    b. Potassium
    c. Calcium
    d. Chloride
79. What is the purpose of a serum biochemistry panel in animals?
    a. To measure blood sugar levels
    b. To evaluate hydration status
    c. To assess enzymes, electrolytes, proteins, and metabolites
    d. To detect specific antigens
80. Which biomarker is used to monitor diabetes in animals over time?
    a. Glucose
    b. Fructosamine
    c. Hemoglobin
    d. Creatinine
81. Which test is used to diagnose Addison's disease in dogs?
    a. Blood Glucose Test
    b. Thyroxine (T4) Test
    c. Cortisol Levels Test
    d. Liver function test
82. What does CBC stand for in medical tests?
    a. Comprehensive Biochemical Check
    b. Complete Blood Count
    c. Cardiovascular Body Check
    d. Chemical Blood Composition
83. Which component of CBC evaluates the oxygen-carrying capacity of blood?
    a. WBC count
    b. Hemoglobin
    c. Platelets
    d. RBC count
84. What is measured in a lipid profile test?
    a. Blood sugar levels
    b. Cholesterol and triglycerides
    c. Liver enzymes
    d. Kidney waste products
85. Which urine test component can indicate diabetes?
    a. Protein
    b. Glucose
    c. Ketones
    d. Blood
86. Elevated levels of which cardiac enzyme are a marker for myocardial infarction?
    a. Troponin
    b. Amylase
    c. ALT
    d. Albumin
87. What does an elevated TSH level with low T4 indicate?
    a. Hyperthyroidism
    b. Hypothyroidism
    c. Normal thyroid function
    d. Pancreatitis
88. What is measured in an electrolyte panel?
    a. Hormone levels
    b. Enzymes
    c. Essential minerals
    d. blood cells
89. Low levels of which protein can suggest malnutrition or liver disease?
    a. Albumin
    b. Hemoglobin
    c. Creatinine
    d. Amylase

90. What technique measures the amount of light absorbed by a sample?
a. Chromatography
b. Mass Spectrometry
c. Spectrophotometry
d. Electrophoresis

91. Mass spectrometry identifies compounds by measuring what?
a. Light absorption
b. Mass-to-charge ratio of ions
c. Electrical resistance
d. Magnetic field strength

92. What does a high C-Reactive Protein (CRP) level indicate?
a. Infection or inflammation
b. Diabetes
c. Liver disease
d. Kidney disease

93. Which diagnostic tool is used for analyzing complex mixtures of chemicals?
a. Chromatography
b. Spectrophotometry
c. Electrophoresis
d. Immunoassays

94. Which hormone is measured to assess reproductive health in males?
a. Estrogen
b. Progesterone
c. Testosterone
d. cortisol

95. Which electrolyte imbalance can indicate dehydration?
a. Low sodium
b. High potassium
c. High calcium
d. High magnesium

96. What does a high LDL level in a lipid profile suggest?
a. Low cardiovascular risk
b. High cardiovascular risk
c. Liver dysfunction
d. Kidney disease

97. What does an increased level of troponin in the blood indicate?
a. Kidney failure
b. Liver disease
c. Myocardial infarction
d. Diabetes

98. What is the primary use of mass spectrometry in biochemistry?
a. Measuring light absorption
b. Quantifying proteins
c. Identifying and quantifying compounds
d. Separating DNA fragments

99. Which method is used for protein and DNA analysis?
a. Chromatography
b. Electrophoresis
c. Mass Spectrometry
d. Spectrophotometry

100. What does ELISA stand for?
a. Electrolyte Ion Assay
b. Enzyme-Linked Immunosorbent Assay
c. Electrophoretic Light Analysis
d. Essential Lipid Immunoassay

101. What does a high hemoglobin A1c level indicate?
a. Good blood glucose control
b. Poor blood glucose control
c. Kidney disease
d. Liver dysfunction

102. What does a high level of bile acids in dogs indicate?
    a. Pancreatitis   b. Liver dysfunction
    c. Kidney disease   d. Diabetes
103. What does a high level of amylase in a dog's blood suggest?
    a. Liver disease   b. Pancreatitis
    c. Kidney disease   d. Hyperthyroidism
104. In dogs, elevated levels of which enzyme can be associated with steroid administration?
    a. CK   b. ALP
    c. AST   d. ALT
105. Which enzyme is commonly elevated in cases of equine rhabdomyolysis?
    a. ALT   b. AST
    c. CK   d. GGT
106. In birds, elevated levels of which enzyme can indicate liver disease?
    a. CK   b. AST
    c. ALT   d. GGT
107. Which enzyme is particularly useful in diagnosing liver fluke infection in sheep?
    a. ALT   b. AST
    c. GGT   d. ALP
108. In cats, which enzyme level is more specific to liver disease compared to ALT?
    a. ALP   b. GGT
    c. CK   d. Amylase
109. Which enzyme is typically measured to monitor muscle damage in working dogs?
    a. CK   b. ALT
    c. GGT   d. ALP
110. What does an elevated level of AST indicate in horses?
    a. Kidney disease   b. Liver or muscle damage
    c. Pancreatitis   d. Bone disease
111. Which enzyme level might be elevated in cattle with fatty liver syndrome?
    a. ALT   b. AST
    c. CK   d. GGT
112. In reptiles, elevated levels of which enzyme can suggest liver disease?
    a. ALT   b. AST
    c. CK   d. ALP
113. Which enzyme is measured to diagnose exocrine pancreatic insufficiency in dogs?
    a. ALT   b. Amylase
    c. Trypsin-like immunoreactivity (TLI)   d. GGT
114. Which enzyme is elevated in birds with muscle damage?
    a. CK   b. ALP
    c. ALT   d. AST

115. In reptiles, elevated levels of which enzyme can indicate metabolic bone disease?
 a. CK b. ALP
 c. ALT d. AST
116. Which enzyme is commonly elevated in cases of canine hypothyroidism?
 a. ALT b. ALP
 c. CK d. GGT
117. What does a low level of trypsin-like immunoreactivity (TLI) indicate in dogs?
 a. Liver disease b. Exocrine pancreatic insufficiency
 c. Kidney disease d. Muscle damage
118. Which of the following is a crucial function of sodium (Na+) in animals?
 a. Bone health b. Muscle contraction
 c. Energy metabolism d. blood clotting
119. Potassium (K+) imbalance in animals can lead to:
 a. Bone diseases b. Cardiac abnormalities
 c. Excessive blood clotting d. Respiratory distress
120. An animal with elevated phosphorus (P) levels may indicate:
 a. Kidney disease b. Dehydration
 c. Hormonal imbalance d. Bone fractures
121. What is the primary purpose of measuring electrolytes in animal diagnostics?
 a. Assessing liver function b. Monitoring fluid therapy
 c. Evaluating lung capacity d. Detecting skin disorders
122. The most common method for measuring electrolytes in animal blood is:
 a. Urinalysis b. Radiography
 c. Blood gas analysis d. Automated analyzer
123. What does a high serum potassium (K+) level indicate in animals?
 a. Cardiac abnormalities b. Hypoglycemia
 c. Iron deficiency d. Hypertension
124. Which enzyme is a marker of tissue damage in the reproductive tract?
 a. Lactate dehydrogenase (LDH) b. Alanine aminotransferase (ALT)
 c. Amylase d. creatine kinase (CK)
125. Which species is particularly susceptible to electrolyte imbalances during endurance events?
 a. Dogs b. Cats
 c. Horses d. Cattle
126. Which electrolyte imbalance is commonly associated with cardiac arrhythmias in animals?
 a. Hyperkalemia b. Hyponatremia
 c. Hypercalcemia d. Hypophosphatemia

127. Which of the following is a biochemical marker used to assess ovarian function in female animals?
   a. Prolactin b. Inhibin
   c. Growth hormone d. Insulin
128. Which electrolyte is most commonly measured in evaluating dehydration in animals?
   a. Calcium (Ca2+) b. Phosphorus (P)
   c. Sodium (Na+) d. Potassium (K+)
129. Which of the following hormones is involved in regulating water and electrolyte balance in animals?
   a. Cortisol b. Aldosterone
   c. Growth hormone d. Thyroid hormone
130. Which electrolyte imbalance is associated with muscle weakness and cardiac arrhythmias?
   a. Hypokalemia b. Hypercalcemia
   c. Hyponatremia d. Hypophosphatemia
131. What is the primary function of the liver in animals?
   a. Digestion of proteins b. Filtration of blood
   c. Production of insulin d. Regulation of body temperature
132. What condition is characterized by low blood protein levels in animals?
   a. Hyperlipidemia b. Hypoproteinemia
   c. Hyperglycemia d. Hypocalcemia
133. Which organ is primarily assessed by measuring serum creatinine levels in animals?
   a. Liver b. Heart
   c. Kidneys d. Pancreas
134. Which test is used to evaluate pancreatic function in animals?
   a. Amylase b. Lipase
   c. Trypsin-like immunoreactivity (TLI) d. Glucose tolerance test
135. Which condition is characterized by an excessive breakdown of muscle tissue?
   a. Rhabdomyolysis b. Osteoporosis
   c. Myopathy d. Hypercalcemia
136. What is the primary reason for collecting cerebrospinal fluid in animals?
   a. To diagnose liver disease
   b. To diagnose neurological disorders
   c. To diagnose cardiovascular disease
   d. To diagnose gastrointestinal disease
137. Which of the following is a common site for cerebrospinal fluid collection in animals?
   a. Jugular vein b. Lumbar cistern
   c. Carotid artery d. Saphenous vein

138. What does an elevated white blood cell (WBccount in CSF typically indicate?

a. Bacterial infection b. Liver disease

c. Kidney disease d. Cardiac disease

139. Which type of cells are most commonly found in normal cerebrospinal fluid?

a. Red blood cells b. Neutrophils

c. Lymphocytes d. Eosinophils

140. What is the normal protein concentration range in cerebrospinal fluid for most animals?

a. 0-10 mg/dL b. 10-45 mg/dL

c. 45-100 mg/dL d. 100-150 mg/dL

141. What is xanthochromia in cerebrospinal fluid?

a. Presence of bacteria b. Yellow discoloration of CSF

c. Increase in red blood cells d. Increase in white blood cells

142. What does an elevated lactate level in CSF indicate?

a. Decreased glucose metabolism b. Increased protein synthesis

c. Decreased oxygenation d. Increased lipid metabolism

143. Which diagnostic test on CSF can help detect the presence of fungal infections?

a. Gram stain b. India ink preparation

c. Wright's stain d. Hematoxylin and eosin stain

144. What is the significance of finding oligoclonal bands in CSF?

a. Indication of multiple sclerosis b. Indication of bacterial meningitis

c. Indication of viral encephalitis d. Indication of parasitic infection

145. What condition might be suspected if the CSF appears cloudy?

a. Hemorrhage b. Infection

c. Dehydration d. Neoplasia

146. Which enzyme is measured in CSF to assess for the presence of neuronal damage?

a. Amylase b. Lipase

c. Lactate dehydrogenase (LDH) d. Creatine kinase (CK)

147. Which immunoglobulin is commonly measured in CSF to evaluate for autoimmune diseases?

a. IgA b. IgG

c. IgM d. IgE

148. What does the presence of red blood cells in CSF typically indicate?

a. Hemorrhage b. Infection

c. Dehydration d. Metabolic disorder

149. How is the cell count in CSF typically measured?

a. Spectrophotometry b. Hemocytometer

c. Flow cytometry d. ELISA

150. Which condition can be diagnosed by the detection of elevated myelin basic protein in CSF?
 a. Multiple sclerosis b. Bacterial meningitis
 c. Viral encephalitis d. Parasitic infection

151. What is the typical appearance of normal cerebrospinal fluid?
 a. Cloudy and viscous b. Clear and colorless
 c. Yellow and turbid d. Red and frothy

152. Which of the following conditions is characterized by increased CSF pressure?
 a. Hypotension b. Hydrocephalus
 c. Dehydration d. Hypoglycemia

153. What does the presence of neutrophils in CSF indicate?
 a. Viral infection b. bacterial infection
 c. Fungal infection d. Parasitic infection

154. What is the significance of elevated CSF immunoglobulin G (IgG) index?
 a. Indication of bacterial infection
 b. Indication of viral infection
 c. Indication of intrathecal synthesis of antibodies
 d. Indication of parasitic infection

155. Which condition is suggested by a high CSF/serum albumin ratio?
 a. Blood-brain barrier dysfunction b. Increased intracranial pressure
 c. Dehydration d. Hypoproteinemia

156. What is the most common reason for performing a CSF culture?
 a. To detect parasites b. To identify bacterial pathogens
 c. To measure protein levels d. To evaluate glucose levels

157. Which of the following can be detected using a CSF cytology exam?
 a. Electrolyte imbalances b. Cellular morphology
 c. Enzyme activity d. Hormone levels

158. What does the presence of eosinophils in CSF suggest?
 a. Parasitic infection b. Viral infection
 c. Fungal infection d.bacterial infection

159. Which protein is often analyzed in CSF to help diagnose Alzheimer's disease in animals?
 a. Tau protein b. C-reactive protein
 c. Albumin d. Hemoglobin

160. What does pleocytosis in CSF refer to?
 a. Decreased white blood cell count b. Increased white blood cell count
 c. Decreased red blood cell count d. Increased protein concentration

Answer Key

1	b	2	d	3	b	4	b	5	b	6	b	7	b
8	a	9	c	10	c	11	b	12	b	13	a	14	a
15	b	16	b	17	a	18	b	19	a	20	a	21	d
22	a	23	a	24	c	25	a	26	b	27	b	28	b
29	b	30	b	31	a	32	b	33	c	34	b	35	c
36	b	37	a	38	d	39	c	40	c	41	b	42	a
43	b	44	b	45	c	46	b	47	b	48	c	49	c
50	d	51	b	52	b	53	c	54	b	55	b	56	c
57	d	58	b	59	a	60	c	61	b	62	b	63	c
64	b	65	c	66	b	67	b	68	a	69	b	70	b
71	b	72	c	73	b	74	b	75	b	76	a	77	a
78	b	79	c	80	b	81	c	82	b	83	b	84	b
85	b	86	a	87	b	88	c	89	a	90	c	91	b
92	a	93	a	94	c	95	b	96	b	97	c	98	c
99	b	100	b	101	b	102	b	103	b	104	b	105	c
106	b	107	c	108	b	109	a	110	b	111	d	112	d
113	c	114	a	115	b	116	b	117	b	118	b	119	b
120	c	121	a	122	b	123	c	124	d	125	a	126	a
127	c	128	a	129	b	130	c	131	b	132	b	133	c
134	c	135	a	136	b	137	b	138	a	139	c	140	b
141	b	142	c	143	b	144	a	145	b	146	d	147	b
148	a	149	b	150	a	151	b	152	b	153	b	154	c
155	a	156	b	157	b	158	a	159	a	160	b		

27

Immunochemistry

Sasmita Barik[1] and Shiv Kumar Yadav[2]

[1]*Department of Veterinary Physiology and Biochemistry, College of Veterinary Sciences and Animal Husbandry, Guru Angad Dev Animal and Veterinary Sciences University, Ludhiana, Punjab*

[2]*KVK, Shahjahanpur, Uttar Pradesh*

Introduction

Immunology deals with the body defence system consisting of various cells and biomolecules that prevents entry of foreign infectious and toxic agents by different mechanisms. The mammalian immune system operates in two ways like innate or non-specific immunity and adaptive or acquired or specific immunity. Innate part constitutes the physical (skin, hair, tears and mucous secretions) containing enzymes that prevents primarily entry of pathogen. It is the first line of defence action, very fast but not adequate. Adaptive form constitutes defensive cells and secreted immunoglobulins. It takes time to develop effectively, especially when the body sees the organism for the first time. Immunoglobulins (Ig) or antibodies are a group of proteins produced from B lymphocytes and plasma cells in response to the presence of any foreign substances. They are 5 basic types like M, A, G, E and D each with specific function. The system can produce antibody molecules, directed to about 1 million different kinds of antigens. All immunoglobulins have a similar basic structure.

The basic structure of all immunoglobulin molecules consists of 4 polypeptide chains linked by disulphide bonds, 2 polypeptide chains are light (L) chains of low molecular weight, 2 polypeptide chains are heavy (H) chains of high molecular weight. Both heavy and light chains have 2 regions like C-terminal constant regions having a constant amino acid sequence within a class or type and N-terminal variable (v) regions with considerable variation in amino acid sequence from molecule to another. Immunoglobulin G (IgG) is a monomer, IgA is a dimer and IgM is a pentamer. Antigen-binding sites on immunoglobulins that combines with antigens. It is formed by a few amino acids in the variable (v) region of H and L chains (dotted lines), at N-terminal ends. There are 2 binding sites per immunoglobulin molecule ie bivalency. There are only 2 major types of L chains in man, the kappa and lambda chains. Either type of light chain can be associated with each of the heavy chain classes. Approximately 70% of the human immunoglobulin molecules carry kappa light chains and 30% carry lambda light chains.The H chain is unique to the class. It is termed gamma chain In IgG, alpha chain in IgA, mu chain in lgM, delta chain in IgD and epsilon chain in IgE. Immunoglobulins contain carbohydrate (CHO) residues (296 to 12 96) like mannose, galactose, fructose, N-acetyl neuraminic a cid or glucosamine. Papain enzyme cleaves immunoglobulins into 2 antibody fragments (Fab. fragments which contain variable fragments and one constant fragment (Fc. (which contains constant fragment.)

Immunoglobulin G (IgG) forms 80% of the immunoglobulins. It is the only immunoglobulin, which has the ability to cross the placent a It is th e major immunoglobulin in secondary immune response with long half- life if compared with other immunoglobulins. It is of low molecular weight formed of one unit only and contains 2-4 % carbohydrate. Immunoglobulin A (Iga. present in the serum as monomer, but it is present in high concentrations in body secretions as dimer where small polypeptide chain called a j chain linked to Fc regions joins the molecules. lgA cannot cross the placent a. IgA contains 5-10 % carbohydrate. The lgA produced in the intestinal wall may either diffuse into the blood stream or binds to a glycoprotein called a secretory component (or secretory piece) to form a complex molecule called secretory lgA, which pass directly into intestinal lumen. Secretory lgA is the predominant immunoglobulin in the intestinal and other secretions. Its secretory component protects IgA from digestion by gastrointestinal proteolytic enzymes. The production of the secretory component is independent of the production of lgA . The function of secretory lgA is to protect body surface against invading microorganisms, since it is the major immunoglobulin in the intestinal, respiratory and urogenital tracts as well as milk, colostrum and tears. lgM is present in serum and has the highest molecular weight amongst all immunoglobulins as it is formed of 5 basic subunits (pentamer). lgM subunits arc joined together by disulfide bonds. Immunoglobulin E (lgE) is present in very low concentration in serum and has the shortest half-life (2 - 3 days). It is largely responsible for immunity against parasites. lgE (through its Fe regions, in the presence of antigen, hinds to mast cells and basophils, causing release of histamine and other substances from mast cells. These substances result in allergic manifestations. Release of histamin and other substances. Immunoglobulin D (lgd. is present in a very low concentration in serum. It cannot cross the placent a. lgD is a cell membrane immunoglobulin found on the surface of B-lymphocytes. It serves in this location as a specific antigen receptor. IgD has activity against thyroid tissue, insulin, penicillin and diphteria toxoid.

Both light and heavy chains are products of multiple genes. Each immunoglobulin light chain is the product of at least 3 separate structural genes, like variable region (VL) gene, joining (J) region gene and a constant region (CL) gene. Each immunoglobulin heavy chain is the product of at least 4 different genes like variable region (VH) gene, a diversity regiond. gene, joining (JH\) region and a constant (CH). There are more than 1 million antibodies derived from 5 basic types (lgG,IgM, lgA, IgE and lgD). The same variable light and heavy chains may combine with the constant chains of immunoglobulin G, A and M. This means that the 3 classes can be directed and combined to the same antigen. Antigens are substances when introduced into the body will stimulate an immune response i.e. antibodies production. Haptens are small molecules that cannot by themselves induce antibody formation but can do so when covalently linked to larger molecules. Proteins with molecular weights greater than 1oo, ooo are the most potent antigens. Under normal conditions, tissues or fluids of the body can be recognized by immune system as self (i.e. own tissues), and do not stimulate immune response. If foreign substances are introduced in the body, immune system recognizes them, as non-self and immune response will occur. A molecule must possess a certain degree of complexity to be antigenic Immunogenicity increases with structural complexity. Proteins, polysaccharides and other synthetic polymers are good antigens. Lipids are not antigenic unless they are combined with proteins polysaccharides. Antigen which can induce an immune response in a particular animal have no effect on another animal. This depends on the genetic constitution of the animal. Initiation of immunoglobulins production requires binding of the antigen to the lymphocyte surface. Antigen receptors are the sites on the surface of lymphocytes that bind the antigen. Antigenic determinant is the portion of antigen that binds with the antigen receptors. Immunopotency is the capacity of the region of the antigenic determinant to induce the formation of specific antibodies.

1. The immunoglobulins are differentiated and also named on the basis of
   a. Electrophoretic mobility
   b. Heat stability
   c. Molecular weight
   d. Sedimentaiton coefficient like 7 S, 19 S etc.
2. The immunoglobulins are classified on the basis of
   a. Light chains b. Heavy chains
   c. Carbohydrate content d. Electrophoretic mobility
3. Skin forms which line of defence
   a. First b. Second
   c. Both d. None
4. The acquired immunity displays which one of the following characters
   a. Antigen specificity b. Recognition diversity
   c. Immunological memory d. All
5. Discrimination between self and non-self is displayed by
   a. Innnate immunity b. Adaptive immunity
   c. Both d. None
6. Which one of the following forms part of innate immunity.
   a. Inflammatory response b. Fever
   c. Both d. None
7. Which cell produces antibodies
   a. T cell b. B cell
   c. Both d. None
8. B-lymphocytes are intimately associated with
   a. Humoral immunity. b. Adaptive immunity
   c. Both d. None
9. Which cell cause cell mediated immunity.
   a. T cell b. B cell
   c. Both d None
10. Which cell mediate the development of T-cells in the thymus.
   a. Inducer T-cells b. Cytotoxic T-cells
   c Helper T-cells d. Suppressor T-cells

11. Which cell recognizes nd kill the infected or abnormal cells
    a. Inducer T-cells
    b. Cytotoxic T-cells
    c. Helper T-cells
    d. Suppressor T-cells
12. Which cell initiate immune responses
    a. Inducer T-cells
    b. Cytotoxic T-cells
    c. Helper T-cells
    d. Suppressor T-cells
13. Which cell mediate the suppression of immune response.
    a. Inducer T-cells
    b. Cytotoxic T-cells
    c. Helper T-cells
    d. Suppressor T-cells
14. The false statement regarding to the immunoglobulin is
    a. The constant regions of H-chains are the same in each class of immunoglobulins
    b. The L-chains are similar in each class of immunoglobulins
    c. IgG is the principle antibody in serum
    d. Ig classes are differentiated from each other by the H-chains
15. MHCs are present on which cell surfaces
    a. T cell
    b. B cell
    c. Both
    d. None
16. The complement system cause which type of reactions
    a. Antibody dependent classical pathway
    b. Antibody independent alternative pathway
    c. Both
    d. None
17. MHC is involved in the recognition of.
    a. Antigens on T-cells
    b. Antigens on B-cells
    c. Both
    d. None
18. Class I MHC molecules are found on which cells
    a. All the nucleated cells
    b. All the non nucleated cells
    c. Both
    d. None
19. Class II MHC molecules are associated only with leukocytes involved in
    a. Cell-mediated immune response.
    b. Humoral response
    c. Both
    d. None
20. Class III MHC molecules include
    a. Tumor necrosis factor
    b. Complement components
    c. Both
    d. None
21. Specific immunity can be acquired either naturally or artificially and involves
    a. All of the below
    b. Antibodies
    c. Antigens
    d. Classical complement pathway

22. Which DOES NOT provide long-term immunity?
    a. Artificially acquired active immunity
    b. Artificially acquired passive immunity
    c. Naturally acquired active immunity
    d. None of the above
23. An epitope is
    a. B-cell.
    b. Hapten.
    c. Antibody
    d. Antigen determinant site
24. An immunoglobulin is a
    a. Carbohydrate
    b. Fatty acid.
    c. Glycoprotein
    d Protein.
25. Isotypes refers to variations in the
    a. Heavy chain constant region
    b. Heavy chain variable region
    c Light chain constant region
    d Light chain variable region.
26. The Fc region mediates all of the below EXCEPT binding to
    a. Antigen
    b. Lysosomes
    c. Phagocytic cells
    d. All
27. Which of the following is the major immunoglobulin in human serum, accounting for 80% of the immunoglobulin pool
    a. IgA
    b. IgD
    c. IgG
    d. IgM
28. Which immunoglobulin is the least prevalent?
    a. IgA
    b. IgD
    c. IgE
    d. IgM
29. Which of the following is useful to STIMULATE antibody production?
    a. An adjuvant
    b. A hapten
    c. Antiserum
    d. Purified antigen
30. Compared to the secondary antibody response, the primary response
    a. Attains a higher IgG titer
    b. Has a longer lag phase
    c. Persists for a longer plateau period
    d. Produces antibodies with a higher affinity for the antigen
31. Monoclonal antibodies are produced by
    a. Hybridomas
    b. Lymphocytes
    c. Myeloma cells
    d. Plasma cells
32. Opsonization refers to
    a. Adherence to mucosal epithelial cells.
    b. Antibody-mediated viral inactivation.
    c. Coating of microorganisms or other particles by antibody and/or complement
    d. Parasitic lysosomal degranulation

33. Pregnancy test detects the presence of which of the following?
    a. Rh
    b. Human Chorionic Gonadotropin (HCG)
    c. Fetal proteins
    d. Agglutination
34. An anamnestic response involves a/an
    a. Effector response
    b. High intensity.
    c. Rapid memory
    d. All of the above
35. Cell-associated differentiation antigens (CDs) are functional cell surface proteins or receptors that can be measured in situ.
    a. Detecting these soluble molecules may help in the management of disease
    b. In normal individuals the concentration of these molecules in serum is always low.
    c. Thousands of CDs have been characterized
    d. All of the above are true
36. The first tenet of clonal selection theory relies specifically on
    a. Combinatorial joinings
    b. Somatic mutations.
    c. Variations in the splicing
    d. B-cell clones
37. B-cells do which of the following?
    a. Act as antigen-processing cells
    b. Respond to antigens by making antibodies
    c. Proliferate and differentiate into plasma cells
    d. All of the above
38. Monoclonal antibodies are routinely used in all of the following EXCEPT
    a. Classification of leukemias
    b. Identification and epidemiological study of infectious microorganisms.
    c. Identification of tumor antigens
    d. Manipulation of the immune response
39. Which of the following DOES NOT play a role in antigen presentation?
    a. MHC class I molecules
    b. MHC class II molecules
    c. MHC class III molecules
    d. None of the above
40. Which of the following is used for typing when a patient is being prepared for an organ transplant?
    a. MHC class I molecules
    b. MHC class II molecules
    c. MHC class III molecules
    d. All of the above
41. Structure of all immunoglobulins is
    a. Y shaped
    b. Z shaped
    c. X shaped
    d. Wshaped

42. All immunoglobulins contain

a. 4 L chains
b. 4 H chains
c. 3 L chains
d. 2 L chains and 2 H chains

43. The immunoglobulin involved in allergic reactions is

a. IgA
b. IgM
c. IgG
d. IgE

44. Which of the following immunoglobulin is a pentamer?

a IgG
b. IgA
c. IgD
d. IgM

45. Which of the following immunoglobulin is a dimer?

a. IgG
b. IgE
c. IgA
d. IgM

46. Glutathione is a

a. Trisaccharide
b. Triglyceride
c. Tripeptide
d Trinucleotide

47. The serum antibody responsible for fighting gram +ve pyogenic bacteria is

a. IgG
b. IgA
c. IgD
d. IgE

48. Decarboxylatin of tyrosine in the intestine will result in the formation of

a. Threonine
b. Histamine
c Pyrimidine
d Tyramine

49. False statement regarding to the immunoglobulins is

a. The two types of light chains are K and λ
b. H-chains present in IgA molecule is two α-chains
c. Each immunoglobulin molecule contains both K and λ chains
d. IgG molecule can pass through placenta

50. Which of the following is an example of IgM?

a. Cold agglutinins
b. Natural anti-A and anti-B
c. Rheumatoid factor
d. All of these

51. The immunoglobulin which contains highest concentration of carbohydrates?

a. IgD
b. IgA
c. IgM
d. IgE

52. The protective effect against malaria is related to

a. Hb-B
b. Hb-F
c. Hb-S
d. All of the above

53. One gram of hemoglobin can carry how much volume of oxygen

a. 1.34 ml
b. 13.4 ml
c. 1.84 ml
d. 3.54 ml

54. An immunoglobulin molecule always contains
   a. 1 κ and 3 λ type of chains   b. 2 κ and 2 λ type of chains
   c. 3 κ and 1λ type of chains   d. 2 κ and 2 λ chains
55. The number of types of H chains identified in human is
   a. 2   b. 4
   c. 3   d. 5
56. The number of hypervariable region in L chain is
   a. 1   b. 3
   c. 2   d. 4
57. The number of hypervariable region in H chain is
   a. 1   b. 3
   c. 2   d. 4
58. Type γ H chain is present in
   a. Ig G   b. Ig A
   c. Ig M   d. Ig D
59. Type α H chain is present in
   a. Ig E   b. Ig A
   c. Ig M   d. Ig D
60. Type μ H chain is present in
   a. Ig E   b. Ig A
   c. Ig M   d. Ig D
61. Type δ δ δ H chain is present in
   a. Ig G   b. Ig A
   c. Ig M   d. Ig D
62. Type ε εε H chain is present in
   a. Ig A   b. Ig M
   c. Ig D   d. Ig E
63. A 'J' chain is present in
   a. Ig D   b. Ig G
   c. Ig M   d. Ig E
64. A secretory protein T chain (T protein) is present in
   a. Ig A   b. Ig M
   c. Ig D   d. Ig E
65. A pentamer immunoglobulin is
   a. IgG   b. Ig A
   c. IgM   d. Ig E
66. The portion of the immunoglobulin molecule that binds the specific antigen is formed by
   a. Variable regions of H and L chains   b. Constant region of H chain
   c. Constant region of L chain   d. Hinge region

67. The class specific function of the different immunoglobulin molecules is constituted by
   a. Variable region of L chain
   b. Constant region of H chain
   c. Variable region of H chain
   d. Constant region particularly CH2 and CH3 of H chain
68. Hinge region, the region of Ig molecule which is flexible and more exposed to enzymes is the
   a. Region between first and second constant regions of H chain (domains CH 1 and CH2)
   b. Region between second and third constant regions of H chain (CH 2 and CH 3)
   c. Variable regions of H chain
   d. Variable regions of L chain
69. The smallest immunoglobulin is
   a. IgG b. IgE
   c. IgD d. IgA
70. The number of sub classes of Ig G is
   a. 2 b. 3
   c. 4 d. 8
71. Most abundant Ig G subclass in the serum is
   a. Ig G1 b. IgG2
   c. Ig G3 d. IgG4
72. The immunoglobulin which can cross the placenta is
   a. IgA b. IgM
   c. IgG d. Ig D
73. The immunoglobulin possessing lowest concentration of carbohydrate is
   a. IgA b. IgE
   c IgM d. Ig G
74. The normal serum level of Ig G is
   a. 1200 mg% b. 500 mg%
   c. 300 mg% d. 200 mg%
75. The half life of Ig G is
   a. 2–8 days b. 1–4 days
   c. 19–24 days d. 6 days
76. Most heat labile immunoglobulin is
   a. IgG b. Ig A
   c. IgM d. Ig D
77. The immunoglobulin possessing highest concentration of carbohydrate is
   a. IgG b. IgM
   c. IgA d. Ig D

78. The normal serum level of Ig D is

a. 1 mg% b. 2 mg%

c 3 mg% d 5 mg%

79. The half life of Ig D is

a. 1 day b. 2–8 days

c. 10–15 days d. 20–24 days

80. The carbohydrate content of Ig M is about

a. 2.8% b. 6.4%

c. 8.0% d 10.2%

81. The immunoglobulin having highest sedimentation coefficient is

a. IgG b. Ig A

c. IgM d. Ig D

82. The immunoglobulin having highest molecular weight is

a. IgG b. Ig M

c. IgE d. Ig A

83. The half life of Ig M is

a. 2 days b. 4 days

c. 5 days d. 8 days

84. The normal serum level of Ig M is

a. 50 mg% b. 120 mg%

c. 200 mg% d. 300 mg%

85. The immunoglobulin associated with reginic antibody is

a. IgE b. IgD

c. IgM d. Ig A

86. The immunoglobulin having least concentration in serum is

a. IgA b. IgM

c. IgD d. Ig E

87. The half life of Ig E protein is

a. 1–6 days b. 2–8 days

c. 10 days d. 20 days

88. The immunoglobulin which provides highest antiviral activity is

a IgD b. IgE

c. IgA d. Ig G

89. The half life of Ig A is

a. 6 days b. 2–4 days

c. 5–10 days d. 12–20 days

90. The normal serum level of Ig A is

a. 100 mg% b. 200 mg%

c. 300 mg% d. 400 mg%

91. All of the following are true concerning IgM ntibodies EXCEPT which one
   a. They are glycoprotein
   b. They fix complement
   c. They mediate allergic reaction
   d. They occur on the surface of lymphocytes
92. All of the following are true concerning IgE molecules, EXCEPT which one
   a. They are involved in mediating anti-parasitic immune responses.
   b. They are the least abundant immunoglobulin in the serum.
   c. They are the principal immunoglobulin class involved in allergic reactions.
   d. They will cross the placenta and fix the complement
93. Which immunoglobulins are generally present in plasma at the highest concentration
   a. IgA b. IgD
   c. IgE d. IgG
94. All of the following are true about antibodies, EXCEPT which one
   a. They are glycoproteins.
   b. They are molecules with a single, defined amino acid sequence
   c. They fix complement
   d. They occur on the surface of B-lymphocyte
95. The major immunoglobulin family to which a particular immunoglobulin belongs can be
   a. Amino terminus of the heavy chain
   b. Amino terminus of the light chain.
   c. Carboxy terminus of the heavy chain.
   d. Carboxy terminus of the light chain.
96. The immunoglobulin Joining chain (J-chain) is
   a. Only produced by T-Cells
   b. Only produced by neutrophils
   c. Associated with only multimeric forms of lgM and IgA
   d. Associated with IgE for histamine release
97. All of the following are true except
   a. an antigenic determinant is a paratope
   b. An epitope is a small portion of a macromolecule
   c. An IgG antibody is bivalent
   d. The class of immunoglobulin is determined by its heavy chain
98. Which immunoglobulin is the principal one found in secretions such as milk?
   a. IgA b. IgD
   c. IgE d. IgG

99. Which of the following statements best characterizes an antibody?
    a. An antibody contains high molecular weight RNA as its basic structure
    b. An antibody is composed of protein and cannot be distinguished from the albumin fraction of the serum proteins.
    c. An antibody is composed of four identical protein subunits, which may be caused to dissociate by treatment with urea
    d. An antibody contains protein as its major chemical component, and its synthesis may be elicited by administering a foreign protein or polysaccharide.
100. The class of an immunoglobulin
    a. Determined by the J-chain
    b. Determined by the carbohydrate attached to the light chain is
    c. Determined by the antigen
    d. Determined by the heavy chain type
101. Complement component C3 is cleaved by
    a. C3b b. C3bBb
    c. Factor B d. Factor D
102. The membrane attack complex in the complement pathway consists of
    a. C3b3b,Bb b. C5b,6,7,8,9
    c. Colicins d. Properdin
103. Complement component C3b
    a. Directly injures bacteria b. Is an anaphylatoxin.
    c. Is chemotactic d. Dpsonizes bacteria.
104. A complement component that is strongly chemotactic for neutrophils is
    a. C3 b. C3b
    c. C5a d. C5b
105. The initial complement component that is bound by complement-fixing antibodies is
    a C1q b. C1s
    c C3b d. C5a
106. Several of the complement components are
    a. Antibodies b. Cytokines
    c. Enzymes d. Glycolipid
107. The classical and alternative pathways meet at complement component
    a. C3 b. C4
    c. C4b d. C5
108. One principal function of complement is to
    a. Bind antibodies attached to cell surfaces and to lyse these cells
    b. Cross-link allergens
    c. Inactivate perforins
    d. Phagocytize antigens

109. The major role of the complement system is to work in conjunction with
 a. Antibodies to lyse cells via the C8 and C9 components
 b. Antibodies to lyse cells via the perforin molecules
 c. Antibodies to opsonize cells
 d. The major histocompatibility complex for cell recognition

110. Complement fixation:
 a. Can be modified by the cholera toxin
 b. Has intrinsic guanylate cyclase activity
 c. Can be desensitized by phosphorylation
 d Is an effector function of IgG and IgM following antigen binding .

111. Naturally acquired active immunity would be most likely acquired through which of the following processes?
 a. Vaccination
 b. Drinkingcolostrum
 c. Naturalbirth
 d. Infection with disease-causing organism followed by recovery

112. Which of the following conveys the longest-lasting immunity to an infectious agent?
 a. Naturally acquired passive immunity
 b. Artificially acquired passive immunity
 c. Naturally acquired active immunity
 d. All of these

113. Which substances will not stimulate an immune response unless they are bound to a larger molecule?
 a. Antigen b. Virus
 c. Hapten d. Antibody

114. B and T cells are produced by stem cells that are formed in
 a. Bone marrow b. The liver
 c. The spleen d. The lymph node

115. B cells mature in the........... while T cells mature in the
 a. Thymus/bone marrow and gut-associated lymphoid tissue (GALT)
 b. Spleen/bone marrow and GALT
 c. Bone marrow and GALT/thymus
 d. Liver/kidneys

116. Which of the following immune cells/molecules are most effective at destroying intracellular pathogens?
 a. T helper cells b. B cells
 c. T cytolytic cells d. Antibodies

117. A living microbe with reduced virulence that is used for vaccination is considered
 a. A toxoid b. Virulent
 c. Denatured d. Attenuated

118. B cells that produce and release large amounts of antibodies are called
   a. Memorycells
   b. Basophils
   c. Plasma cells
   d. Killer cells
119. The specificity of an antibody is due to
   a. Its valence
   b. The heavy chains
   c. The Fc portion of the molecule
   d. The variable portion of the heavy and light chain
120. In agglutination reactions, the antigen is a________ and in precipitation reactions, the antigen is a___________
   a. whole-cell/solublemolecule
   b. Soluble molecule/whole-cell
   c. Bacterium/virus
   d. Protein/carbohydrates
121. B Cells are activated by Bacterium/viru
   a. Complement
   b. Antibody
   c. Interferon
   d. Antigen
122. Fusion between a plasma cell and a tumor cell creates a
   a. Myeloma
   b. Natural killer cell
   c. Lymphoma
   d. Hybridoma
123. Monoclonal antibodies recognize a single:
   a Antigen
   b. Bacterium
   c. Epitope
   d. Paratope
124. Cell-mediated immunity is carried out by_________while humoral immunity is mainly carried out by______________
   a. B cells/T cells
   b. Epitopes/antigens
   c. T cells/B cells
   d. Antibodies/antigens
125. The ability of the immune system to recognize self-antigens versus non-self antigen is an example of
   a. Specific immunity
   b. Self-tolerance
   c. Antigenic immunity
   d. Humoral immunity
126. Which of the following antibody is an important host defense against encapsulated bacteria?
   a IgG1
   b. IgG2
   c. IgG3
   d. IgG
127. Which of the following immunoglobulin is the most abundant immunoglobulin in new borns?
   a. IgA
   b. IgM
   c. IgG
   d. IgD
128. Which of the following immunoglobulin is produced early in the primary response to infection?
   a. IgE
   b. IgA
   c. IgG
   d. IgM

129. Which of the following immunoglobulin is the primary host defense against parasitic infections?

a. Secretory IgA b. IgG

c. IgM d. IgE

130. Which of the following immunoglobulin has the highest avidity of the immunoglobulins?

a. IgA b. IgM

c. IgE d. IgG

131. The order of percent of total immunoglobulin in serum is

a. IgM, IgA, IgG, IgD, IgE b. IgG, IgA, IgM, IgE, IgD

c. IgG, IgA, IgM, IgE, IgD d. IgG, IgA, IgM, IgD, IgE

132. Which of the following antibody is a prominent antigen receptor expressed on B Cells?

a. IgG b. IgA

c. IgM d. IgE

133. The antibody which is found in secretions is:

a. IgD b. IgE

c. IgG d. IgA

134. Which of the following antibodies directly participate in the opsonization process?

a. IgM b. IgG

c. IgA d. IgE

135. Complement fixation is one of the most crucial host defenses against infections. The complement is activated by

a. IgM Only

b. IgG only

c. both IgM and IgG

d. all five classes of antibodies activate complements.

136. Which type of antibody is most effective in activating complement?

a. IgG1 b. IgG2

c. IgG3 d. IgM

137. Most abundant Ig G subclass in the serum is

a. Ig G1 b. Ig G2

c. Ig G3 d. Ig G4

138. The immunoglobulin which can cross the placenta is

a. Ig A b. Ig M

c. Ig G d. Ig D

139. The immunoglobulin possessing lowest concentration of carbohydrate is

a. Ig A b. Ig E

c. Ig M d. Ig G

140. Type γ H chain is present in
   a. Ig G   b. Ig A
   c. Ig M   d. Ig D
141. Type α H chain is present in
   a. Ig E   b. Ig A
   c. Ig M   d. Ig D
142. Type μ H chain is present in
   a. Ig E   b. Ig A
   c. Ig M   d. Ig D
143. Type δ δ δ H chain is present in
   a. Ig G   b. Ig A
   c. Ig M   d. Ig D
144. An immunoglobulin is a
   a. Carbohydrate   b. Fatty acid.
   c Glycoprotein   d. Protein.
145. Isotypes refers to variations in the
   a. Heavy chain constant region   b. Heavy chain variable region
   c. Light chain constant region   d. Light chain variable region.
146. The Fc region mediates all of the below EXCEPT binding to
   a. Antigen   b. Lysosomes.
   c. Phagocytic cells   d. All
147. Which of the following is the major immunoglobulin in human serum, accounting for 80% of the immunoglobulin pool
   a. IgA   b. IgD
   c IgG   d IgM
148. Which immunoglobulin is the least prevalent?
   a. IgA   b. IgD
   c. IgE   d. IgM
149. The immunoglobulin associated with reginic antibody is
   a. Ig E   b. Ig D
   c. Ig M   d. Ig A
150. The immunoglobulin having least concentration in serum is
   a. Ig A   b. Ig M
   c. Ig D   d. Ig E

Answer Key

1	d	2	b	3	a	4	a	5	b	6	c	7	b
8	a	9	a	10	a	11	b	12	c	13	d	14	a
15	a	16	a	17	a	18	a	19	a	20	a	21	a
22	b	23	d	24	c	25	a	26	a	27	c	28	c
29	a	30	b	31	a	32	c	33	b	34	d	35	d
36	d	37	d	38	d	39	c	40	a	41	a	42	d
43	d	44	d	45	c	46	c	47	a	48	d	49	c
50	d	51	a	52	c	53	a	54	d	55	d	56	c
57	d	58	a	59	b	60	c	61	d	62	d	63	b
64	a	65	c	66	a	67	d	68	a	69	a	70	c
71	a	72	c	73	d	74	a	75	c	76	d	77	d
78	c	79	b	80	d	81	c	82	b	83	c	84	b
85	a	86	d	87	a	88	c	89	a	90	b	91	c
92	d	93	d	94	b	95	c	96	c	97	a	98	a
99	d	100	d	101	c	102	b	103	e	104	c	105	a
106	c	107	a	108	a	109	a	110	b	111	d	112	c
113	c	114	a	115	c	116	c	117	d	118	c	119	d
120	a	121	d	122	e	123	c	124	c	125	b	126	b
127	c	128	d	129	d	130	b	131	d	132	c	133	d
134	b	135	c	136	d	137	a	138	c	139	d	140	a
141	b	142	c	143	d	144	c	145	a	146	a	147	c
148	c	149	a	150	d								

28

Collection of Biological Fluids

Syed Ashaq Hussain and Rahil Razzak Bhat

Faculty of Veterinary Sciences and Animal Husbandry, Sher-e-Kashmir University of Agricultural Sciences and Technology of Kashmir-190 006, Jammu and Kashmir

Introduction

Biological fluids refer to any liquid substances found within living organisms that play essential roles in physiological functions. These fluids can include blood, urine, cerebrospinal fluid, saliva, digestive juices, rumen fluid, peritoneal fluid, pleural fluid, pericardial fluid, synovial fluid, amniotic fluid, milk etc.

Collection of biological fluids refers to the process of gathering various types of bodily fluids from animals for scientific study or medical purposes. This collection often involves techniques like blood draws, urine collection, cerebrospinal fluid sampling, saliva collection, etc., depending on the specific fluid and the research or diagnostic needs. These fluids are valuable for understanding the health, metabolism, genetics, and other aspects of animal biology. Collecting and analyzing these biological fluids is crucial for understanding health and disease processes, diagnosing illnesses, monitoring treatment effectiveness, and advancing medical and scientific research.

1. Collection of blood

For all purposes blood samples should be collected aseptically. Venous blood can be collected from the following sites with the help of a hypodermic needle.

Site of Collection	Advantage/ Comments	Disadvantages
Cattle		
Jugular vein$^+$	Large volume collected	Risk to collector
Coccygeal vein$^\pm$	Handling ease	Small volume
Cephalic vein $^£$	Possibly easier in calf	-
Sheep		
Jugular vein$^+$	Moderate to large volume collected	
Cephalic vein $^+$	Small volume collected	
Lateral saphenous vein$^\pm$	Small volume collected	
Goat		
Jugular vein$^+$	Convenient	
Cephalic vein $^£$		

Horse		
Jugular vein⁺	Convenient and large volume is collected	
Pig		
Cranial Vena Cava⁺	Large volume collected	Sedation require d.
Marginal Ear vein ⁺	Small volume	
Jugular vein±	Moderate volume	
Dog/Cat		
Cephalic vein ⁺	Small to moderate volume collected	
Jugular vein⁺	Large volume of blood collected	
Median saphenous vein±	Small to moderate volume collected	
Femoral vein £	Small to moderate volume collected	
+ Preferred; ± Acceptable; £ Possible		

2. Collection of Urine

Methods commonly used for urine collection in veterinary practice are free capture, that is, spontaneous micturition and manual urinary bladder compression, catheterization, and cystocentesis. Cystocentesis requires the use of sterile needles and syringes to extract bladder urine. The process of catheterization extracts urine samples straight from the urethra. Free pick involves hand gathering urine samples directly from the pet's voluntary urination. Every approach has its benefits and disadvantages.

3. Collection of Cerebrospinal Fluid (CSF)

Cerebrospinal fluid is derived from the blood plasma and therefore it has qualitatively the same composition, but the discrepancies between the ionic concentration in cerebrospinal fluid and blood plasma indicate that the fluid is not a simple filtrate but a product of active secretary mechanism. Functionally CSF protects and nourishes the parenchyma and maintains homeostasis. Diagnosis of diseases of CNS pose a challenge to the clinician and confirmation of tentative diagnosis requires cytological and biochemical examination of CSF. The CSF can be collected by from the following sites. The puncture must be performed under sterile conditions after cleaning, shaving and disinfecting the site, and using a sterile needle, in order to prevent the introduction of infection into subarachnoid space.

Species	Site of collection
Bovines	Post-occipital or lumbar puncture. In lateral recumbency post-occipital method is more suitable
Ovines	Post-occipital puncture
Porcines	Lumbo-sacral puncture
Equines	Post-occipital puncture
Dogs	Cistrena magna or atlanto-occipital puncture. Lumbar puncture is extremely difficult due to the lumbar vertebral arches and the small subarachnoid area.

4. Collection of Rumen Fluid

Rumen fluid can be collected via orogastric tube or by puncture of ventral sac of rumen. In orogastric collection, volume of fluid is more but there are chances of salivary contamination. To avoid salivary contamination, discard a small quantity of fluid.

Rumen puncture increases the chances of peritoneal contamination. Sample should be preferably collected in air tight container and should be evaluated as soon as possible because cooling and exposure to air alters the protozoan and bacterial activity.

5. Collection of Peritoneal Fluid

Abdominocentesis in cattle: The choice of sites for paracentesis is a problem because the rumen covers such a large portion of the ventral abdominal wall and avoiding penetration of it is difficult. Cattle have a low volume of peritoneal fluid, and failure to obtain a sample is not unusual. The most profitable sites are those that, on an anatomical basis, consist of recesses between the forestomachs, abomasum, diaphragm and liver. These are usually

a. Caudal to the xiphoid sternum and 4-10 cm lateral to the midline
b. Left of the midline, 3-4 cm medial and 5-7 cm cranial to the foramen for the left subcutaneous abdominal vein.
c. Just anterior to base of udder on right side

Abdominocentesis in horses: In the horse the recommended site for paracentesis is on the ventral midline, 25 cm caudal to the xiphoid (or midway between the xiphoid and the umbilicus). Following surgical preparation and subcutaneous infiltration of an anesthetic, a stab incision is made through the skin and subcutaneous tissues and into the linea albaa 9 cm long blunt-pointed bovine teat cannula, or similar metal catheter, with the tip wrapped in a sterile swab to avoid blood and skin contamination, is inserted into the wound and manipulated and with a quick thrust the cannula is pushed into the peritoneal cavity. A 'pop' is often heard on entry into the peritoneal cavity. In most horses (about 75%) a sample of fluid is readily obtained. In others it takes a moment or two before the fluid runs out, usually spurting synchronously with the respiratory movements. Applying suction with a syringe may yield some fluid if there is no spontaneous flow.

Abdominocentesis in dog: Place the dog in left lateral recumbency. Prepare 1-3 inch area between bladder and umbilicus to the right of midline. Distended bladder should be emptied before paracentesis. Abdominal puncture is made with 18-20 G needle. Do not change the position of patient as it may cause laceration of abdominal viscera. Peritoneal fluid examination in dog is diagnostic to ascertain the cause of ascites and neoplasm in peritoneal or abdominal viscera and peritonitis.

6. Collection of Pericardial Fluid

Pericardiocentesis is the technique of removing fluid from the pericardial space. In most cases this is done to relieve the life threatening pressure caused by progressive pericardial effusion (cardiac tamponade). The 4th, 5th or 6th intercostal space are preferred, however best method is to guide the needle via use of ultrasound.

7. Collection of Pleural Fluid

Pleurocentesis (Thoracocentesis) is the paracentesis of the pleural cavity and is of value when the presence of fluid in the pleural sac is suspected. The withdrawal of pleural fluid can provide symptomatic relief in an animal with large quantities of pleural effusion. For this the needle is inserted at 6th or 7th intercostal space. The aspirated fluid is examined grossly and microscopically for any alteration.

8. Transtracheal Aspirate

The collection and evaluation of tracheobronchial secretions is useful for assessing lower airways disease. Although detection of secretion is a very sensitive indicator of pulmonary disease, cytological and bacteriological analysis is usually required to determine its etiology. Percutaneous transtracheal aspiration is a practical method in horse, cattle, sheep and goat.

9. Bronchoalveolar lavage (BAL)

It is a safe and relatively simple technique for harvesting cells from distal airways and alveoli. Examination of BAL fluid for cytology has proved to be invaluable in the investigation of equine pulmonary diseases, particularly chronic pulmonary disease, and is considered the most sensitive method for diagnosis of COPdbAL cytology is easier to examine and interpret than tracheal cytology and also correlates well with pulmonary histopathology.

Multiple Choice Questions

1. Which of the following is an indication for collection of cerebrospinal fluid in dogs
   a. As therapeutic measure to remove certain amount of CSF
   b. To introduce opaque substance for conducting X-ray studies
   c. Both of the above
   d. Neither a nor b
2. Which of the following statements is not true for cerebrospinal fluid (CSF)
   a. It is derived from the blood plasma
   b. The composition of CSF is same as that of the blood
   c. The fluid is a product of active secretary mechanism.
   d. CSF nourishes the parenchyma and maintains homeostasis.
3. Which of the following is the most sensitive method for diagnosis of chronic obstructive pulmonary disease in horses
   a. Radiography
   b. Hematological examination
   c. Examination of transtracheal aspirate
   d. Examination of bronchoalveolar lavage
4. The preferred vein for collection of blood in cattle is
   a. Jugular vein b. Cephalic vein
   c. Lateral saphenous vein d. Ear vein
5. The preferred vein for collection of blood in dog is
   a. Jugular vein b. Cephalic vein
   c. Lateral saphenous vein d. Ear vein
6. The preferred vein for collection of blood in pig is
   a. Jugular vein b. Cephalic vein
   c. Lateral saphenous vein d. Cranial vena cava

7. The preferred veins for collection of blood in sheep are
   a. Jugular vein and Cephalic vein
   b. cephalic vein and Ear vein
   c. Lateral saphenous vein and cephalic vein
   d. Ear vein and jugular vein
8. A blood culture sample may be rejected if it:
   a. Is not labelled correctly
   b. has too little blood in the bottle
   c. Has not been requested correctly
   d. all of the above
9. The top of the blood culture sample bottle should be:
   a. Washed with water prior to use once the cap has been removed
   b. Washed with soap and water prior to use once the cap has been removed
   c. Wiped with a chlorhexidine wipe prior to use once the cap has been removed
   d. Used immediately once the cap has been removed
10. If other blood samples are required at the same time as the blood culture samples, you should:
   a. Take these before the blood culture samples are taken
   b. Take these after the blood culture samples are taken
   c. Take the samples in any order
   d. None of the above
11. Which of the following blood cells play an important role in blood clotting?
   a. Thrombocytes
   b. Neutrophils
   c. Leucocytes
   d. Erythrocytes
12. Serum differs from blood as it lacks
   a. Antibodies
   b. Clotting factors
   c. Albumins
   d. Globulins
13. Which of the following is correct?
   a. Serum contains blood and fibrinogen
   b. Plasma is blood without lymphocytes
   c. Blood comprises plasma, RBC, WBC and platelets
   d. Lymph is plasma with RBC and WBC
14. This plasma protein is responsible for blood coagulation
   a. Fibrinogen
   b. Globulin
   c. Serum amylase
   d. albumin
15. Lymph differs from blood in having
   a. No plasma
   b. More rbcs and less wbcs
   c. More wbcs and no rbcs
   d. Plasma without proteins
16. Retro-orbital bleeding without anesthesia is used for blood collection in
   a. Rats
   b. Mice
   c. guinea pigs
   d. all of the above
17. Cardiac puncture with anesthesia is used for blood collection in
   a. Rats
   b. Rabbits
   c. Ferrets
   d. All of the above

18. Which electrolyte is helpful in blood clotting?
    a. Na b. K
    c. Ca d. Phosphorus
19. Subcutaneous solid mass of blood at the site of venepuncture?
    a. Sarcoma b. Hematoma
    c. Bleeding d. Hemolysis
20. Use of excess amount of EDTA in blood sample causes
    a. Swelling of platelets b. Shrinking of WBC & RBC
    c. A & B d. None
21. Which anticoagulant is used in ESR westergren's method?
    a. EDTA b. Heparin
    c. 3.8% tri sodium citrate d. any of the above
22. What are the function of anticoagulant agent?
    a. Preserving cell morphology b. Preventing clot
    c. A & B d. None
23. Which of the following anticoagulant tube need to collect sample for HbA1C?
    a. Sodium fluoride b. EDTA
    c. Heparin d. Sodium oxalate
24. Colour code used for EDTA anticoagulant vial
    a. Green b. Grey
    c. Purple d. Red
25. In Leishman's staining fixation is done by
    a. Eosin b. Methyl alcohol
    c. Distilled water d. acetone
26. As soon as the CSF reaches the laboratory note its ________
    a. Emergency b. Appearance
    c. Volume d. Patient
27. Urine osmolality is related to:
    a. pH b. Filtration
    c. Specific gravity d. Volume
28. The most commonly reagent use in occult blood?
    a. Rothera's b. benedict's
    c. Fouchet's d. benzidine
29. Presence of RBC in urine is detected by:
    a. Physical examination b. Chemical examination
    c. Microscopic examination d. all of the above
30. Which of the following crystals may be found in acidic urine?
    a. Calcium carbonate b Calcium oxalate
    c. Calcium phosphate d. Triple phosphate

31. Urine specimen become cloudy due to
    a. Bacteria b. RBC
    c. Pus cell d. All options
32. The principle of the reagent strip test for bilirubin is the:
    a. Diazo reaction b. Ehrlich reaction
    c. Greiss reaction d. Peroxidase reaction
33. Ketone bodies sin urine are identified by:
    a. Heat coagulation test b. Benzidine test
    c. Rothera'a test d. Fouchet's test
34. For estimating urea and bicarbonate, the preferred specimen of choice is:
    a. White blood corpuscles b. Whole blood
    c. Plasma d. Red blood corpuscles
35. Which of the following is not a test of LFT
    a. Serum Bilirubin b. SGPT
    c. Albumin d. Urea
36. Which of the following substances is not present in normal urine?
    a. Creatinine b. Bicarbonate
    c. Glucose d. Urea
37. In which of the following conditions the patient serum or plasma appears in milky or cloudy?
    a. Jaundice b Anemia
    c. Lipemia d. Proteinemia
38. If sample is taken in EDTA tube, which of the following biochemistry test result will affect?
    a. Glucose b. Urea
    c. Cholesterol d. Calcium
39. The liquid portion of blood is reffered to as:
    a. Whole blood b. Haematocrit
    c. Plasma d. Serum
40. Which needle gauge corresponds with the smallest needle size?
    a. 18 b. 20
    c. 22 d. 23
41. Normal urine primarily consists of:
    a. Water, protein, and sodium b. Water, urea, and protein
    c. Water, urea, and sodium chloride d. Water, urea, and bilirubin
42. Cessation of urine flow is defined as:
    a. Azotemia b. Dysuria
    c. Diuresis d. Anuria

43. In small animal patients, free-catch urine samples that are positive for white cells, bacteria, and protein will necessitate sampling via

a. Cystocentesis b. Catheterization

c. Either a or b d. Neither a nor b

44. __________is the preferred method of urine collection when evaluating the significance of cells or bacteria in the urine.

a. cystocentesis b. catheterization

c. Either a or b d. Neither a nor b

45. In cats, orange-red urine discoloration can occur after treatment with

a. Clofazimine b. Rifampicin

c. Enrofloxacin d Penicillin

46. Urine specific gravity is measured by

a. Barometer b. Refractometer

c. Urinometer d. None of these

47. Urine specific gravity in healthy cat range within

a. 1.001-1.085 b. 1.001-1.075

c. 1.001-1.040 d. 1.001-1.060

48. Urine specific gravity in healthy dogs range within

a. 1.001-1.085 b. 1.001-1.075

c. 1.001-1.040 d. 1.001-1.060

49. Which of the following statements about the use of urinary chemical strip (urinary dipstick) in small animal practice is false

a. pH, protein calcium, caffeine, ketones, hemoglobin/occult blood, bilirubin, etccan be conveniently and reliably tested with the use of urinary dipstick

b. Analysis of dipstick is always reliable in dogs and cats

c. Strips for urine specific gravity, urobilinogen, nitrite, and leukocytes are not used for animal species

d. All of the above

50. Which of the following can be conveniently and reliably tested in house with the use of urinary chemical strip (urinary dipstick)

a. Nitrite and leukocytes

b. Urine specific gravity and urobilinogen

c. Protein and calcium

d. All of the above

51. The normal urinary pH range of dog and cat is

a. 5.5-6 b. 6-7.5

c. 5.3-6.2 d. 7-7.5

52. Which of the following animals commonly has a cloacal opening for urine excretion?

a. Dog b. Cat

c. Bird d. Rabbit

53. Urine collection from fish typically involves sampling from which part of the fish's anatomy?

a. Gills b. Cloaca

c. Mouth d. Dorsal fin

54. Which species has a unique urine collection method involving the use of a trained pan or tray under a wire-bottom cage?

a. Rabbit b. Guinea pig

c. Ferret d. Hamster

55. Urine collection from reptiles often involves collecting from which part of their anatomy?

a. Vent b. Tail

c. Mouth d. Scales

56. Which species commonly has a urine collection method involving environmental sampling of feces and urine together?

a. Koala b. Sloth

c. Kangaroo d. Elephant

57. Which urine collection method involves manually expressing the bladder through abdominal palpation?

a. Catheterization b. Free-catch

c. Cystocentesis d. Bladder massage

58. Which method is often used for urine collection in laboratory rodents like mice and rats?

a. Catheterization b. Cystocentesis

c. Free-catch d. Metabolic cage

59. Which method is used for urine collection in dolphins and other marine mammals?

a. bladder massage b. Free-catch from water

c Catheterization d. blowhole collection

60. Which method is used for urine collection in domestic cats and dogs in veterinary clinics?

a. Automatic collection method b. Catheterization

c. Bladder expression d. Jugular vein puncture

61. Which species commonly has a urine collection method involving naturally occurring urine trails on tree bark or leaves?

a. Squirrel b. bear

c. beaver d. deer

62. Which method is typically used for urine collection in elephants in zoos or wildlife parks?

a Catheterization b. Free-catch from ground

c. Bladder massage d. Trained collection pan

63. Which method is commonly used for urine collection in horses during veterinary examinations?

a. Free-catch b. Catheterization

c. Bladder expression d. Metabolic cage

64. Which method is often used for urine collection in bats in research settings?
    a. Metabolic cage b. bladder massage
    c Free-catch from roost d Cloacal wash
65. Which species has a urine collection method involving marking territory with urine scent glands?
    a. Lion b. Wolf
    c. Tiger d. all of the above
66. Which method is typically used for urine collection in sea turtles during rehabilitation or research?
    a. cloacal wash b. Free-catch from water
    c. Jugular vein puncture d. blowhole collection
67. Which anatomical site is typically used for CSF collection in domestic dogs and cats?
    a. Jugular vein b. Lateral ventricle
    c. cisterna magna d. bladder
68. Which of the following is a common indication for CSF collection in domestic animals?
    a. Routine health check b. diagnosis of neurological disease
    c. Vaccination protocol d. Monitoring kidney function
69. Which of the following positions is commonly used during CSF collection in domestic animals to facilitate access to the cisterna magna?
    a. Lateral recumbency (lying on the side)
    b Ventral recumbency (lying on the belly)
    c. Dorsal recumbency (lying on the back)
    d. Standing position
70. Which of the following complications is a potential risk associated with CSF collection in domestic animals?
    a. Increased appetite b. Nerve damage
    c. Skin rash d. Hair loss
71. Which laboratory test is commonly performed on collected CSF samples to assess neurological conditions?
    a. Complete blood count (CBC) b. Urinalysis
    c. Protein analysis d. Liver enzyme panel
72. Which factor is crucial to consider before performing CSF collection in domestic animals?
    a. Recent meal intake b. Lack of exercise
    c Overhydration d. administration of pain medications
73. Which of the following CSF collection methods involves inserting a needle into the subarachnoid space between the vertebrae?
    a. Ventricular puncture b. Lumbar puncture
    c. Cisterna magna puncture d. Nasal swab

74. Which species may require sedation or anesthesia during CSF collection to minimize stress and ensure safety?

a. Rabbit
b. Sheep
c Chicken
d. Fish

75. Which of the following is a common method used for rumen fluid collection in cattle?

a. Venipuncture
b. Cystocentesis
c. Abdominocentesis
d. Rumenocentesis

76. Rumen fluid is primarily collected for the study of:

a. Kidney function
b. digestive enzymes
c. Microbial fermentation
d. Respiratory diseases

77. What is the preferred site for rumen fluid collection in cattle?

a. Right paralumbar fossa
b. Left paralumbar fossa
c. Pamamedian site
d. Ventral abdomen

78. During rumen fluid collection, the cow is typically in which position?

a. Standing
b. Lying on the back
c. Lateral recumbency
d. Hanging upside down

79. Which of the following is NOT a potential complication of rumen fluid collection?

a. Rumen perforation
b. Infection
c. Nerve damage
d. Increased milk production

80. Which technique involves the insertion of a needle and syringe directly into the rumen to collect fluid?

a. Trocarization
b Rumenocentesis
c Abdominocentesis
d. Cystocentesis

81. Which species other than cattle might require rumen fluid collection for research or diagnostic purposes?

a. Dog
b. Horse
c. Sheep
d. Cat

82. Which test is commonly performed on rumen fluid samples to assess microbial populations and fermentation parameters?

a. Electrolyte analysis
b. Culture and sensitivity
c. Volatile fatty acid analysis
d. Blood glucose measurement

83. Which factor should be considered before rumen fluid collection to ensure accurate results?

a. Recent feed intake
b. Age of the animal
c. coat color
d. Weight gain

84. Which method allows continuous monitoring of rumen fluid without repeated collection?

a. Ultrasound imaging
b. Metabolic cage
c. Rumen cannulation
d. Electrocardiogram

85. In rumenocentesis, the needle is typically inserted into which part of the rumen?

a. Dorsal sac
b. Ventral sac
c. Cranial sac
d. Rumen Pillar

86. Which instrument is typically used for performing abdominocentesis in veterinary practice?

a. Scalpel
b. Otoscope
c Ultrasound probe
d. Syringe and needle

87. Which of the following techniques involves inserting a needle through the body wall into the abdominal cavity to collect fluid?

a. Cystocentesis
b. Arthrocentesis
c. Abdominocentesis
d. Venipuncture

88. Which condition might prompt a veterinarian to perform abdominocentesis in a dog or cat?

a. Heartworm disease
b. Chronic arthritis
c. Abdominal distension
d. Skin infection

89. Which of the following is a potential complication of abdominocentesis in veterinary patients?

a. Increased appetite
b. Nerve damage
c. Hair loss
d. Improved coat condition

90. Which laboratory test is commonly performed on abdominal fluid collected via abdominocentesis?

a Blood glucose measurement
b. complete blood count
c. Protein analysis
d. Electrocardiogram (ECG)

91. In horses, which technique is commonly used for abdominocentesis?

a. Standing with sedation
b. Lying down in lateral recumbency
c. Hanging upside down
d. Underwater collection

92. What precaution should be taken before performing abdominocentesis to reduce the risk of contamination?

a. Administering antibiotics
b. Clipping and cleaning the area
c. Providing sedation
d. Applying a bandage

93. Which of the following is an indication for performing abdominocentesis in a small animal emergency?

a. Routine vaccination
b. Suspected gastrointestinal foreign body
c. Chronic skin rash
d. Long-term weight loss

94. In which situation might abdominocentesis be used to guide therapeutic procedures, such as draining excess fluid?

a. Routine physical examination
b. Post-surgical monitoring
c. Emergency trauma cases
d. Chronic joint pain

95. What role does abdominocentesis play in managing cases of suspected organ rupture or bleeding in small animal practice?

a. Monitoring temperature changes
b. Assessing eye conditions
c. Providing pain relief
d. Diagnosing and relieving pressure

96. Which of the following conditions might necessitate thoracocentesis in canine practice?

a. Dental disease
b. Renal failure
c. Heartworm infection
d. Skin rash

97. Which condition might be indicated by the presence of blood in pleural fluid collected via thoracocentesis?

a. Pancreatitis
b. Respiratory infection
c. Kidney stones
d. Internal bleeding

98. Which of the following is a potential complication of thoracocentesis in veterinary patients?

a. Improved appetite
b. Pneumothorax
c. Weight gain
d. Clear nasal discharge

99. Which of the following is an indication for performing thoracocentesis in a veterinary emergency?

a. Routine vaccination
b. Suspected fracture
c. Chronic ear infection
d. Acute respiratory distress

100. Which technique involves inserting a needle through the body wall into the pleural cavity to collect fluid?

a. Cystocentesis
b. Arthrocentesis
c. Thoracocentesis
d. Venipuncture

101. Pleural fluid collected from domestic animals is primarily analyzed to detect:

a. Blood sugar levels
b. Microbial infections
c. Digestive enzymes
d. Synovial fluid abnormalities

102. Pericardiocentesis is primarily performed to relieve pressure caused by:

a. Kidney stones
b. Excessive gas accumulation
c. Accumulation of fluid around the heart
d. Bone fractures

103. Which type of fluid is typically collected during pericardiocentesis in cases of pericardial effusion?

a. Synovial fluid
b. Pleural fluid
c. Blood
d. Pericardial fluid

104. Which condition might be indicated by the presence of blood in pericardial fluid collected via pericardiocentesis?

a. Dental disease
b. Respiratory infection
c Cardiac tamponade
d. Liver disease

105. In which situation might pericardiocentesis be used as a life-saving procedure in small animal medicine?

a. Treatment of arthritis
b. Routine dental cleaning
c. Management of heart failure with cardiac tamponade
d. Control of skin allergies

106. Which species might require pericardiocentesis for the diagnosis and management of conditions like pericardial effusion?

a. Rabbit b. Horse

c. Bird d. Cat

107. Which of the following is an indication for performing pericardiocentesis in a veterinary emergency?

a. Routine vaccination

b. Suspected fracture

c. Chronic ear infection

d. Cardiac tamponade causing respiratory distress

108. Which technique involves inserting a needle through the body wall into the pericardial sac to drain fluid?

a Cystocentesis b. Arthrocentesis

c. Pericardiocentesis d. Venipuncture

109. Which of the following equipments is not needed to perform a pericardiocentesis:

a. Scissors b. Clippers

c. Surgical scrub d. Intravenous catheters

110. The most common complication of pericardiocentesis is

a. Cardiac arrhythmia b. Cardiac puncture

c. Respiratory distress d. None of the above

111. A pericardiocentesis is often done to remove excess fluid from the pericardial space caused by a pericardial effusion or _____.

a. Pleural effusion b. Endocarditis

c. cardiac tamponade d. catheterization

112. Typically ---------ml of Synovial fluid is collected from most equine joints

a. 0.5 b. 1.0

c. 2.0 d. 5.0

113. Which of the following is not a part of laboratory analysis of equine synovial fluid

a. Viscosity

b. Protein concentration

c. Total and differential nucleated cell counts

d. None of the above

114. For best results, synovial fluid should be analyzed

a. After storage at 4°C for up to 24 hours b. As quick as possible.

c. After freeze drying d After storage at 8°C for 8 hours

115. Synovial fluid analysis is also recommended in disorders characterized by

a. Persistent or fluctuating fever of unknown origin

b. Shifting leg lameness

c. Generalized malaise in which arthralgia is suspected

d. All of these

116. Which of the following is not a feature of normal synovial fluid in the dog and cat
   a. Clots on standing b. Is clear, colorless
   c. Is Viscous d. Is free of flocculent debris
117. Joint aspiration in most dogs or cats yields less than --------ml of synovial fluid
   a. 0.6-1.0 b. 0.4-0.5
   c. 0.1-0.25 d. 1-1.5
118. After milking a cow, the cows teats should be dipped ___________
   a. After 2 minutes b. After 1 minute
   c. After 30 seconds d. Immediately
119. Milk from a cow with mastitis will have__________
   a. Abnormal freezing point
   b. A high somatic cell count
   c. Both abnormal freezing point and a high somatic cell count
   d. Abnormal boiling point
120. The most common measurement of milk quality and udder health in cattle is
   a. Electrical conductivity b. Somatic cell count
   c. Protein concentration d. Udder size
121. In healthy lactating cattle mammary gland, total somatic cell count are often
   a. $<10^5$/ml of milk b. $<10^6$/ml of milk
   c $<10^7$/ml of milk d $<10^8$/ml of milk
122. Which of the following does not constitute milk somatic cells?
   a. Lymphocytes b. Macropahges
   c. Fibroblasts d. Epithelial cells
123. What is the purpose of collecting milk samples from cows for laboratory analysis?
   a. To determine the cow's breed b To measure milk yield only
   c. To assess milk quality and composition d. To determine the cow's age
124. How should milk samples be stored before being sent to the laboratory for analysis?
   a. Refrigerated b. Frozen
   c. Room temperature d. Sun-dried
125. Which of the following factors can affect the composition of milk?
   a. Time of day b. cow's diet
   c. Weather conditions d. all of the above
126. Why is it important to collect milk samples from each quarter separately in some cases?
   a. To reduce labor costs
   b. To ensure accurate testing of mastitis
   c. To compare milk yield
   d. To determine cow health
127. Which method is used to detect somatic cell count in milk samples?
   a. Microscopic examination b. Visual inspection
   c. Smell test d. Taste test

128. What does the term "composite sample" mean in milk sampling?
  a. A sample composed of milk from several cows
  b. A sample mixed with water
  c. A sample taken from the top layer of milk
  d. A sample mixed with preservatives
129. Why is it important to agitate milk samples before analysis?
  a. To improve taste
  b. To mix preservatives
  c. To prevent cream separation
  d. To accelerate testing
130. What is the purpose of testing for bacterial count in milk samples?
  a. To determine milk yield
  b. To assess milk quality and freshness
  c. To detect lactose intolerance
  d. To measure milk acidity
131. Which method is used to determine the presence of antibiotics in milk samples?
  a. Taste test
  b. Microbial assay
  c. Spectrophotometry
  d. Chromatography
132. What is the primary purpose of testing for aflatoxin in milk samples?
  a. To assess milk quality
  b. To detect bacterial contamination
  c. To detect mycotoxin contamination
  d. To determine milk acidity
133. How does high somatic cell count in milk affect its quality?
  a. It improves milk taste
  b. It reduces milk yield
  c. It indicates potential mastitis
  d. It increases milk fat content
134. Which method is commonly used for collecting saliva samples from animals?
  a. Squeezing the animal's cheeks
  b. Saliva collection tubes
  c. Swabbing the mouth
  d. Licking collection pads
135. Why is collecting saliva from animals useful for research?
  a. To assess dental health only
  b. To measure hormone levels, genetic material, and health indicators
  c. To determine breed characteristics
  d. To study eating habits
136. How should saliva samples be stored for laboratory analysis?
  a. Room temperature
  b. Frozen
  c. Refrigerated
  d. Exposed to sunlight
137. What equipment is commonly used to collect saliva samples non-invasively from animals?
  a. Needles and syringes
  b. Collection bags
  c. Swabs or sponges
  d. Petri dishes
138. Which factors can affect the composition of saliva samples from animals?
  a. Time of day
  b. Animal's age
  c Diet
  d All of the above

139. Why is it important to collect saliva samples in a stress-free environment?
   a. To prevent contamination
   b. To avoid saliva degradation
   c. To ensure accurate results
   d. To reduce collection time

140. Which analytes are commonly measured in saliva samples from animals?
   a. DNA and RNA
   b. Blood glucose levels
   c. Bone density
   d. Muscle mass

141. What is the primary advantage of using non-invasive methods for collecting saliva from animals?
   a. Lower cost
   b. Faster collection time
   c. Reduced stress for animals
   d. Higher sample volume

142. Which type of animals can saliva collection methods be used on?
   a. Only domesticated animals
   b. Only carnivorous animals
   c. both domesticated and wild animals
   d. Only herbivorous animals

143. Which biological fluid is useful for assessing kidney function in animals?
   a. Blood
   b. Saliva
   c. Urine
   d. Tears

144. Which biological fluid is useful for assessing respiratory infections in animals?
   a. Blood
   b. Tears
   c. Mucus
   d. Urine

145. Which biological fluid is useful for detecting reproductive hormones in animals?
   a. Blood
   b. Sweat
   c. Tears
   d. Mucus

146. Which biological fluid is useful for assessing electrolyte balance in animals?
   a Sweat
   b. blood
   c. Tears
   d. Urine

147. How does the method of collecting biological fluids vary between different animal species?
   a. It doesn't vary; the same method applies to all species
   b. Larger animals require less frequent collection
   c. Small animals require more frequent collection
   d. different species may require different collection techniques and volumes

148. What is the primary purpose of collecting semen from dogs?
   a. To assess sperm count only
   b. To diagnose reproductive diseases
   c. To freeze for future breeding
   d. To measure testosterone levels

149. Which technique is used to assess sperm motility in collected semen samples from dogs?
   a. Microscopic examination
   b. Spectrophotometry
   c. DNA analysis
   d. Chromatography

150. What is the primary advantage of using artificial insemination with frozen semen in dogs?
   a. Lower success rate
   b. Higher genetic diversity
   c. Reduced risk of disease transmission
   d. Shorter breeding season

151. Which of the following is a common method for collecting blood from cattle for biochemical analysis?

a. Venipuncture b. Intramuscular injection

c. Subcutaneous injection d. catheterization

152. What is the primary purpose of conducting blood biochemical analysis in cattle?

a. To measure heart rate

b. To diagnose skin conditions

c. To assess metabolic status and overall health

d. To evaluate lung capacity

153. Which blood component is commonly measured to assess liver function in cattle?

a. Albumin

b. Urea

c. Bilirubin

d. Gamma-glutamyl transferase (GGT)

154. What does the measurement of blood urea nitrogen (BUN) in cattle indicate?

a. Kidney function b. Muscle condition

c. bone density d. Liver function

155. Which blood enzyme is often elevated in cases of muscle damage or injury in cattle?

a. Amylase b. Creatine kinase (CK)

c. Lipase d. Lactate dehydrogenase (LDH)

156. Which blood parameter is crucial for assessing mineral metabolism in cattle?

a. Iron b. Sodium

c. calcium d. chloride

157. What does the measurement of blood albumin levels indicate in cattle?

a. Liver function b. Protein status

c. Kidney function d. Glucose levels

158. Which blood parameter is indicative of lipid metabolism in cattle?

a. Triglycerides b. Uric acid

c. Potassium d. Hemoglobin

Answer Key

1	c	2	b	3	d	4	a	5	b	6	d	7	a
8	d	9	c	10	b	11	a	12	b	13	c	14	a
15	c	16	d	17	a	18	c	19	b	20	c	21	c
22	c	23	b	24	c	25	b	26	b	27	c	28	d
29	c	30	b	31	d	32	a	33	c	34	c	35	d
36	c	37	c	38	d	39	d	40	d	41	c	42	d
43	c	44	a	45	b	46	b	47	a	48	b	49	b
50	b	51	c	52	c	53	b	54	a	55	a	56	b
57	d	58	d	59	b	60	b	61	b	62	d	63	b
64	c	65	d	66	b	67	c	68	b	69	a	70	b
71	c	72	a	73	b	74	a	75	d	76	c	77	b
78	a	79	d	80	b	81	c	82	c	83	a	84	c
85	a	86	d	87	c	88	c	89	b	90	c	91	a
92	b	93	b	94	c	95	d	96	c	97	d	98	b
99	d	100	c	101	b	102	c	103	d	104	c	105	c
106	c	107	d	108	c	109	a	110	a	111	c	112	b
113	d	114	b	115	d	116	a	117	c	118	d	119	c
120	b	121	a	122	c	123	c	124	a	125	d	126	b
127	a	128	a	129	c	130	b	131	d	132	c	133c	
134	c	135	b	136	b	137	c	138	d	139	c	140	a
141	c	142	c	143	c	144	c	145	a	146	b	147	d
148	c	149	a	150	c	151	a	152	c	153	d	154	a
155	b	156	c	157	b	158	a						

29

Biochemical Pathology of Urine

P.C. Prabu[1], K.R. Sangavi[2], T. Sarath[3] and G. Selvam[4]

[1]*Department of Veterinary Pathology, Veterinary College and Research Institute Orathanadu, Tamil Nadu.*

[2]*Division of Veterinary Pathology, Indian Veterinary Research Institute, Izatnagar*

[3]*Department of Veterinary Clinical Complex, Veterinary College and Research Institute, Salem, Tamil Nadu*

[4]*Department of Pathology, Bioscience Research Foundation, Chennai, Tamil Nadu*

Introduction

Urinalysis, the examination of normal and abnormal components of urine, is one of the most important aspect of clinical pathology that aids in accurate and timely diagnosis in veterinary practice. Urine is considered as one of the most accessible bio-fluid that can be collected using non- invasive techniques in adequate quantities. It includes the evaluation of colour, odour, turbidity, volume, pH, specific gravity, protein and glucose content, ketone bodies, blood, erythrocytes, leukocytes, epithelial cells, casts, crystal, micro-organisms, etc. Urinalysis gives us valuable information regarding the several important attributes of renal function. For example, specific gravity of urine gives valuable insights over the potential of the Henle's loop to dilute urine and the distal convoluted tubules to concentrate urine after ruling out the extra-renal factors affecting the urine specific gravity. It is highly useful to evaluate the different types of urogenital diseases and it also provides significant information regarding several systemic disorders. It is comparatively quicker to perform and is relatively a low-cost test that could be easily done in most clinical setups.

Glomerular function that is usually evaluated based on serum or plasma biochemical tests, can also be assessed by detecting proteinuria, especially albuminuria that is indicative of altered glomerular barrier function. Proteinuria in spite of normal specific gravity and glucosuria with normal blood glucose levels suggest possible proximal tubular disease. Dipstick analysis is a valuable test to assess the potential of proximal convoluted tubules with respect to resorption of *normally* filtered low molecular weight substances like proteins and glucose. Examination of urine sediment aids in detecting tubular injury through the identification of cellular, granular and other casts. At times, other conditions including haemorrhage, infections, inflammation, neoplasia, metabolic disorders also can be diagnosed through urinalysis.

Collection and storage

Urine is generally collected by cystocentesis, urethral catheterization or during voiding. An early morning sample is regarded to be ideal as it contains the components of diagnostic importance. This is because of the reason that water consumption during the day time can dilute urine resulting in decreased specific gravity and loss of integrity of cells and other constituents. The initial stream of urine is not recommended because it will have cell debris, WBCs and fluids flushed from the uro- genital tract. A mid-stream collection of urine is ideal as it will have the least contamination with bacteria. Proper catheterization is essential to avoid trauma and subsequent haemorrhage. If a catheter is used, presence of sloughed off transitional epithelial cells greater than normal should be expecteddue care should be taken for sterile collection of the sample. Cystocentesis is considered to be the ideal and cleanest method of collection of urine. However, if any tissue injury occurs during collection, it can result in microscopic hematuria although the urine collected will be normal colour. More than 100 erythrocytes per high power field can be seen in samples confusing with a true hematuria. Urine should be at room temperature at the time of analysis for accurate evaluation of specific gravity and other chemical evaluations.

Delay in analysis after sample collection needs to be avoided. Otherwise, it can end up in increased pH, increased microbial content, degradation / degeneration of cells and casts, degradation of chemical substances present (bilirubin, ketone bodies), etc affecting the diagnosis. In case, if evaluation cannot be done immediately i.e., within half an hour, then the sample has to be refrigerated to improve preservation of the cells and to decrease the bacterial growth. However, the evaluation needs to be completed within 12 hours of collection. Beyond this duration, the cells will undergo lysis as urine is a toxic environment for cells to survive and a good environment for the microbes to proliferate. Further, artefacts can develop because of storage. For example, calcium oxalate and magnesium ammonium phosphate crystals develop with increased storage time. In case, if cytology of urine samples has to be done, then a preservative, e.g. a few drops of 10% formalin, can be added to the sample.

Renal function tests are helpful to identify the presence of kidney diseases, to monitor the response of kidneys to treatment and to determine the progression of kidney diseases. In addition, they also can give valuable information on whether the renal disease is acute or chronic. Several tests aid in the investigation and evaluation of renal function. Most of the renal function tests assess the glomerular filtration rate (eGFR) and estimate proteinuria / albuminuria. The best overall indicator of the glomerular function is the glomerular filtration rate (GFR). GFR is the rate in milliliters per minute at which substances in plasma get filtered through the glomerulus. Direct tests of renal function are dependent on the elimination kinetics of certain markers of glomerular filtration, renal blood flow, tubular reabsorption / secretion, etcdirect tests aid in earlier diagnosis of decreased renal function. However, it is difficult and time consuming to perform direct tests. Kidney function can be assessed indirectly, based on the levels of plasma or urine constituents. These indirect markers of kidney function can be easily and rapidly quantified. However, the sensitivity of such markers is low and they usually remain unchanged till around 75% of the kidney function is affected. Other diseases of renal tubular function, can be identified using more detailed renal function tests, especially urine amino acids, glucose, phosphate, etc.

1. In most of the species, the number of nephrons increases progressively during fetal development. For which species the number of nephrons increases during few months after birth?
   a. Sheep b. Dog
   c. Goat d. Rat
2. Kidney receives__________ percentage of cardiac output.
   a. 10 b. 20
   c. 45 d. 55
3. In glomerulus, the fenestrated endothelium of capillaries has an approximate pore size of __________.
   a. 25 to 55nm b. 50 to 100nm
   c. 110 to 155nm d. 150 to 200nm
4. The glomerular basement membrane is made of 90% water and____________
   a. Positively charged methylated triglycerides
   b. Negatively charged methylated triglycerides
   c. Positively charged sulphated glycosaminoglycans
   d. Negatively charged sulphated glycosaminoglycans
5. The filtration slits between the foot-like processes of podocytes are of________nm.
   a. 25 b. 35
   c. 45 d. 55
6. Denotes the presence of renal tubular casts in the urine sediment.
   a. Pollakiuria b. cylinduria
   c. Azoturia d. Pyuria
7. What is the net effective filtration pressure for dogs and cats?
   a. 10 to 15mmHg b. 20 to 25mmHg
   c. 30 to 35mmHg d. 40 to 45mmHg
8. Neutral molecules of less than____________nm diffuse freely across the glomerulus.
   a. 1 b. 1.5
   c. 2 d. 2.5
9. Because of the high concentration ofat the surface of endothelial cells and in the glomerular basement membrane, the filtration slit tends to repel negatively charged molecules.
   a. Methylated glycosaminoglycans b. Alkylated glycosaminoglycans
   c. Sulfated glycosaminoglycans d. Chlorinated glycosaminoglycans
10. The portion of nephron where most of the solutes and water are reabsorbed is
   a. PCT b. Descending loop of Henle
   c. Ascending loop of Henle d. DCT

11. Which among the following has long loops of nephrons?
    a. Pigs
    b. Sheep
    c. Dogs
    d. Humans
12. The cells in the macula densa respond to by releasing renin.
    a. Hypernatremia
    b. Hyponatremia
    c. Hyperphosphatemia
    d. Hypophosphatemia
13. Which of the following statement is false?
    a. The driving force is the hydrostatic pressure in the capillary, which is opposed by hydrostatic pressure within Bowman's space and oncotic pressure in the capillary.
    b. Average urine is more concentrated in dogs and cats than in humans or swine.
    c Reabsorption is dominant in healthy animals and mainly occurs in the descending loop of Henle by active and passive transport.
    d Excretion in distal tubule is controlled by hormones, so that the final urine is usually more concentrated than the ultrafiltrate.
14. Glucose reabsorption is permitted by_______transporter in the apical membrane of PCT.
    a. SGLT1
    b. Na/K-ATPase
    c. GLUT2
    d. Aquaporin2 channel
15. Sodium concentration is kept low in tubule cells by_______in the basolateral membrane of PCT.
    a. SGLT1
    b. Na/K-ATPase
    c. GLUT2
    d. aquaporin2 channel
16. Maximal tubular reabsorption (Tm) is attained when plasma glucose concentration (P-Glucose) is ________________________mmol/lit in dogs.
    a. 25
    b. 20
    c. 15
    d. 12
17. Identify the false statement-
    a Glucose, amino acids, and low-molecular-weight protein are mostly secreted into the proximal tubule from the interstitial fluid
    b. The extent of reabsorption can be estimated from the fractional excretion (FE) of solutes
    c. Urea transporters are present at the thin extremity of the descending loop of Henle and corresponding segments of the *vasa recta*
    d. Final absorption of Na ions in the distal part of the nephron is hormonally controlled by aldosterone and natriuretic peptides
18. Reabsorption of phosphates in the proximal tubule by a sodium co-transporter is inhibited by which hormone?
    a. Natriuretic peptides
    b. Aldosterone
    c. Thyroxine
    d. Parathyroid hormone

19. The maximum rate of transport (Tm) for phosphate reabsorption is higher in which species?
    a. Ruminants b. Canines
    c. Felines d. Porcines
20. Which species excrete significant amounts of calcium ions in the urine under normal conditions?
    a. Rabbit b. Goat
    c. Cattle d. Cat
21. Reabsorption of calcium ions occurs mostly by
    a. Adsorptive transcytosis b. Transcellular route
    c. Paracellular route d. None of the above
22. Which among the following statement is true?
    a. Most magnesium reabsorption occurs in the proximal convoluted tubule.
    b. Most water (75%) is reabsorbed passively in the ascending loop of Henle along with ions and small hydrophilic molecules.
    c. Kidney plays a major role in acid-base regulation by involving in the elimination of carbon dioxide.
    d. Potassium is secreted by the distal tubule and cortical collecting duct, mainly during hyperkalemia.
23. Major hormones produced by the kidneys are
    a. Erythropoietin and aldosterone b. Erythropoietin and calcitrol
    c. Clairol and parathormone d. Aldosterone and parathormone
24. Which of the following is a direct test for kidney function?
    a Creatinine estimation b. Urea estimation
    c. Cystatin Cestimation d. Fractional excretion of ions
25. The main determinant of specific gravity in dog urine is___
    a. Renin b. Water
    c. Urea d. Cystatin C
26. Which protein secreted by the distal convoluted tubule is the major constituent of proteinaceous casts?
    a. Tamm-horsfall b. Urokinase
    c. Immunoglobin A d. Angiotensin II
27. Proteinuria is observed in which of the following pre-renal conditions?
    a. Intense exercise b. Glomerulonephritis
    c. Urinary tract infection d. Cystolithiasis
28. Pyrogallol red method is used for determining which constituent in urine?
    a. Glucose b. Calcium
    c. Ketone bodies d. Protein
29. Collecting duct requires the action of which hormone to absorb water?
    a. Parathormone b. ADH
    c. Calcitrol d. Prolactin

30. Which stream of urine is ideal for urine analysis?
    a. Initial stream   b. Mid stream
    c. End stream   d. Both a and c

31. Supernatant portion of urine after centrifugation is not clear and is reddish brown in which of the following conditions?
    a. Haemoglobinuria   b. Myoglobinuria
    c. Hematuria   d. Both a and b

32 Decreased urinary specific gravity is observed in which of the following conditions?
    a. Hyperadrenocortism   b. Dehydration
    c. Decreased water intake   d. Extreme heat

33. Which of the following statement is false?
    a. Glucosuria can be seen in excited or scared animals, particularly cats.
    b. False positive results for ketone bodies can occur in calves with polioencephalomalacia.
    c. Renal threshold for glucose in cattle is 260mg/dL.
    d. An ammonium sulphate test can be performed to distinguish myoglobin from haemoglobin.

34. Renal threshold of glucose for dogs and cats are
    a. 110mg/dL and 220mg/dL, respectively
    b. 220mg/dL and 110mg/dL, respectively
    c. 180mg/dL and 280mg/dL, respectively
    d. 280mg/dL and 180mg/dL, respectively

35. Tests available to more accurately confirm the presence of proteinuria are
    a. Urine protein-creatinine ratio   b. Microalbumin estimation
    c. Both a and b   d. None of the above

36. Refers to the maximal concentration of a given substance that the renal tubules can reabsorb.
    a. Renal clearance   b. Renal threshold
    c. Fractional clearance   d. Tubular maximum

37. Which ketone body is most sensitive to dipstick method?
    a. Acetone   b Acetoacetate
    c. Beta hydroxy butyrate   d. Albumin

38 Alkaline picric acid method of Jaffe is commonly used for detection of_______.
    a. Creatinine   b. Blood urea nitrogen
    c. Albumin   d. Calcium

39. p-aminohippuric acid clearance is used for the determination of_______.
    a. Aldosterone concentration in DCT   b. Vasopressin levels
    c. Osmotic pressure of capillaries   d. Renal blood flow

40. Which of the following is not involved in urea formation?
    a. Ornithine   b. Citrulline
    c. Arginase   d. Inulin

41. Urine volume is not dependent on which of the following variables?
   a. Diet b. Fluid intake
   c. Environmental temperature d. Sialolith

42. Urine volume is inversely related to specific gravity with the exception in which condition?
   a. diabetes insipidus b. diabetes mellitus
   c. both a and b d. None of the above

43. _____ is a condition that results due to deficiency of ADH causing decreased reabsorption of water in DCT.
   a. Methemoglobinuria b. Rheumatoid arthritis
   c. Diabetes insipidus d Lipemia

44. The usage of which urine preservative most commonly can cause false positive results with the sulphosalicylic acid test?
   a. Thymol b. boric acid
   c. Chloroform d. Formalin

45. The common preservative used for estimation of vitamin C in urine is
   a. Toluene b. Thymol
   c. boric acid d. Metaphosphoric acid

46. Dark yellow coloured concentrated urine with a high specific gravity not seen in which of the following?
   a. Hemoglobinuria b. diminished intake of fluids
   c. Prolonged vomiting or diarrhea d. Fever

47. Which of the following method is not used for determining specific gravity of urine?
   a. Microalbumin test b. dipstick method
   c. Urinometer d. Refractometer

48. What does a positive result for Robert's test indicate?
   a. Presence of increased ketone bodies b. Presence of increased protein
   c. Increased presence of bile salts d. Increased presence of magnesium

49. After which of the following drug administration, the resulting urine is acidic in nature
   a. Sodium citrate b. Sodium lactate
   c. Ammonium chloride d. Potassium nitrate

50. Hemoglobinuria is commonly seen in which of the following conditions?
   a. Sweet clover poisoning b. copper poisoning
   c. Photosensitization d. both a and b

51. Wallace-Diamond test is used for identifying which of the following?
   a. Calcium b. Urobilinogens
   c. Magnesium d. Hemoglobin

52. Presence of indican in urine is detected by which of the following test?
   a. Obermayer's test b. Sulkowitch test
   c. Ross test d. Watson method

53. Presence of sulphonamide in urine can be found by which test?
    a. Hay's test b. Lignin test
    c. Xylidyl test d. Benzedrine test
54. Which type of cast is commonly seen in renal graft rejection?
    a. Hyaline cast b. Granular cast
    c. Waxy cast d. Fatty cast
55. Which of the following factors increases GFR?
    a. Increased nephroliths b. Reduced renal blood flow
    c. Increased blood pressure d. both a and b
56. Which of the following is correct regarding urinary filtration rate (UFR)?
    a. UFR= reabsorption rate + secretion rate – filtration rate
    b. UFR= filtration rate + reabsorption rate – secretion rate
    c. UFR= filtration rate – reabsorption rate + secretion rate
    d. UFR= secretion rate – filtration rate + reabsorption rate
57. How does kidney respond to decreased calcium ion concentration?
    a. Increased secretion of calcium ions
    b. Decreased excretion of phosphorus
    c. Formation of active form of vitamin D
    d. both a and b
58. Which of the following is not true about role of angiotensin II in urine regulation?
    a. Inhibits aldosterone secretion by adrenal cortex
    b. Arteriolar constriction which increases the blood pressure
    c. Stimulates ADH secretion
    d. Reabsorption of NaCl by PCT
59. Renal plasma flow cannot be quantitated by which of the following methods?
    a. Plasma renin assay b. Inulin clearance
    c. Diodrast clearance d. PAH clearance
60. White or pink cloud in acid urine upon standing or when chilled is due to_______
    a. Calcium carbonates b. Hippuric acid
    c Amorphous urates d. Amorphous phosphates
61. What is the role of kidney in acid-base disturbances?
    a. Compensates for primary metabolic disturbances
    b Compensates for primary respiratory disturbances
    c Compensates for both primary metabolic and respiratory disturbances
    d Compensates for secondary respiratory disturbances
62. Albumin concentration of primitive urine is___.
    a. ~ 10mg/l b. ~ 25mg/l
    c. ~ 40mg/l d. 0

63. Which among the following is false?
    a. Creatinine is the product of creatine breakdown.
    b. Creatinine levels in urine is proportional to muscle mass.
    c. Creatinine is produced from creatine phosphate.
    d. Creatinine levels in urine are independent of the diet in carnivores.
64. Creatinine is not reabsorbed or secreted in the renal tubules in_.
    a. Horse b. Ponies
    c. Sheep d. Goat
65. Tamm-Horsfall protein in the urine originates from which part of the nephron and causes what type of cast commonly?
    a. PCT and hyaline cast b. DCT and waxy cast
    c. Loop of Henle and hyaline cast d. Loop of Henle and fatty cast
66. All the following conditions causes increased anion gap except
    a Rhabdomyolysis b. Ethylene glycol toxicity
    c. Hypoalbuminemia d. Diabetic ketoacidosis
67. Which of the following significantly causes elevated GFR?
    a. Protein meal b. Carbohydrate meal
    c. Fatty meal d. High fibre diet
68. In addition to kidney failure, which of the following also elevates serum BUN levels?
    a. Diabetes mellitus b. Osteodystrophy
    c. Following estrus d. Upper GI bleeding
69. Prostaglandins in kidneys is produced by
    a. Tubular epithelial cells b. Medullary interstitium
    c. Both a and b d. None of the above
70. Bicarbonate secretion occurs in
    a. Type A intercalated cells b. Type B intercalated cells
    c. Mesangial cells d. Principal cells
71. Species which lack loop of Henle among the following is
    a. Birds b. Mammals
    c. Reptiles d. None of the above
72. Which part of the nephron is majorly involved in creating and maintaining renal medullary hypertonicity?
    a. Glomerulus b. PCT
    c. DCT d. Loop of henle
73. ADH primarily acts at____________________.
    a. PCT b. DCT
    c. Loop of Henle d. Collecting duct
74. Nephrogenic diabetes mellitus is due to mutation of which channel?
    a. $Na^+K^+ATPase$ b. SGLT 2
    c. GLUT 1 d. Aquaporin 2

75. Which of the following contributes to the negative charge of membrane in glomeruli?
   a. Podocytes
   b. Bowmans capsule
   c. Sulphated glycosaminoglycans
   d. Mesangial cells
76. CKD causes what type of anaemia?
   a. Microcytic and hypochromic
   b. Macrocytic and hypochromic
   c. Microcytic and hypochromic
   d. Normocytic and normochromic
77. An increase in levels of urinary indicans is suggestive of_______________.
   a. SIBO
   b. Chronic kidney disease
   c. Acute renal failure
   d. Exocrine pancreatic insufficiency
78. If the pH of blood is high and the PCo2 and HCO3- are also higher than the normal range, what is the primary acid-base disturbance?
   a. Respiratory alkalosis
   b. Metabolic alkalosis
   c. Respiratory acidosis
   d. Metabolic acidosis
79. A Novel renal biomarker is_______________.
   a. NT – Pro BNP
   b. SDMA
   c. CTnl
   d Creatinine
80. Which of the following is more significantly associated with early renal failure stage?
   a. Isosthenuria
   b. Hyposthenuria
   c. Hyperthenuria
   d. Proteinuria
81. Fanconi like syndrome causes which type of renal calculi?
   a. Silica
   b. Cysteine
   c. Struvite
   d. Oxalate
82. Weddellite kidney stones that can occur as an artifact in stored urine is composed of
   a. Calcium carbonate
   b. Struvite
   c. Calcium oxalate
   d. Cysteine
83. The urine concentration mechanism is mainly contributed by which part of nephron in camels?
   a. PCT
   b. DCT
   c. Long loop of Henle
   d. collecting duct
84. Erythropoietin is secreted by_______________.
   a. Loop of Henle
   b. Peritubular capillary endothelium
   c. Juxtaglomerular cells
   d. DCT
85. Most of the H^+ proton secretion occurs at_____.
   a. DCT
   b. Collecting tubule
   c. PCT
   d. Loop of Henle
86. Titration acidosis occurs in all except ________
   a. Secretory diarrhea
   b. Diabetic ketoacidosis
   c. Hypovolemia
   d. Lactic acidosis
87. Macrophages of kidney are
   a. Mesangial cells
   b. Polkissen cells
   c. Lacis cells
   d. All the above

88. The additional clinic-pathologic abnormality observed in nephrotic syndrome that is not seen in nephrotic tendency is

a. Hypoalbuminemia
b. Hypercholesterolemia
c. Edema
d. Proteinuria

89. Nephrotic syndrome is characterized by the following abnormalities except______.

a. Hypoalbuminemia
b. Proteinuria
c. Edema
d. Hypocholesterolemia

90. Hypercholesterolemia seen in protein losing nephropathy is due to _____

a. Lipoprotein – X
b. Cholesterol
c. Proteinuria
d. Fatty acids

91. Which of the following causes secondary urinary tract infection?

a. TCC
b. Hypoadrenocorticism
c. Hyperadrenocorticism
d. Hyperthyroidism

92. Best method to collect urine sample for culture is___________

a. Free catch
b. Catheterization
c. Cystocentesis
d. Voided urine

93. Increased bile pigment in urine is seen in which of the following conditions?

a. Hepatitis
b. Hemolytic jaundice
c. Obstruction of bile passage
d. a and b

94. Ideal time to analyze a urine sample is within _.

a. 30 minutes of collection
b. 2 hours of collection
c. 12 hours of collection
d. 24 hours after refrigeration of the sample

95. Which among the following species voids cloudy urine normally?

a. Camel
b. Horse
c. Rabbit
d. b and C

96. Which of the following ketone body is most sensitive to Rothera's test?

a. Acetone
b. Acetoacetate
c. Beta hydroxybutyrate
d. All the above

97. CKD in a cachectic animal can cause which of the following?

a. Elevated BUN and creatinine levels in serum
b. Elevated BUN and normal creatinine
c. Elevated creatinine and normal BUN
d. Decreased BUN and elevated creatinine

98. In large animals, which of the following is the most reliable serum parameter to estimate glomerular function?

a. Creatinine
b. Protein
c. BUN
d. Urea

99. Which of the following statement is true?
    a. All azotemic patients are uremic
    b. All uremic patients are azotemic
    c. Both are true
    d. Both are false

100. Comparing the concentration of a substance in urine to concentration of the same substance in serum is called as_____________.
    a. Renal clearance
    b. Fractional clearance
    c. GFR
    d. Renal plasma flow

101. Excretion of urine above which level is considered as polyuria in cats?
    a. >30ml/kg/day
    b. >40ml/kg/day
    c. >50ml/kg/day
    d. >60ml/kg/day

102. Storing the urine sample for prolonged period causes all of the following artifacts except?
    a. ↑ pH
    b. ↑ bacteria
    c. ↓ pH
    d. ↓ bacteria

103. Bence-Jones protein is seen in which of the following conditions and is caused because of ______and ____________________________, respectively.
    a. Essential thrombocythemia and it is due to heavy chain of Ig
    b. Multiple myeloma and it is due to heavy chain of Ig
    c. Essential thrombocythemia and is due to light chain of Ig
    d. Multiple myeloma due to excretion of light chain

104. Ammonium urate crystals are formed in which pH?
    a. Acidic
    b. Neutral
    c. Basic
    d. Both a and b

105. What is the shape of calcium oxalate crystals?
    a. Dumb bell shaped
    b. Picket – fence shaped
    c. Hemp seed shaped
    d. All the above

106. Which of the following statement is true?
    a. Amyloid deposition is primarily seen in renal tubules in canines.
    b. Amyloid deposition is primarily seen in glomerulus in felines.
    c. Amyloid deposition is primarily seen in glomerulus in canines.
    d. None of the above.

107. In saturated ammonium sulfate precipitation test, if no precipitation occurs in urine, it is indicative of
    a. Hemoglobinuria
    b. Proteinuria
    c. Hematuria
    d. Myoglobinuria

108. Which type of cast is predominantly found in chronic interstitial nephritis?
    a. Epithelial
    b. Granular
    c. Hyaline
    d. Waxy

109. Bilirubin crystals in urine are relatively normal in which of the following species?
   a. Cats
   b. Dogs
   c. Horse
   d. Ruminants
110. Ammonium biurate crystalluria is associated with__
   a. Ethylene glycol toxicity
   b. artifacts
   c. Urinary tract infections
   d. Porto-systemic shunt
111. Paradoxic aciduria is seen in which condition?
   a. Chronic diarrhea
   b. Displaced abomasum
   c. Hyperadrenocorticism
   d. Vagal indigestion
112. Which parasitic egg excreted in the urine of cats looks similar to *Trichuris spp* egg?
   a. Capillaria spp
   b. *Dioctophyma renale*
   c. *Stephanurus dentatus*
   d. Microfilaria of *Dirofilaria immitis*
113. Which of the following does not cause ADH release?
   a. Hypoosmolarity
   b. Hypovolemia
   c. Hypotension
   d. Hyperosmolarity
114. Which of the following factors do not elevate the serum BUN concentration?
   a. Fever
   b. Exercise
   c. Hypoadrenocorticism
   d. Hyperadrenocorticism
115. The following stimulates renin release except________________.
   a. Hypotension
   b. Sympathetic tone
   c. Hyponatremia
   d. Parasympathetic tone
116. Comparing the concentration of a substance in urine to its concentration in the initial glomerular filtrate is_____________________.
   a. Fractional clearance
   b. GFR
   c. Renal clearance
   d. Renal plasma flow
117. Which of the following is best measured to diagnose uroabdomen?
   a. Protein
   b. BUN
   c. Creatinine
   d. Sodium
118. What is the most accurate method to detect pH?
   a. pH meter
   b. Dipstick technique
   c. Litmus paper
   d. Refractometer
119. If the urine is collected after a meal, which of the following is most likely to occur?
   a. Bacteriuria
   b. Crystalluria
   c. Post prandial acid tide
   d. Post prandial alkaline tide
120. Which of the following crystals is not formed in alkaline urine?
   a. Calcium carbonate
   b Amorphous phosphate
   c. Amorphous urate
   d. Struvite
121. Strenuous exercise is most likely because which of the following?
   a. Hyaline cast
   b. Waxy cast
   c. Granular cast
   d. Fatty cast

122. *In vivo* iatrogenic crystalluria is not caused by which of the following?

 a. Prolonged storage of urine b. Sulfamethoxazole administration

 c. Radiocontrast media d. Allopurinol

123. The following serves as countercurrent multiplier and countercurrent exchanger, respectively

 a. Loop of Henle and PCT b. Loop of Henle and capillaries

 c. PCT and DCT d. DCT and collecting duct

124. Which of the following is a pathologic cause of polyuria and not a non-pathogenic cause?

 a. Increased water consumption b. Administration of parenteral fluids

 c. Intake of excess salty foods d. Pyometra

125. _____is the normal urine output of an adult healthy dog.

 a. 10-11 ml/kg/hr b. 5-6 ml/kg/hr

 c. 1-2 ml/kg/hr d. 0.25-0.5 ml/kg/hr

Answer Key

1	d	2	b	3	b	4	d	5	a	6	b	7	a
8	d	9	c	10	a	11	c	12	b	13	c	14	a
15	b	16	d	17	a	18	d	19	a	20	a	21	c
22	d	23	b	24	d	25	d	26	c	27	a	28	d
29	d	30	b	31	d	32	a	33	c	34	c	35	c
36	b	37	b	38	a	39	d	40	d	41	d	42	d
43	c	44	a	45	d	46	a	47	a	48	b	49	c
50	c	51	b	52	a	53	b	54	c	55	c	56	c
57	d	58	a	59	a	60	c	61	c	62	b	63	d
64	b	65	c	66	c	67	a	68	d	69	c	70	b
71	c	72	d	73	b	74	d	75	c	76	d	77	a
78	b	79	b	80	a	81	b	82	c	83	c	84	b
85	a	86	a	87	d	88	c	89	d	90	a	91	c
92	c	93	c	94	a	95	a	96	a	97	b	98	a
99	b	100	a	101	b	102	d	103	d	104	d	105	d
106	c	107	d	108	b	109	b	110	d	111	b	112	a
113	a	114	d	115	d	116	a	117	c	118	a	119	c
120	c	121	a	122	a	123	b	124	d	125	c		

References

1. Clinical Biochemistry of Domestic Animals, 6th Edition, Academic Press. Jiro Jerry Kaneko, John W. Harvey and Michael L. Bruss, 2008.
2. Outline of Veterinary Clinical Pathology, 6th edition, Kalyani Publishers, Maxine M. Benjamin, 2013.
3. Veterinary Clinical Pathology Secrets, Elsevier Inc. Rick L. Cowell, 2004.

30

Quantitative Estimation

Rahil Razzak Bhat and Syed Ashaq Hussain

Faculty of Veterinary Sciences and Animal Husbandry, Sher-e-Kashmir University of Agricultural Sciences and technology of Kashmir-190 006, Jammu and Kashmir

Introduction

Biochemistry is branch of life science which deals with the study of chemical reactions occurring in the living cells and organisms. The term biochemistry was first introduced by German chemist Carl Neuberg in 1903. Since biochemistry is associated with the biological reactions and energy changes associated with these reactions or transformations within the living cell, biochemistry may thus be treated as a discipline in which biological phenomenon are analysed in terms of chemistry. The branch of biochemistry for the same reason has been variously named as "Biological Chemistry" or "Chemical Biology". Modern biochemistry has two branches descriptive and dynamic biochemistry. Descriptive biochemistry deals with qualitative and quantitative characterization of the various chemical components of cell and the dynamic biochemistry deals with the elucidation of the nature and the mechanism of reactions involving these chemical cell components.

Qualitative analysis of biological sample deals with the examination of the organic or inorganic cell associated components in order to determine its composition. It denotes the presence of various biomolecules, elements or groups of elements that are present in the sampling population. It is possible to determine whether a particular component is present or absent in a sample by performing a qualitative analysis of the sample. Qualitative analysis is the identification of elements, species and/or compounds present in a sample.

Quantitative analysis in biochemistry is a branch of life science that is concerned with the amounts of different cell associated organic and inorganic components present in a biological sample obtained from living organism. The quantity can be expressed as a mass, a volume, a concentration, a relative abundance, or any combination of these. A variety of **chemical methods** like chemical reactions (oxidation, reduction, precipitation, and neutralisation), titration procedures, gravimetric procedures and combustion analysis procedures and **physical methods** like spectroscopy- AES (Atomic emission spectroscopy), x-ray fluorescence spectroscopy, and mass spectroscopy) are employed in the process of quantitative analysis.Most of the time, qualitative and quantitative analytical techniques are used in conjunction with one another (Ex: use qualitative analysis followed by quantitative analysis).

In many diseases, health abnormality is reflected changes in the composition of tissues or biological fluids like blood, CSF or urine from normal. Such changes if measured quantitatively can be used in diagnostic and prognostic purposes. By normal value, it is meant the amount of a particular constituent present in the body fluids or tissue of clinically healthy individuals. The normal value is affected by a number of factors such as age, sex, type of the individual, genetic make-up etc. Hence we usually use the term **normal ranges or reference ranges.** These investigations or biochemical assays which help to reach at a clinical diagnosis constitute what is meant by **clinical chemistry.** Usually the samples used for routine analysis in a disease are blood, urine, CSF, pleural and peritoneal fluidcareful attention is needed in all stages of investigation from the collection of samples to the estimation of constituents to avoid false results. Interpretation of results requires information regarding complaints, management and the conditions under which samples are collected and the method of assay. Quantitative analysis gives an exact amount of the substance present in the sample unlike qualitative tests which only give information of the presence or absence of a compound in the given sample. Semi-quantitative tests (e.g. Benedict's test, Heat coagulation test) on the other hand give an idea or approximation on the range of substance present in the sample, like glucose in urine present between 0.5 – 1.0 gm/100 ml in Benedict's test.

Quantification of components in body fluids are measured as their ratio. The precise expression of this can be achieved via concentration units. In liquid-state solutions, it is usually a certain quantity of the solution to which the quantiti(es) of its component(s) are compared, depending on the concentration unit. For instance, in the case of molar concentration (molarity, M, mol/dm^3 or mol/L), the most widely used concentration unit in biochemistry, we refer to the number of moles of a given substance in one litre of solution. (For instance, 0.2 M means 0.2 moles of a substance in one litre of solution.) Various percentage forms (%, reference to 100 units of something) are also widely used in biochemistry, although they are not SI units. In the case of weight-by-volume and volume-by-volume percentages (w/v% and v/v%, respectively) we refer to 100 mL of solution, whereas in the case of weight by-weight percentage (w/w%) we refer to 100 g of solution. In the case of v/v% the volume of the solute, while in the case of w/v% and w/w% the weight of the solute is the basis of reference. (For example, a 15 w/v% solution contains 15 g of solute in 100 mL of solution.). During conversions from or into w/v%, one must also consider the density of the solution (unless it is one g/mL). The density of dilute solutions (up to several %) generally deviates only negligibly from that of the solvent. Therefore, the w/w% and w/v% values of such solutions are practically identical (i.e. 3 w/v% corresponds to c. a. 3 w/w %). It is important to note that, for practical reasons, the "biochemical" concentration units mg/mL and µg/mL are also used in the case of protein and other macromolecular solutions.

Vocabulary

Analysis: the procedural steps performed to determine the kind or amount of analyte in a specimen.

Analyte: Compound that is measured.

Bias: Difference between the average (strictly the expectation) of the test results and an accepted reference value

Matrix All components of a material system except the analyte.

Measurand: The "quantity" that is actually measured (e.g., the concentration of the analyte). For example, if the analyte is glucose, the measurand is the concentration of glucose. For an enzyme, the measurand may be the enzyme activity or the mass concentration of enzyme.

Reference material (RM): A material or substance, one or more properties of which are sufficiently well established to be used for the calibration of a method or for assigning values to materials.

Test: in a clinical laboratory, a test is a qualitative, semiqualitative, quantitative or semiquantitative procedure for detecting the presence or measuring the quantity of an analyte in a biological sample.

1. Which of the following is said to be spectral
   a. Colour b. Voltage changes
   c. Elasticity d. Phosphorescence
2. Which of the following could be said to be a quantitative result?
   a. The test is positive
   b. The sample contains more than 5g of glucose
   c. The sample contain 0.3g of glucose
   d. The sample contains both glucose and lactose.
3 Which of the following is the qualitative method?
   a. Colorimetry b. Calorimetry
   c. Weighing d. Mass spectrophotometry
4. Which of the following are acceptable SI units?
   a. g/100mL b. mol sec^{-1}
   c. KgL^{-1} d. Both b & c
5. Which of the following concentration expression terms is least used now a days
   a. Molarity b. Normality
   c. Formality d. ppm.
6. A_______solution contains 1 gm mol. wt. (mole) of solute in one litre of solution.
   a. Molar b. Molal
   c. Normal d. Formal.
7. Molarity of a solution of 2 litres containing 58.5 gm. NaCl dissolved
   a. 0.01 b. 0.1
   c. 1 d. 10
8. A 10% W/W solution contains
   a. 10 gm of solute in 90 gm of solvent
   b. 10 gm of solute in 100 gm of solution
   c. 10 gm of solute in 100gm of solvent
   d. Both a & b
9 A 10% V/V solution contains
   a. 10 ml of the concentrate per 100 ml of solution
   b. 10 ml of the concentrate per 90 ml of solution
   c. 10 ml of the concentrate per 1000 ml of solution
   d. 10 ml of the concentrate per 10 ml of solution

10. A 10% W/V solution contains
    a. 10 gm of solute dissolved in final volume of 100 ml of solution
    b. 10 gm of solute dissolved in final volume of 1000 ml of solution
    c. 10 gm of solute dissolved in final volume of 10 ml of solution
    d. 10 gm of solute dissolved in final volume of 100 ml of solvent
11. A normal solution contains 1 gm equivalent Wt. (eq.) of solute dissolved in
    a. One litre of solution. b. One litre of solvent.
    c. 100mL of solution. d. 100 gm of solution.
12. Normality of a solution of 2 litres containing 180 gm of glucose.
    a. 0.1N b. 0.00N1
    c. 0.5N d. 0.005N
13. Unlike normality and molarity, the following parameter of expressing the concentration is independent of temperature
    a. Formality b. Ppm
    c. Molality d. W/V percentage
14. The pH range of Methyl yellow (Topfer's reagent) indicator is
    a. 2.9 - 4.0 b. 5.9 - 7.0
    c. 7.1 - 12.0 d. 7.0 - 14.0
15. Gillespie's drop method is used to
    a. Determine buffer capacity of biological fluids
    b. Determine the pH of solutions
    c. Determine the molarity of biomolecules in blood
    d. All of the above.
16. The general test for detection of carbohydrates is
    a. Iodine test b. Molisch test
    c. barfoed test d. Osazone test
17. The purple ring of Molisch reaction is due to
    a. Furfural b. Furfural + α-Naphthol
    c. α-Naphthol d. Furfural + α-Naphthol + H_2SO_4
18. Choose the correct option given below
    a. Quantitative analysis gives an exact amount of the substance present in the sample
    b. Qualitative tests which only give information of the presence or absence of a compound in the given sample
    c. Semi-quantitative tests give an idea or approximation on the range of substance present in the sample.
    d. All of the above
19. Colour code for the vacutainer required for the determination of ammonia from blood
    a. Red b. Yellow
    c. Green d. Purple

20. The anticoagulant used in purple coloured vacutainer for haematology study is
    a. K3 EDTA
    b. Heparin
    c. Sodium lithium
    d. Sodium citrate.
21. The analytical results of the biochemical tests are subjected to various types of errors which may be either:
    a. Random error
    b. Systemic error
    c. Gross error
    d. All of the above.
22. Random error can be assessed
    a Empirically
    b Statistically
    c Experimentally
    d By performing sensitivity analysis.
23. The error which occurs if the checking of an instrument is not correctly aligned with the direction of desired measurement is called:
    a. Characteristic error
    b. Alignment error
    c. Environmental error
    d. Reading error
24. Errors that occur due to carelessness of operator is called
    a. Random
    b. Observational
    c. Environmental
    d. Instrumental
25. The errors that are due to conditions external to measuring device
    a. Random
    b. Observational
    c. Instrumental
    d. Environmental
26. According to the International Organization for Standardization (ISO) 15189:2012,the phase of biochemical testing which involves the collection of specimen/sample, transport and processing is known as
    a. Analytical
    b. Preanalytical
    c. Post analytical
    d. Microanalytical
27. Results transmission, interpretation, follow up and retesting are performed under
    a. Preanalytical phase
    b. Postanalytical phase
    c. Analytical phase
    d. Microanalytical phase
28. Technique that is used to detect & correct errors before they result in a defectiveproduct or service
    a. Measuring analysis
    b. Transferring the staff
    c. Quality control
    d. Strengthening the financial status of laboratory
29. ____________indicates how close test measurements to each other when the same test is run on the same sample repeatedly.
    a. Quality of test
    b. Accuracy
    c. Precision
    d. Sensitivity

30. Substance of constant composition of sufficient purity to be used for comparison purpose.
    a. Analytical reagen
    b. Molecular reagent
    c. Standard
    d. Sample
31. ____________is a sample i.e. chemically & physically similar to the unknown specimen.
    a. Primary standard
    b. Control
    c. Reagent and distilled water
    d. Secondary standard.
32. Intrinsic errors that are due to an imprecise & inaccurate methods can be eliminated by
    a. Selecting precise & accurate method only
    b. by using fresh batches of reagents
    c. Both of these
    d. None of the these
33. Systemic errors in the biochemistry laboratory can be eliminated by
    a. Using different concentration of primary standard
    b. Analyzing control serum
    c. Both of these
    d. All of these
34. Multi control QC rules on laboratory quality control was given by
    a. Robert Boyer
    b. Neil Bohr
    c. Leiberg
    d. James Westgard
35. Which of the following is not included in post analytical error
    a. Incorrect calculation
    b. Unit of measurement
    c. Delay in delivering the result
    d. Wrong labelling of containers
36. The aim of QC is to evaluate the errors in prenalytical, analytical and postanalytical phase
    a. Before test results are reported
    b. After test results are reported
    c. While analysis is carried out in machine
    d. After interpretation of results
37. Which of the following statement below is incorrect
    a. Laboratory investigations are one of the major contributors to most clinical decisions and one of the indispensible tool in the modern healthcare
    b. Quality control is one of the components of quality assurance which is a statistical way to monitor and evaluate the analytical process
    c. While reporting results, laboratories should have well-established reference ranges based on physiological parameters such as age, the period of gestation, gender
    d. Reliability of the results is independent on evaluationand implementation of analytical methods for investigations.

38. Choose the correct statement below:
    a. Internal quality control is run everyday or every time the test is performed
    b. Internal quality control checks the correct execution of the procedure
    c. External quality control is comparing the performances of different laboratories And is performed once a Month
    d. All of these are correct
39. The purity of an isolated protein can be tested by employing various methods.
    a. Solubility curve
    b. Molecular weight
    c. Ultra Centrifugation
    d. Immuno Reactivity
40. Diphenylamine method is employed in the quantitation of
    a. Nucleic acid
    b. RNA
    c. DNA
    d. Proteins
41. Orcinol method is employed in the quantitation of
    a. Nucleic acid
    b. DNA
    c. RNA
    d. Proteins
42. Document describing in detail, exactly how a measurement is performed to give a valid result is known as
    a. Training log book
    b. Analyser maintenance log book
    c. Standard operating procedures
    d. Calibration log books.
43. ______________of any assay describes its ability to detect only patients with a particular disease process.
    a. Clinical sensitivity
    b. Clinical specificity
    c. Clinical predictive value
    d. Range check
44. ____________________ is defined as the range of values for a clinical test within which 95% of the healthy population fall.
    a. Delta checks
    b. Range checks
    c. Reference range
    d. Absolute precision
45. In 1993 the NHS defined ________________ as 'a quality improvement process that seeks to improve patient care through review of care against explicit criteria and the implementation of change'.
    a. Internal quality control program
    b. External quality control program
    c. Audit
    d. Turnaround time
46. Which of the following is (are) post analytical step(s)?
    a. Centrifugation
    b. Recapping
    c. Sample storage & sample retrieval
    d. Decapping
47. Range of analyte concentrations that can be directly measured without dilution, concentration, or other pre-treatment
    a. Clinically reportable range
    b. Analytic measurement range
    c. Standard deviation index
    d. Limit of quantitation

48. If 6.3 mL of acetone are dissolved in a water solution such that the total volume of solution is 500.0 mL, what is the concentration of the acetone expressed as a volume percent?

a. 0.13% b. 1.3%

c. 0.013% d. 13%

49. What is the weight/volume percent concentration of a solution if 2.48 g of solute are dissolved in 600.0 mL of solution?

a. 0.1 b. 0.2

c. 0.3 d. 0.4

50. What is the molarity of a solution of NaOH that has 0.491 g dissolved in 400.0 mL of solution?

a. 0.001M b. 0.02M

c. 0.03M d. 0.0001M

51. How many milliliters of concentrated HCl (12 M) are needed to prepare 250.0 mL of a 0.15 M solution of HCl?

a. 1.11 b. 2.14

c. 3.12 d. 3.01.

52. For preparation of 100 mL of a 5.0-ppm (parts per million) copper solution from a 1000-ppm copper solution, what quantity of 1000ppm solution is required to prepare desired solution?

a. 0.3 b. 0.4

c. 0.5 d. 0.1.

53. In gel filteration, biomolecules are separated according to:

a. The net charge

b. The difference in molecular weight

c. Ability of diffusion through porous membranes

d. Polarity

54. The following technique is the most suitable for the separation of a mixture of the 20 amino acids

a. Two dimensional electrophoresis b. Gel filtration

c. Affinity chromatography d. Dialysis

55. The following method is used only to detect RNA and can be used to measure the difference in levels of specific mRNA in different tissues:

a. Northern blot analysis

b. Polymerase chain reaction

c. Restriction fragment length polymorphism linkage analysis

d. DNA fingerprint analysis.

56. ELISA
   a. Is a separation technique
   b. Involves use of radioisotopes
   c. Is ideal for quantitative measurements of hormones
   d. Involves change of color in enzymaticreactions

57. Ninhydrin with evolution of CO2 forms a blue complex with
   a. Peptide bond
   b. α-Amino acids
   c. Serotonin
   d. Histamine

58. Sanger's reagent contains
   a. Phenylisothiocyanate
   b. Dansyl chloride
   c. 1-Fluoro-2, 4-dinitrobenzene
   d. Ninhydrin

59. The useful reagent for detection of amino acids is
   a. Molisch reagent
   b. Dichlorophenol Indophenol
   c. Ninhydrin
   d. Biuret

60. The amino acid which gives yellow colour with Ninhydrin in paper chromatography is
   a. Tyrosine
   b. Proline
   c. Tryptophan
   d. Alanine

61. Which of the followings gives a positive test for Ninhydrin
   a. Reducing sugars
   b. Triglycerides
   c. Alpha aminoacids
   d. Esterified Fats.

62. Ninhydrin reaction gives a purple colour and evolves CO_2 with
   a. Peptide bonds
   b. Histamine
   c. Ergothioneine
   d. Aspargine

63. N-terminal amino acids of a polypeptide are estimated by
   a. Edmann reaction
   b. Sanger's reagent
   c. Formaldehyde test
   d. Ninhydrin reaction

64. Primary structure of proteins can be determined by the use of
   a. Electrophoresis
   b. Chromatography
   c. Ninhydrin
   d. Sanger's reagent

65. Which of the following is used as an indicator in the titration of a strong acid and a weak base?
   a. Methyl orange
   b. Phenolphthalein
   c. Thymol blue
   d. Fluorescein

66. The ideal indicator for the titration of strong acid and weak base should have a pH range between ________
   a. 3-5
   b. 4-6
   c. 6-8
   d. 7-9

67. Find the concentration of HCl, if 10 ml of 0.5 M Ca(OH)2 is required to titrate 50 ml of HCl.

a. 1/10M b. 1/5M

c. 5M d. 10M

68. What is the concentration of the sulphuric acid solution, if 100 ml of the solution is neutralised by 50 ml of 0.5 M Ba(OH)2 solution?

a. 0.25M b. 50M

c. 1/10m d. 0.5m

69. If 30 ml of acid is neutralised by 15 ml of 0.2 N alkali, then the concentration of acid is ______.

a. 0.1N b. 0.2N

c. 0.3N d. 0.4N

70. Which of the following is used as an indicator in the titration of a weak acid and a strong base?

a. Methyl orange (3 to 4.6) b. Bromothymol blue (6 to 7.5)

c. Phenolphthalein (8 to 9.6) d. Methyl red (5 to 6.9)

71. What is the molarity of the solution of barium hydroxide, if 35 ml of 0.1 M HCl is used in the titration of 25 ml of the barium hydroxide solution?

a. 0.28 b. 0.21

c. 0.70 d. 0.07

72. Which of the following titrations will have the equivalence point at a pH more than 8?

a. CH_3COOH and NaOH b. HCl and NaOH

c. CH_3COOH and NH_3 d. HCl and NH_3

73. The titre is the ____________ of liquid delivered by the burette during a titration

a. Volume b. Mass

c. Mole d. Concentration

74. The process of adding known concentration until it complete thereaction with known volume is called as

a. Titrant b. Analyte

c. Titration d. Titrend

75. Exactly required concentration can be prepared from chemical reagent is called as

a. Primary standard b. Secondary standard

c. Both d. None of the above

76. Normality of an acid is

a. Molarity ×acidity b. Molarity ×basicity

c. Molality ×acidity d. Molality × basicity

77. A positive Seliwanoff's test is obtained with

a. Glucose b. Fructose

c. Lactose d. Maltose

78. ADH test is based on the measurement of
   a. Specific gravity of urine
   b. Concentration of urea in urine
   c. Concentration of urea in blood
   d. Volume of urine in ml/minute

79. Addis test is the measure of
   a. Impairment of the capacity of the tubule to perform osmotic work
   b. Secretory function of liver
   c. Excretory function of liver
   d. Activity of parenchymal cells of liver.

80. Specific test for ketohexoses:
   a. Seliwanoff's test
   b. Osazone test
   c. Molisch test
   d. None of these

81. In Thymol turbidity test the protein involved is mainly
   a. Albumin
   b. α1-Globulin
   c. α2-Globulin
   d. β-Globulin

82. Millon's test is for identification of
   a. Tyrosine
   b. Tryptophan
   c. Proline
   d. Arginine

83. Hopkins-Cole test is for identification of
   a. Tyrosine
   b. Tryptophan
   c. Arginine
   d. Cysteine

84. In Nitroprusside test, amino acid cysteine produces
   a. Blue colour complex
   b. Red colour
   c. Yellow colour
   d. Purple colour

85. Group that reacts in the Biuret test
   a. Peptide
   b. Amino group
   c. Carboxylic group
   d. Aldehyde group

86. The purity of an isolated protein can be tested by employing various methods.
   a. Solubility curve
   b. Molecular weight
   c. Ultra Centrifugation
   d. ImmunoRactivity

87. Xanthoproteic test is positive in proteins containing
   a. Sulphur amino acids
   b. α-Amino acids
   c. Aromatic amino acids
   d. Aliphatic amino acids

88. Guanidine group of argentine gives positive test with
   a. Lead acetate
   b. Sakaguchi reagent
   c. Tricholoroacetic acid
   d. Molisch's reagent

89. Biuret test is specific for
   a. Two peptide linkage
   b. Phenolic group
   c. Imidazole ring
   d. None of these

90. Salkowski test is performed to detect
   a. Glycerol b. Cholesterol
   c. Fatty acids d. Vitamin D
91. Impaired galactose tolerance test suggests
   a. Defect in glucose utilisation b. Liver cell injury
   c. Renal defect d. Muscle injury
92. The best known and most frequently used test of the detoxicating functions of liver is
   a. Hippuric acid test b. Galactose tolerance test
   c. Epinephrine tolerance test d. Rose Bengal dye test
93. Urea clearance test is used to determine the
   a. Glomerular filtration rate
   b. Renal plasma flow
   c. Ability of kidney to concentrate the urine
   d. Measurement of tubular mass
94. Average maximum urea clearance is
   a. 30mL b. 50mL
   c. 75mL d. 90mL
95. Glomerular filtration rate can be measured by
   a. Endogenous creatinine clearance b. Para-aminohippurate test
   c. Addis test d. Mosenthal test
96. The normal values for creatinine clearance varies from
   a. 20–40 mL/min b. 40-60mL/min
   c. 70-85mL/min d. 90-105ml/min
97. Creatinine EDTA clearance is a test to measure
   a. Renal plasma flow b. Filtration fraction
   c. Glomerular filtration rate d. Tubular function
98. Phenolsulphonephthalein excretion test is an indicator of
   a. Glomerular filtration b. Tubular secretion
   c. Tubular reabsorption d. Renal blood low
99. Para-amino hippurate excretion test is an indicator of
   a. Glomerular filtration b. Tubular secretion
   c. Tubular reabsorption d. Renal plasma flow
100. Among the following, a test of Glomerular function is
   a. Urea clearance b. PSP excretion test
   c. PAH clearance d. Hippuric acid excretion test
101. The number of milliliters of 0.1 N KOH required to neutralize the insoluble fatty acids from 5 gms of fat is called
   a. Acid number b. Acetyl number
   c. Halogenation d. Polenske number

102. Acrolein Test is positive for

a. Glycerol
b. Prostaglandins
c. Carbohydrates
d. Proteins

103. Pyridoxine deficiency can be diagnosed by measuring the urinary excretion of xanthurenic acid following a test dose of

a. Glycine
b. Histidine
c. Tryptophan
d. Pyridoxine

104. deficiency of vitamin B_{12} can be diagonised by

a. Carr-Price reaction
b. Ames assay
c. Watson-Schwartz test
d. Schilling test

105. An early diagnosis of vitamin C deficiency can be made by

a. Measuring plasma ascorbic acid
b. Measuring urinary ascorbic acid
c. Ascorbic acid saturation test
d. All of these

106. The most useful test for the diagnosis of acute hemorrhagic pancreatitis during the first few days is

a. Urinary lipase test
b. Serum calcium
c. Urinary amylase
d. Serum amylase

107. The best test for acute pancreatitis in the presence of mumps is

a. A serological test for mumps
b. Serum amylase
c. Urinary amylase
d. Serum lipase

108. If results of the serum bilirubin, serum ALP, LDH and AST determinations suggest obstructive jaundice, the best confirmatory test would be the estimation of

a. Serum ALT
b. Serum 5' nucleotidase
c. Serum Pseudo cholinesterase
d. None of these

109. 5 HIAA test is negative if patient is taking

a. Aspirin
b. Colchicine
c. Phenothiazone
d. Methotrexate

110. Radioactive iodine uptake by thyroid gland 24 hours of a test dose is

a. 1.5–15% of the test dose
b. 15–20% of the test dose
c. 20–40% of the test dose
d. 50–70% of the test dose

111. What is the actual weight of a supply of concentrated HCl whose label reads specific gravity 1.19 with an assay value of 37%?

a. 0.44g/mL of HCl
b. 0.55g/mL of HCl
c. 0.34g/mL of HCl
d. 1.44g/mL of HCl

112. What is the dilution factor needed to make a 100 mmol/L sodium solution from a 3,000mmol/L stock solution?

a. 1:30 (1 part of stock and 29 parts of diluent)
b. 1:40 (1 part of stock and 39 parts of diluent)
c. 3: 17 (3 parts of stock and 14 parts of diluent)
d. 3: 19 (3 parts of stock and 16 parts of diluent)

113. The ΔA per minute for an enzyme reaction is 0.250. The product measured has a molar absorptivity of 12.2×10^3 at 425 nm at 30°c. The incubation and reaction temperature are also kept at 30°c. The assay calls for 1 mL of reagent and 0.050 mL of sample. What is the enzyme activity results in international units:

a. 420 U
b. 425 U
c. 430 U
d. 330 U

114. The biuret protein assay is very stable and follows Beer's law. Rather than make up a completely new standard graph, one standard (6 g/dL) was assayed. The absorbance of the standard was 0.400, and the absorbance of the unknown was 0.350. The concentration of the unknown in g/dL is :

a. 5.45
b. 5.25
c. 4.44
d. 4.54

115. When selecting quality control reagents for measuring an analyte in urine, the medical technologist should select:

a. Quality control reagent prepared in a urine matrix.
b. Quality control reagent prepared in a serum matrix.
c. Quality control reagent prepared in deionized water.
d. The matrix does not matter; any quality control reagent as long as the analyte of measure is chemically pure.

116. A patient's serum sample was placed on the chemistry analyzer and the output indicated 'out of range' for the measurement of creatine kinase (CK) anzyme. A dilution of the patient serum was required. Which of the following should be used to prepare a dilution of patient serum?

a. Deionized water
b. Tap water
c. Another patient's serum with confirmed, low levels of CK
d. Type I water

117. Which of the following containers is calibrated to hold only one exact volume of liquid?

a. Volumetric flask
b. Erlenmeyer flask
c. Griffin beaker
d. Graduated cylinder

118. Which of the following errors is NOT considered a preanalytical error?

a. during a phlebotomy procedure, the patient is opening and clenching his fist multiple times.
b. The blood was not permitted to clot and spun in a centrifuge after 6 minutes of collection.
c. The patient was improperly identified leading to a mislabelled blood sample.
d. The serum sample was diluted with tap water.

119. Using the Henderson-Hasselbalch equation, give the ratio of salt to weak acid for a Veronal buffer with a pH of 8.6 and a pKa of 7.43.

a. 14.7/1
b. 1/8.6
c. 1.17/1
d. 1/4.3

120. The pKa for acetic acid is 4.76. If the concentration of salt is 5 mmol/L and that of acetic acid is 10 mmol/L, what is the expected pH?

a. 4.4
b. 6.1
c. 104
d. 56

121. If two methods agree perfectly in a method comparison study, the slope equals and the y-intercept equals.

a. 1.0, 0.0
b. 0.0, 1.0
c. 1.0, 1.0
d. 0.0, 0.0.

122. For a data value set that is Gaussian distributed, what is the likelihood (%) that a data point +1 or -1 SD from the mean?

a. 68%
b. 99%
c. 95%
d. 100%

123. The pipette is designed to drain by:

a. Tapping it against the container
b. Gravity
c. Forcing air into the opening
d. Rapidly moving it up & down.

124. Which of the following calibration devices is used to verify the accuracy of laboratory thermometers?

a. Refractometer
b. Tachometer
c. SRM 1968 gallium melting-point cell
d. Holnium oxide filter

125. Which of the following techniques has the highest potential sensitivity?

a. Chemiluminescence
b. Fluorescence
c. Turbidimetry
d. Nephelometry.

126. Which of the following procedures is not currently or routinely used for point-of-care testing devices?

a. Polymerase chain reaction
b. Immunochromatography
c. Biosensors
d. Colorimetric detection

127. In which of the following components of a chromatography instrument does selective separation of a mixture occur?

a. Sample injection port
b. Column
c. Spectrometer
d. Quadrupole.

128. Mass spectrometry identifies analytes based on:

a. Mass to charge ratio
b. Retention factor
c. Density of the band
d. Molecular weight

129. Which of the following is NOT a driving force for more automation?

a. Increased use of chemistry panels
b. High-volume testing
c. Fast turnaround time
d. Expectation of high-quality, accurate results

130. Which of the following types of analyzers offers random-access capabilities?

a. Discrete analyzers
b. Continuous-flow analyzers
c. Centrifugal analyzers
d. None of these

131. All of the following are primary considerations in the selection of an automated chemistry analyzer EXCEPT
   a. How reagents are added or mixed
   b. The cost of consumables
   c. Total instrument cost
   d. The labor component

132. Isoelectric focusing is the type of electrophoresis used to phenotype for α1-antitrypsin deficiencies. When the protein iselectrophoresed, it migrates to:
   a. The site where the pH is the same as its pI.
   b. The site where the molecular weight of the protein correlates with the pI.
   c. The site where the protein's net charge exceeds the pI.
   d. The site where the protein's net charge is less than the pI. e. The site where the gel pore size inhibits further migration.

133. An urea N result of 9 mg/dL is obtained by a technologist. What is the urea concentration?
   a. 3.2 mg/dL
   b. 4.2 mg/dL
   c. 18.0 mg/dL
   d. 19.3 mg/dL

134. Enzyme reaction rates are increased by increasing temperatures until they reach the point of denaturation at
   a. 40-60°C
   b. 25-35°C
   c. 100°C
   d. 37°C

135. The sample of choice for measuring blood osmolality is:
   a. Serum
   b. Plasma
   c. Whole blood
   d. Serum or plasma may both be used

136. The anticoagulant of choice for arterial blood gas measurements is in the state.
   a. Lithium heparin; dry
   b. EDTA; dry
   c. Potassium oxalate; liquid
   d. Sodium citrate; dry

137. Measuring serum ammonia levels has the potential to be fraught with preanalytical errors that may interfere with achieving an accurate result. Of the following preanalytical steps, which is incorrect?
   a. After phlebotomy, the patient's blood should be immediately placed on ice.
   b. The blood should be collected in a red clot tube without anticoagulant.
   c. Hemolyzed samples should be rejected as this interferes by falsely increasing ammonia levels.
   d. Lipemia may also interfere with plasma ammonia measurements.

138. Calculate creatinine clearance, given the following information: serum creatinine, 1.2 mg/dL; urine creatinine, 120 mg/dL; urine volume, 1750 mL/24h; body surface area, 1.80 m^2.
   a. 117mL/min
   b. 119mL/min
   c. 117L/min
   d. 1.17 μL/hr

139. Which of the following is not considered a recognized discipline in laboratory medicine?
   a. Immunology
   b. Physiology
   c. Microbiology
   d. Hematology
   e. Clinical chemistry
140. Which of the following is not an important driver in transforming laboratory data to information and knowledge?
   a. Application of evidence-based medicine
   b. Application of information management technology
   c. Data mining
   d. Technology-driven laboratory medicine
141. Which of the following analytes would be most affected for arterialized capillary blood sample if the site is not appropriately warmed?
   a. pH
   b. PCO_2
   c. PO_2
   d. PO2 and PCO_2
142. Which of the following analytes does not exhibit a difference in composition between heparin plasma and serum?
   a. Cholesterol
   b. Total protein
   c. Glucose
   d. Lactate dehydrogenase
   e. Potassium
143. Which of the following analytes exhibits the greatest difference in composition between capillary and venous serum?
   a. Phosphate
   b. Urea
   c. Glucose
   d. Potassium
   e. calcium
144. Identify the correct order of tubes in which blood should be collected for multiple specimens:
   a. Yellow (no additive), Gold/ red (serum), Green (heparin), Lavender (EDTA), Gray (Sodium fluoride)
   b. Gold/ red (serum), Yellow (no additive), Green (heparin), Lavender (EDTA), Gray (Sodium fluoride)
   c. Gray (Sodium fluoride), Lavender (EDTA), Green (heparin), Gold/ red (serum), Yellow (no additive)
   d. Yellow (no additive), Gold/ red (serum), Green (heparin), Gray (Sodium fluoride), Lavender (EDTA)
   e. Green (heparin), Yellow (no additive), Gold/ red (serum), Gray (Sodium fluoride), Lavender (EDTA)
145. What is the concentration of nicotinamide adenine dinucleotide (NADH) in a solution if the absorbance at 340nm in a 1-cm cuvette is 0.1? Use the NADH molar absorptivity 6220 L$\times$ mol^{-1} $\times$cm^{-1}.
   a. 1.6 μM
   b. 16μM
   c. 6.2μM
   d. 62μM

146. Which of the following techniques is used to determine total protein concentration?
    a. Jaffe Method
    b. Watson-Schwartz Method
    c. Jendrassik-Grof Method
    d. Biuret Method
147. Which of the following best describes appropriate use for most serum tumor marker measurements?
    a. Diagnosing or excluding a diagnosis of malignancy
    b. Providing definitive information about likely prognosis in individual patients
    c. Monitoring treatment effectiveness and the course of disease
    d. Identifying the primary cancer by testing panels of serum tumor markers
148. The distribution of laboratory data from healthy individuals is often
    a. Gaussian
    b. Skewed to the right
    c. Wider than Gaussian
    d. Bimodal
149. In a patient whose calcium is significantly below thelower reference limit, which of the following tests wouldbe expected to be outside conventional reference limits?
    a. Alanine aminotransferase
    b. Bilirubin
    c. Parathyroid hormone
    d. Cortisol
150. Which of the following would most likely be used asan exclusion criterion for a reference interval study forserum iron?
    a. Age
    b. Ethnicity
    c. Body mass index
    d. Recent transfusion

Answer Key

1	a	2	c	3	c	4	d	5	d	6	a	7	c
8	d	9	a	10	a	11	a	12	c	13	c	14	a
15	b	16	b	17	b	18	d	19	c	20	a	21	d
22	b	23	b	24	b	25	d	26	b	27	b	28	c
29	c	30	c	31	b	32	c	33	c	34	d	35	d
36	a	37	d	38	d	39	c	40	c	41	c	42	c
43	a	44	c	45	c	46	c	47	b	48	b	49	d
50	c	51	c	52	c	53	b	54	a	55	a	56	c
57	b	58	c	59	c	60	b	61	c	62	d	63	a
64	d	65	a	66	b	67	b	68	a	69	a	70	a
71	d	72	a	73	d	74	c	75	a	76	a	77	b
78	a	79	a	80	a	81	d	82	a	83	b	84	b
85	a	86	a	87	c	88	b	89	a	90	b	91	b
92	a	93	a	94	c	95	a	96	a	97	c	98	d
99	d	100	d	101	d	102	a	103	c	104	d	105	c
106	d	107	d	108	b	109	c	110	c	111	a	112	a
113	c	114	b	115	d	116	d	117	a	118	d	119	a
120	a	121	a	122	a	123	d	124	c	125	a	126	a
127	b	128	a	129	a	130	a	131	a	132	a	133	d
134	a	135	a	136	a	137	b	138	a	139	b	140	d
141	c	142	a	143	c	144	a	145	b	146	a	147	c
148	b	149	c	150	d								

31

Colorimetry

Rahil Razzak Bhat and Syed Ashaq Hussain

Faculty of Veterinary Sciences and Animal Husbandry, Sher-e-Kashmir University of Agricultural Sciences and technology of Kashmir 190 006, Jammu and Kashmir

Introduction

Colorimetry is a scientific technique widely used across various fields to quantify the concentration of substances based on their color intensity. Colorimetry is a branch of analytical chemistry that focuses on measuring the absorbance or transmission of light by colored solutions. It utilizes the principles of optics and spectroscopy to determine the concentration of a substance in a solution based on its color intensity. This technique relies on the Beer-Lambert law, which states that the absorbance of light by a solution is directly proportional to its concentration and path length.

Principles of Colorimetry

The fundamental principle of colorimetry lies in the interaction of light with matter. When light passes through or is reflected off a substance, certain wavelengths are absorbed, while others are transmitted or reflected. The color we perceive is due to the wavelengths of light that are reflected back to our eyes. In colorimetry, a photometric measurement is made using a colorimeter or spectrophotometer, which quantifies the intensity of light absorbed or transmitted by a sample.

Colorimeter and its Components

A colorimeter is a device that helps specific solutions to absorb a particular wavelength of light. The colorimeter is usually used to measure the concentration of a known solute in a given solution. The colorimeter was invented in the year 1870 by Louis J Duboscq. A colorimeter typically consists of a light source, filters or monochromators to select specific wavelengths, a sample holder or cuvette, and a detector (photodetector or photocell). The light source emits a specific wavelength of light, which passes through the sample. The detector measures the amount of light absorbed or transmitted, which is then converted into a numerical value that correlates with the concentration of the substance being analyzed.

Applications of Colorimetry

1. **Environmental Analysis:** Colorimetry is extensively used in environmental monitoring to measure pollutants such as heavy metals, organic compounds, and nutrients in water and soil samples. For example, the determination of nitrate levels in groundwater using colorimetric assays helps assess water quality and potential environmental impact.

2. **Clinical Diagnostics:** In clinical settings, colorimetry plays a crucial role in diagnostic tests to detect biomarkers, enzymes, hormones, and metabolites in biological fluids like blood, urine, and other body fluids. It enables rapid and quantitative analysis, aiding in disease diagnosis, monitoring of treatment efficacy, and patient health management.
3. **Food and Beverage Industry:** Quality control in the food and beverage industry relies on colorimetry to analyze components such as sugars, proteins, fats, vitamins, and additives. This ensures compliance with regulatory standards, maintains product consistency, and verifies nutritional content labels.
4. **Pharmaceutical Analysis:** Pharmaceutical laboratories use colorimetry for drug development, formulation analysis, and quality control. It assists in determining the concentration of active ingredients, assessing stability, and detecting impurities in drug formulations.
5. **Education and Research:** Colorimetry is an essential tool in educational laboratories for teaching principles of spectroscopy, light absorption, and quantitative analysis. In research, it facilitates studies on chemical reactions, kinetics, and molecular interactions by providing precise measurements of concentration changes over time.

Advancements in Colorimetry

1. **Nanotechnology Integration:** Recent advancements in colorimetry involve integrating nanomaterials such as gold nanoparticles or quantum dots (QDs) into assays. These nanostructures enhance sensitivity, enable multiplexed detection, and offer rapid analysis capabilities for point-of-care diagnostics and field testing.
2. **Smartphone-Based Colorimetry:** The development of smartphone-based colorimetric assays has democratized access to analytical testing. Mobile apps coupled with inexpensive attachments or integrated sensors allow users to perform quantitative analyses remotely, making healthcare diagnostics and environmental monitoring more accessible in resource-limited settings.
3. **Machine Learning and Data Analysis:** Machine learning algorithms are being applied to colorimetric data to improve accuracy in complex sample analysis. These techniques automate data interpretation, pattern recognition, and outlier detection, enhancing the reliability and efficiency of colorimetric assays in diverse applications.

Challenges and Future Directions

Despite its versatility, colorimetry faces challenges such as interference from sample matrix effects, limited sensitivity for low-concentration analytes, and the need for standardization across instruments and methodologies. Future research aims to overcome these challenges through advancements in sensor technology, signal amplification strategies, and computational methods for data analysis.

In conclusion, colorimetry is a powerful analytical technique that continues to evolve with technological advancements and interdisciplinary applications. From environmental monitoring to clinical diagnostics and beyond, its ability to provide rapid, quantitative results makes it indispensable in modern scientific research, industry, and education. As innovations in nanotechnology, mobile technology, and data analytics expand its capabilities, colorimetry remains at the forefront of analytical chemistry, driving progress and enabling new discoveries in diverse fields.

1. What is the primary principle behind colorimetry?
   a. Light emission
   b. Light absorption
   c. Light reflection
   d. Light refraction
2. Which law governs the relationship between absorbance, concentration, and path length in colorimetry?
   a. Avogadro's law
   b. Boyle's law
   c. Lambert-Beer law
   d. Newton's law of motion
3. What is the purpose of using a colorimeter or spectrophotometer in colorimetry?
   a. To emit light of specific wavelengths
   b. To measure light absorption or transmission by a sample
   c. To reflect light off a sample
   d. To refract light through a sample
4. Which component of a colorimeter selects specific wavelengths of light for analysis?
   a. Photodetector
   b. Sample holder
   c. Filter or monochromator
   d. Light source
5. What does a higher absorbance value indicate in colorimetry?
   a. Higher sample concentration
   b. Lower sample concentration
   c. No relationship to concentration
   d. Higher light intensity
6. Which factor does not affect the absorbance measurement in colorimetry?
   a. Concentration of the sample
   b. Path length of light through the sample
   c. Temperature of the sample
   d. Color of the light source
7. In colorimetry, what is transmittance?
   a. The ratio of light absorbed by a sample to the incident light intensity
   b. The ratio of light transmitted through a sample to the incident light intensity
   c. The ratio of reflected light from a sample to the incident light intensity
   d. The ratio of refracted light through a sample to the incident light intensity
8. Which colorimetric assay is commonly used to measure blood glucose levels?
   a. Enzyme-linked immunosorbent assay
   b. Hexokinase assay
   c. Bradford assay
   d. PCR assay
9. What is the role of a standard curve in colorimetric analysis?
   a. To calibrate the colorimeter
   b. To measure the intensity of light
   c. To determine the path length
   d. To correlate absorbance values with known concentrations

10. Which parameter is not typically controlled during a colorimetric assay?
    a. Temperature b. pH
    c. Light intensity d. Pressure
11. Which type of light source is commonly used in modern colorimeters?
    a. Incandescent bulb b. Fluorescent tube
    c. Light-emitting diode d. Laser
12. What is the purpose of using a blank sample in colorimetry?
    a. To provide a reference for light intensity
    b. To absorb excess light
    c. To calibrate the instrument
    d. To correct for background absorbance
13. Which substance is commonly used as a reference standard in colorimetric assays?
    a. Potassium dichromate b. Sodium chloride
    c. Potassium permanganate d. Water
14. What is the relationship between absorbance (aand transmittance (T) in colorimetry?
    a. A = log(T) b. A = -log(T)
    c. A = T^2 d. A = T/2
15. Which unit is commonly used to express absorbance in colorimetry?
    a. Joules (J) b. Molar (M)
    c. Tesla (T) d. Absorbance units (AU)
16. What is the purpose of using a cuvette in a colorimeter?
    a. To measure light intensity b. To hold the sample
    c. To filter specific wavelengths d. To generate light
17. Which type of analysis does not typically use colorimetry?
    a. Blood glucose testing b. Water quality assessment
    c. DNA sequencing d. Protein quantification
18. Which substance is commonly measured using a Bradford assay in colorimetry?
    a. Glucose b. Proteins
    c. Lipids d. Nucleic acids
19. Which parameter does not affect the accuracy of a colorimetric measurement?
    a. Sample turbidity b. Quality of cuvette
    c. Instrument calibration d. Time of day
20. What is the primary limitation of colorimetry in quantitative analysis?
    a. Limited sample size
    b. Interference from background color
    c. High cost of instruments
    d. Low sensitivity
21. What is colorimetry primarily concerned with?
    a. Measuring light intensity b. Measuring color
    c. Measuring temperature d. Measuring pressure

22. In colorimetry, what does the Beer-Lambert law describe?
    a. The relationship between absorbance, concentration, and path length
    b. The relationship between light intensity and wavelength
    c. The relationship between light reflection and absorption
    d. The relationship between color intensity and temperature
23. Which instrument is commonly used for colorimetric measurements?
    a. Spectrophotometer b. Microscope
    c. pH meter d. Voltmeter
24. What is the purpose of using a monochromator in a colorimeter?
    a. To measure light intensity
    b. To select specific wavelengths of light
    c. To calibrate the instrument
    d. To convert absorbance to transmittance
25. What does a colorimeter measure?
    a. absorption of light by a sample b. Reflection of light from a sample
    c. Refraction of light through a sample d. dispersion of light by a sample
26. Which parameter does the Beer-Lambert law relate to absorbance?
    a. Temperature b. Concentration
    c. pH d. Pressure
27. Which factor is important to control during a colorimetric assay?
    a. Atmospheric pressure b. Humidity
    c. pH of the solution d. Time of day
28. Which parameter is crucial for ensuring accuracy in a colorimetric measurement?
    a. Sample temperature b. Sample viscosity
    c. Sample turbidity d. Sample homogeneity
29. Which statement is true about the relationship between absorbance and concentration in colorimetry?
    a. Absorbance is inversely proportional to concentration
    b. Absorbance is directly proportional to concentration
    c. Absorbance is not related to concentration
    d. Absorbance is proportional to temperature
30. What is the purpose of using a reference standard in colorimetric analysis?
    a. To filter light b. To measure light intensity
    c. To calibrate the instrument d. To heat the sample
31. Which type of sample is unsuitable for colorimetric analysis?
    a. Transparent b. Colored
    c. Opaque d. Homogeneous

32. Which substance is commonly measured using a colorimeter in water quality testing?
   a. Sodium chloride b. Ammonia
   c. Calcium carbonate d. Potassium iodide
33. What is the advantage of using a colorimeter over visual assessment of color?
   a. Higher sensitivity b. Faster analysis
   c. Lower cost d. All of the above
34. Which statement is true about the path length in colorimetry?
   a. Path length affects the color of the sample
   b. Path length is not related to absorbance
   c. Longer path length increases absorbance
   d. Shorter path length decreases transmittance
35. The most important and extensively used assay technique in biochemistry is
   a. Titrimetric analysis b. Gravimetric analysis
   c. Spectrophotometry d. all of the above
36. __________the generic name that means light-measurements, includes absorption spectrophotometry (a subset of which is colorimetry), fluorometry, flame photometry, and atomic absorption.
   a. HPLC b. Atomic absorption spectroscopy
   c. Photometry d. LED
37. Spectrophotometric measurements are ordinarily made in the spectral range
   a. 100-200nm b. 200-300nm
   c. 290-800nm d. 500-926nm
38. Colorimetric analyses are made in the
   a. Visible range b. Infra red range
   c. Ultraviolet range d. Any one of the above.
39. Spectrophotometric analysis usually implies analysis in the
   a. Visible range b. Infra red range
   c. Ultraviolet range d. Any one of the above.
40. The glass ware used to carry analysis of sample in colorimeter is known as
   a. Cuvette/absorption cell b. Erlynmeyer flask
   c. Microcolour tube d. Spectrotubule
41. Which of the following is used as the indicator of the concentration of the solution in the cuvette while performing colorimetry
   a. Transmitted light b. Absorbed light
   c. Both of these d. Reflected light
42. Using the Beer Lambert`s law the relationship between concentration of solutions (this is what we are after) and absorbance is
   a. Parabolic b. Hyperbolic
   c. Exponential d. Linear

43. Colorimetric analysis are made in the range of
   a. 380-750 nm
   b. Below 380nm
   c. Above 800 nm
   d. Any of the above
44. Beer lambert`s law is applicable only under following condition(s)
   a. Incident light on the substance of interest is monochromatic
   b. The solvent absorption is insignificant compared with the solute absorbance
   c. Absence of optical interference and the absence of chemical reaction between the molecule of interest and another solute or solvent molecule
   d. All of the above.
45. Double beam spectrophotometer instrument includes all the components of single beam in duplex except
   a. Light source
   b. Entrance slit
   c. Detector
   d. Cuvette
46. The device that converts light into an electric signal that is proportional to the number of photons striking its photosensitive surface is known as
   a. Fibre optics
   b. Photoradiater
   c. Photodetector
   d. Readout devices
47. Most of the cuvette path length is
   a. 100mm
   b. 10mm
   c. 10cm
   d. 100cm
48. Choose the correct statement given below:
   a. Cuvettes may be square, rectangular or round, and are constructed from quartz, glass or plastic
   b. Borosilicate glass cuvettes are used for measurements in the visible portion of spectrum (colorimetry)
   c. Quartz cuvette is used for measurements in the UV portion of spectrum (spectrophotometry)
   d. All of the above are correct
49. The unit of absorbance is :
   a. Mol L-1
   b. Mol-1 L-1 cm-1
   c. Mol L-1 cm-1
   d. None of the above
50. Unit of molar absorptivity of any substance is
   a. LMol-1cm-1
   b. Mol L-1
   c. MolL-1cm-1
   d. It is unit less.
51. Choose the correct statement below:
   a. Colorimetric analysis mainly means estimation of colourless substances by causing them to form a coloured complex quantitatively
   b. Thecoloured complex produced during colorimetry analysis can be measured in the visible wavelengths in a colorimeter.
   c. Colourless substances can be measured in UV region provided they have absorbance in the UV region
   d. All of the above.

52. Biomolecules show absorbance of incident light due to presence of :
    a. Transition of electrons between the two closely spaced d-orbitals of transition elements
    b. Conjugated double-bond systems
    c. High affinity to reagent
    d. High content of carbon, oxygen and hydrogen atoms
53. Deoxyribonucleic acid(DNaand ribonucleic acid (RNaabsorb light in the UV region, maximally at
    a. 260nm b. 270nm
    c. 280nm d. 277nm
54. Proteins show maximum UV absorption at
    a. 250nm b. 260nm
    c. 280nm d. 279nm
55. The ODmax of proteins at 280nm (A280) is due
    a. Peptide bonds b. Aliphatic amino acids
    c. Aromatic amino acids d. Tertiary protein structure
56. A260/A280 for pure DNA solution is
    a. 1 b. 100
    c. 1.8 d. 1.1
57. DNA sample with A260/A280ratio less than 1.8 generally indicate contamination by
    a. RNA b. B type DNA
    c. Proteins d. MicroRNA
58. cuvette of 1 cm path length, containing the DNA sample shows A260 of 1.00, the establishedconcentration of DNA in samples is
    a. 100µg/mL b. 50 µg/mL
    c. 30µg/mL d. 1 µg/mL
59. 1.0 mL of a glucose solution (of unknown concentration) was assayed by a standard colorimetric method along with 1.0 mL of a 200 µg/mL standard glucose. OD,unknown = 0.2 OD, std = 0.2, Concentration of the unknown is
    a. 202µg/mL b. 200 µg/mL
    c. 102 µg/mL d. 201 µg/mL
60. In the Somogyi–Nelson colorimetric method, 1 mL 200 µg/mL glucose gave an absorbance of 0.38. What absorbance would you expect for 1 mL 100 µg/mL xylose under identical conditions?
    a. 0.228 b. 0.456
    c. 200 d. 0.38

61. A glucose solution of unknown concentration was diluted 1 in 500 and 1 mL assayed by the Somogyi–Nelson method. The standard (1 mL of 1 mmol/L) gave an optical densityreading of 0.51; the unknown 0.17. What is the concentration of the original glucose solution?

a. 167 mol/L
b. 30 g/L
c. Both of these
d. None of these

62. Glucose and an unknown sugar-like substance containing C H O only and one oxidisable group were assayed by the Somogyi–Nelson method. Each at identical concentrations (100 μg/mL) gave optical density readings of 0.40 and 0.35, respectively. Calculate Mr of the unknown. Mr of glucose 180 Ar C 12 O 16 H 1

a. 20.6
b. 206
c. 103
d. 10.3

63. A mixture known to contain galactose, glucose, and fructose was assayed by different colorimetric methods. Calculate the concentrations of each of galactose, glucose, and fructose, giving your answers in mmol/L.

a. 278, 139, 92.3
b. 278, 92.3, 139,
c. 139, 92.3, 278,
d. 92.3, 278, 139,

64. 1.33 mmol/L NADH is diluted 1:15 and read in a spectrophotometer at 340 nm. What would be the absorbance? εNADH 6.22 × 103

a. 0.552
b. 6.25
c. 0.656
d. 0.655

65. In the Warburg-Christian protein estimation method, the following absorbencies were recorded:A280= 0.426, A260 = 0.413. Calculate protein concentration in g/100 mL.(correction factor =0.81).

a. 35 mg/dL
b. 45mg/dl
c. 45.6mg/dl
d. 55.6 mg/dl

66. The technique involved in the study of wavelength, frequency of radiation absorbed or emitted by an atom or molecule that gives information about its identity is known as:

a. Qualitative spectroscopy
b. Quantitative spectroscopy
c. Atomic absorbtion spectroscopy
d. Laser guided spectroscopy

67. What describes the radiation with a wavelength of 340nm?

a. UV radiation
b. Visible radiation
c. Near infrared radiation
d. Far infrared radiation

68. UV radiation will frequently induce which of the following molecular transition?

a. Inner shell electronic transition
b. Valence electronic transition
c. Molecular vibrational transition
d. Molecular rotational transition

69. Which of the following statements are true about the absorption of radiation?

a. The amount of radiation is proportional to the incident radiation
b. absorbance is reciprocal of transmittance
c. The Beer lambert`s law is valid only at maximum absorption
d. absorbance is dependent on concentration of analyte

70. Calculate the molar concentration of compound X, which has absorbance of 1.2 at 350nm. The molar absorption coefficient of compound X is 0.5 ×103Lmol-1cm-1at 350nm. Which of the following is the correct answer?

a. 2.4mmol-1 b. 4.2 mmol-1

c. 6 mmol-1 d. 2.4 mol L-1

71. Beer's law states that the intensity of light decreases with respect to______

a. Concentration b. Distance

c. Composition d. Volume

72. Laminar flow burner used in Flame photometers is also known as ________

a. Turbulent burner b. Premix burner

c. Total consumption burner d. Nozzle mix burner

73. Bolometer, a type of detector, is also known as __________

a. Resistance temperature detector (RTD) b. Thermistor

c. Thermocouple d. Golay cell

74. Lambert's law states that the intensity of light decreases with respect to __________

a. Concentration b. Distance

c. Composition d. Volume

75. In Michelson's interferometer, the __________ of the detector output will depend upon the intensity of incoming radiation.

a. Velocity b. Frequency

c. Amplitude d. Phase

76. In Flame emission photometers, the measurement of _____________ is used for qualitative analysis.

a. Colour b. Intensity

c. Velocity d. Frequency

77. In Flame emission photometers, the measurement of _____________ is used for quantitative analysis.

a. Colour b. Intensity

c. Velocity d. Frequency

78. In Michelson's interferometer, the frequency of the detector output can be determined by translating the _________ of movable mirror and the ___________ of monochromatic radiation.

a. Velocity, wavelength b. Thickness, intensity

c. Length, velocity d. angle, intensity

79. In the most widely used beam splitter, a thin film of ________ is sandwiched between two plates of low refractive index solid. Fill the blank with a suitable option.

a. Mylar b Silicon carbide

c Ferrous oxide d. Silver chloride

80. Beer Lambert's law gives the relation between which of the following?
   a. Reflected radiation and concentration
   b. Scattered radiation and concentration
   c. Energy absorption and concentration
   d. Energy absorption and reflected radiation
81. The representation of Beer Lambert's law is given as A = abc. If 'b' represents distance, 'c' represents concentration and 'A' represents absorption, what does 'a' represent?
   a. Intensity
   b. Transmittance
   c. Absorptivity
   d. Admittance
82. Which of the following is the wavenumber of UV and Visible radiation?
   a. 1 x 106 to 1.3 x 104 m-1
   b. 1 x 106 to 1.3 x 104 m
   c. 13 – 27 m-1
   d. 1 x 106 to 1.3 x 104 m2
83. Spectroscopy deals with interaction of electromagnetic radiation with matter. What is the speed of this radiation in vacuum in m/s?
   a. 6 x 108
   b. 5 x 108
   c. 7 x 108
   d. 3 x 108
84. Which of the following is not a limitation of Beer Lambert's law, which gives the relation between absorption, thickness and concentration?
   a. Concentration must be lower
   b. Radiation must have higher bandwidth
   c. Radiation source must be monochromatic
   d. Does not consider factors other than thickness and concentration that affect absorbance
85. Which of the following is not true about Absorption spectroscopy?
   a. It involves transmission
   b. Scattering is kept minimum
   c. Reflection is kept maximum
   d. Intensity of radiation leaving the substance is an indication of a concentration
86. Which of the following is not a property or parameter of electromagnetic radiation?
   a. Wavelength
   b. Voltage
   c. Wave number
   d. Amplitude
87. In which of the following ways, absorption is related to transmittance?
   a. Absorption is the logarithm of transmittance
   b. Absorption is the reciprocal of transmittance
   c. Absorption is the negative logarithm of transmittance
   d. Absorption is a multiple of transmittance
88. Which of the following is the wavelength of microwave radiation?
   a. 10 – 780nm
   b. 0.78 – 30μm
   c. 0.6 – 10 m
   d. 0.75 – 3.75 mm

89. Which type of Quantum Transition takes place in Ultra Violet and Visible spectroscopy?
    a. Rotation of molecules
    b. Nuclear
    c. Bonding electrons
    d. Spin of nuclei in a magnetic field
90. Which of the following is not a type of Spectroscopy?
    a. Gamma ray
    b. X ray
    c. Nuclear magnetic resonance
    d. Sound
91. Transmittance is given as T = I/Io. If Io is the power incident on the sample, what does I represent?
    a. Radiant power transmitted by the sample
    b. Radiant power absorbed by the sample
    c. Sum of powers absorbed and scattered
    d. Sum of powers transmitted and reflected
92. Which of the following is false about the wavelengths of electromagnetic radiation?
    a. Radiation with short wavelengths have high energies
    b. Energy does not depend on wavelength
    c. Radiation with long wavelengths have low energies
    d. Energy depends on wavelength
93. Which of the following is not an advantage of Laminar flow burner used in Flame photometry?
    a. Noiseless
    b. Stable flame for analysis
    c. Efficient atomization of sample
    d. Sample containing two or more solvents can be burned efficiently
94. How is the wave number of electromagnetic radiation related to wavelength?
    a. It is the reciprocal of wavelength
    b. It is directly proportional to wavelength
    c. It is not related to wavelength
    d. It is equal to wavelength
95. Which of the following is not a detector used in Flame emission photometers?
    a. Photronic cell
    b. Photovoltaic cell
    c. Photoemissive tube
    d. Chromatogram
96. Which of the following is the principle of Flame emission photometers?
    a. Radiation is absorbed by non-excited atoms in vapour state and are excited to higher states
    b. Medium absorbs radiation and transmitted radiation is measured
    c. Colour and wavelength of the flame is measured
    d. Only wavelength of the flame is measured

97. Which of the following is the advantage of prism monochromators?
   a. Dispersion is non-overlapping
   b. Dispersion occurs in non-linear manner
   c. Dispersion is overlapping
   d. Dispersion occurs in a linear manner

98. Which of the following is not an application of Flame emission photometers?
   a. Analysis of biological fluids
   b. Determination of sodium, potassium in soil
   c. Determination of metals such as Mn, Cu
   d. Analysis of complex mixtures

99. Which of the following is the advantage of grating monochromators?
   a. Dispersion is non-overlapping
   b. Dispersion occurs in non-linear manner
   c. Dispersion is overlapping
   d. Dispersion occurs in a linear manner

100. Which of the following is not an advantage of a photovoltaic cell which is used as a detector in Flame emission photometers?
   a. Portable
   b. No external supply
   c. Robust in construction
   d. Does not show fatigue

101. In Atomic Absorption Spectroscopy, which of the following is the generally used radiation source?
   a. Tungsten lamp
   b. Xenon mercury arc lamp
   c. Hydrogen or deuterium discharge lamp
   d. Hollow cathode lamp

102. Which of the following is the principle of Atomic Absorption Spectroscopy?
   a. Radiation is absorbed by non-excited atoms in vapour state and are excited to higher states
   b. Medium absorbs radiation and transmitted radiation is measured
   c. Colour is measured
   d. Colour is simply observed

103. Which of the following is the function of the chopper in Atomic Absorption Spectroscopy?
   a. To split the beam into two
   b. To break the steady light into a pulsating light
   c. To filter unwanted components
   d. To reduce the sample into atomic state

104. In Atomic Absorption Spectroscopy, with what material is the cathode in Hollow cathode lamp constructed?
   a. Tungsten
   b. Quartz
   c. Element to be investigated
   d. Aluminium

105. How can the intensity of radiation be increased in Hollow cathode lamp?
    a. Addition of non-conductive protective shield of mica
    b. Addition of nitrogen to neon or argon in the lamp
    c. Increasing the pressure of the filling gas
    d. Changing the metal of the anode
106. Which of the following is the function of the Flame or Emission system in Atomic Absorption Spectroscopy?
    a. To split the beam into two
    b. To break the steady light into pulsating light
    c. To filter unwanted components
    d. To reduce the sample into atomic state
107. Which of the following is not a component of the emission system in Flame photometer?
    a. Burner
    b. Atomiser
    c. Fuel gases and their regulation
    d. Chopper
108. Which of the following is not a fuel used in flame photometry?
    a. Acetylene
    b. Propane
    c. Hydrogen
    d. Camphor oil
109. Which of the following options explains the process of 'sputtering' that occurs in Hollow Cathode Lamp?
    a. Positive ions collide with cathode surface and metal atoms from cathode are ejected
    b. Negative ions collide with cathode surface and metal atoms from anode are ejected
    c. Positive ions collide with negative ions and metal atoms from anode are ejected
    d. Positive ions collide with negative ions and photons are ejected
110. Which of the following is not the requirement of a good flame in flame photometer?
    a. Liquid sample must be evaporated to form solid residue
    b. Solid residue must decompose to form atoms
    c. Atoms must be produced such that they have the ability to get excited to higher states
    d. Atoms must be produced such that they are in stable state
111. Which of the following detectors is used to detect light intensities which are very weak?
    a. Photomultiplier tube
    b. Photovoltaic cell
    c. Photoemissive tubes
    d. Photo reflector

112. Instead of glass filters, why gelatin filters could not be used for a long period while both are Absorption filters?
   a. Gelatin tends to evaporate and hence they deteriorate
   b. Gelatin is affected by humidity in the environment
   c. They deteriorate due to absorption of heat leading to changes in gelatin
   d. Gelation is affected by temperature in the environment
113. Which of the following could be used as the layer of dielectric in interference filters used in Absorption Spectroscopy?
   a. Graphite
   b. MgF2
   c. Fe
   d. AgNO3
114. How is Tungsten Halogen lamp differs from normal Tungsten filament lamp used in absorption spectroscopy?
   a. It has a tungsten filament and is filled with inert gas
   b. Iodine is added to normal filling gas
   c. Iodine is coated on tungsten filament
   d. Iodine is added to inert gas
115. How does continuous wedge filter differ from normal interference filter used in absorption spectroscopy?
   a. It permits continuous selection of different wavelength
   b. It allows a narrow band of wavelengths to pass
   c. It has two semi-transparent layers of silver
   d. Space layer is made of a substance having low refractive index
116. How can stability of radiation be achieved in incandescent or discharge source used in Absorption Spectroscopy?
   a. Using filters
   b. Using monochromators
   c. Using slits
   d. By controlling the source voltage
117. Which of the following statement is false about double beam absorption instruments?
   a. It is similar to single beam instruments except two beams are present
   b. Tungsten bulb is used as a source
   c. Reference beam must have a higher intensity than sample beam
   d. Both the beams after they pass through respective samples are compared
118. Which of the following is the purpose of balance indicator in double beam photometer or colorimeter?
   a. Selects a particular wavelength
   b. Splits the wavelength selected into two equal beams
   c. Detects and indicates the amount of light falling on it
   d. Indicates the difference between the output of two photometers
119. Which of the following is not a reason for laser not being generally used as a source of radiation for UV, Visible Spectroscopy?
   a. High cost
   b. Limited range of wavelength
   c. Less intensity
   d. Complex to work with

120. Which of the following statements is false about single beam absorption instruments?
    a. Tungsten bulb is used as a source
    b. Beam splitter is used to get parallel beam
    c. Test tube is used as sample holder
    d. Photovoltaic cell as detector
121. Which of the following is not an application of colorimeter?
    a. Paints
    b. Inks
    c. Cosmetics
    d. Composition detection
122. To tolerate high operating temperatures, which of the following has to be done in incandescent or tungsten filament lamps?
    a. Alloys must be used
    b. Nitrogen be used instead of inert gas
    c. Envelope is fabricated with quartz
    d. Envelope is fabricated with copper
123. In photometers, the readings of the specimen are initially obtained in the form of which of the following parameters?
    a. Transmittance
    b. Absorption
    c. Wavelengths
    d. Volume
124. Which of the following is the purpose of the beam splitter in double beam photometer or colorimeter?
    a. Splits beam into two equal intensity beams
    b. Splits beam in such a way that sample beam has higher intensity
    c. Splits beam in such a way that a reference beam has higher intensity
    d. Merge two equal intensity beams into single beam
125. Colorimeters are used in applications where great accuracy is required.
    a. The above statement is true
    b. The statement is false
    c. Colorimeter is valid for only biomolecules
    d. Colorimeter is sensitive as well as accurate
126. Choose the correct statement given below
    a. Colorimeters are used to determine the concentration of solutions.
    b. Atomic Absorption Spectroscopy is used for the analysis of metals.
    c. The function of pressure regulators in the emission system of flame photometer is to have a steady flame which is free from flickers.
    d. All of the Above
127. Choose the incorrect statement below:
    a. Computer accepts analog signals directly.
    b. In Total consumption burner, only samples of particular droplet size will enter the burner.
    c. Electromagnetic radiation can travel through a vacuum.
    d. Both a & b are incorrect

128. Choose the correct statements below:
    a. Atomic absorption spectroscopy is also called as Absorption Flame Photometry.
    b. Phototubes are more sensitive than photovoltaic cells.
    c. Velocity of electromagnetic radiation is more in a vacuum than in any medium.
    d. All of these

129. Calorimetry is performed with the help of
    a. Calorimeter
    b. Colorimeter
    c. Photothermometer
    d. Calography

130. Which part of the spectrophotometer is adjusted to select the desiredwavelength?
    a. Filter
    b. Light source
    c. Sample
    d. photodetector

131. In spectrophotometric experiments, the blank contains
    a. Solute
    b. Solvent
    c. Light source
    d. absorption spectrum

132. Which of the following statement is incorrect regarding UV-visibles pectrophotometry?
    a. It gives a measure of the amount of light absorbed by a sample
    b. The sample is exposed to UV-visible light of different wavelengths
    c. It is used to determine the concentration of a compound in solution
    d. The amount of UV-visible light absorbed by a sample during UV-visiblespectrophotometry is called its absorbance

133. The distance travelled by light as it passes through a cuvette is called
    a. Sample width
    b. Focal length
    c. Field length
    d. Path length

134. Which of the following statements is incorrect with respect to Beer-Lambert law?
    a. The amount of light absorbed is proportional to concentration of absorbing substance
    b. Io/I give transmittance
    c. Transmittance measures the amount of light transmitted after passing through the medium
    d. Intensity of transmitted light decreases exponentially with increase in concentration of absorbing substance

135. The plot of absorption verses wavelength for a particular compound is referred to as the
    a. Path length
    b. Emission spectrum
    c. Absorption spectrum
    d. None of these

136. Which of the following is not a limitation of Beer- Lambert law?
   a. Light must be of a narrow wavelength range and preferably monochromatic
   b. At high concentration, molecules may polymerize and thereby affecting absorption of solution
   c. Presence of fluorescent molecule in solution may interfere in the final absorbance of solution
   d. Beer- Lambert law does not form the quantitative basis for all types of absorption spectroscopy
137. The photomultiplier tube is a widely used ---------------in UV-Vis spectroscopy
   a. Wavelength selector   b. Detector
   c. Signal processor   d. Cuvette
138. Which of the following is the correct relationship between absorbance and transmittance of a solution at a given wavelength :
   a. $A = \log (1/T)$ b. $A = \log 100 - \log T$
   c. $A = =2\text{-}\log T$ d. All of these
139. Choose the correct statement below:
   a. "Colorimetry is the measurement of intensityof color in a solution
   b. The concentration of colorless biochemicalcompounds and metabolites can be estimated by colorimeter if theyare converted into colored compounds usingchemical reactions under defined conditions.
   c. A standard solution or Calibrator refers to the solution ofthe same substance as of the test but of known concentration.
   d. All of these
140. One of the disadvantage of colorimeter is
   a. It is cost ineffective.
   b. It is not easily transportable.
   c. It is well applicable only for quantitative analysis ofnatural colored compounds.
   d. Cannot be used for colorless compounds, does notwork in UV and IR ranges.
141. The ratio of the radiant power transmitted by a sample to the radiant power incident on the sample is known as
   a. Absorbance   b. Transmittance
   c. Optical density   d. Photometric concentration
142. If absorbance is plotted graphically against concentration, the graph is
   a. Parabola   b. Increasing
   c. Straight line   d. Decreasing
143. Which of the following statement is false about double beam absorption instruments?
   a. It is similar to single beam instruments except two beams are present
   b. Tungsten bulb is used as a source
   c. Reference beam must have a higher intensity than sample beam
   d. Both the beams after they pass through respective samples are compared

144. Deviation of Beers law is due to:
   a. Use of monochromatic beam of light
   b. Homogenous medium of solution
   c. Heterogeneous beam of light
   d. Stable supply of voltage

145. If absorbance of solution is less than expected the solution shows
   a. + deviation
   b. – deviation
   c. Obey Beer`s law
   d. None

146. Sample cell/ cuvette utilized in spectrophotometer is made of:
   a. Glass
   b. Quartz
   c. Stainless steel
   d. Cupper

147. Hyperchromic shift is
   a. Increase in intensity of absorption
   b. Decrease in intensity of absorption
   c. Shift to shorter wavelength
   d. Shift to longer wavelength

148. Bathochromic or red shift is
   a. Increase in intensity of absorption
   b. decrease in intensity of absorption
   c. Shift to shorter wavelength
   d. Shift to longer wavelength

149. Hypsochromic or blue shift is
   a. Increase in intensity of absorption
   b. Decrease in intensity of absorption
   c. Shift to shorter wavelength
   d. Shift to longer wavelength

150. Absorbance is
   a. Constitutive property
   b. Additive property
   c. Extensive property
   d. Intensive property

Answer Key

1	b	2	c	3	b	4	c	5	a	6	d	7	b
8	b	9	d	10	d	11	c	12	d	13	a	14	b
15	d	16	b	17	c	18	b	19	d	20	b	21	b
22	a	23	a	24	b	25	a	26	b	27	c	28	c
29	b	30	c	31	c	32	b	33	c	34	b	35	c
36	c	37	c	38	a	39	c	40	a	41	c	42	d
43	a	44	d	45	a	46	c	47	b	48	d	49	d
50	a	51	d	52	d	53	a	54	c	55	c	56	c
57	c	58	b	59	b	60	a	61	c	62	b	63	a
64	a	65	a	66	a	67	a	68	b	69	d	70	a
71	a	72	b	73	b	74	b	75	c	76	a	77	b
78	a	79	a	80	c	81	c	82	a	83	d	84	b
85	c	86	b	87	c	88	d	89	c	90	d	91	a
92	a	93	d	94	a	95	d	96	c	97	a	98	d
99	d	100	d	101	d	102	a	103	b	104	c	105	c
106	d	107	d	108	d	109	a	110	d	111	a	112	c

113	b	114	b	115	a	116	d	117	d	118	d	119	c
120	b	121	d	122	d	123	a	124	a	125	b	126	d
127	d	128	d	129	a	130	a	131	b	132	b	133	d
134	b	135	c	136	d	137	b	138	d	139	d	140	d
141	b	142	c	143	c	144	c	145	a	146	b	147	a
148	d	149	c	150	b								